American Medical Association
Physicians dedicated to th

EVIDENCE-BASED PRACTICE

LOGIC AND CRITICAL THINKING IN MEDICINE

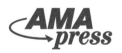

MILOS JENICEK ▪ DAVID L. HITCHCOCK

AMA Press

Vice President, Business Products: Anthony J. Frankos
Publisher: Michael Desposito
Director, Production and Manufacturing: Jean Roberts
Senior Acquisitions Editor: Barry Bowlus
Developmental Editor: Katharine Dvorak
Copy Editor: Kathleen Louden
Director, Marketing: J. D. Kinney
Marketing Manager: Amy Postlewait
Senior Production Coordinator: Rosalyn Carlton
Senior Print Coordinator: Ronnie Summers

Internet address: www.ama-assn.org

Additional copies of this book may be ordered by calling 800 621-8335 or from the secure AMA Press Web site at www.amapress.org. Refer to product number OP842204.

ISBN 1-57947-626-0

Library of Congress Cataloging-in-Publication

Jenicek, Milos, 1935-
    Evidence-based practice : logic and critical thinking in medicine / Milos Jenicek, David L. Hitchcock.
        p. ; cm.
    Includes bibliographical references and index.
    ISBN 1-57947-626-0 .
    1. Evidence-based medicine. 2. Medical logic. 3. Critical thinking. 4. Medicine—Philosophy.
    [DNLM: 1. Evidence-Based Medicine. WB 102 J51e 2005] I. Hitchcock, David, 1942- II. Title.
    R723.7.J463 2005
    616—dc22

                                                                    2004007858

"Tree Diagram" in *Critical Thinking: An Introduction to the Basic Skills* by William Hughes. Broadview Press, 2000 (3/e), p. 99. ISBN: 1551112515. Copyright © 2000 William Hughes. Reprinted with permission of Broadview Press.

BP87:04-P-032:09/04

Contents

Part 1
Theory and Methodological Foundations

CHAPTER 4   **Critical Thinking in a Nutshell**
What Is "Critical" and What Is Not? 99

Part 2

Practical Applications

ILLUSTRATIONS

Figures

Tables

PHILOSOPHER'S FOREWORD

It was with great delight that I learned that Drs Jenicek and Hitchcock were doing a book on logic and critical thinking in medicine. Although all critical thinking dispositions, abilities, and principles apply in a large number of areas, including medicine, there are very few detailed attempts to exhibit the explicit application of these general aspects of critical thinking in a field of study or practice. Jenicek and Hitchcock are to be congratulated for this pioneering detailed work.

As someone who has specialized for over 50 years in the nature and assessment of critical thinking, as the author of a general critical thinking textbook and co-author of several critical thinking tests, and also as a medical consumer, I am strongly attracted by several features of this book:

1. its emphasis on seeking "all the relevant justified obtainable information," and the inevitably concomitant need for alertness for alternative hypotheses, explanations, points of view, and interpretations;

2. its attention to the importance of, but also the problems and criteria involved in, securing expert opinion (the credibility of sources);

3. its attention to some contexts that are usually ignored in critical thinking books, such as the legal context (in which physicians might be testifying or challenged, as in connection with worker compensation boards), the context of consultation with medical consumers like myself, the context of challenge to their approach to the field (that is, the challenge to what they call "evidence-based medicine" by "complementary and alternative medicine"), and the context of communicating with the outside world in electronic and printed media;

4. its attention to the complexities of the concept of causation; and

5. the glossary at the end and the amazingly large number of citations of useful sources.

In providing these features, as well as many others, Drs Jenicek and Hitchcock have set a standard that people in other fields, as well as the field of medicine, will have to strive to meet. I urge them to try. As critical thinking becomes more widely dispersed and exemplified (by physicians among others) in a variety of human activities, the more likely it is that, like a developing snowball, critical thinking will be employed and exemplified, making it more likely that our decisions about what to believe and do will be justified. That will include physicians' decisions, which are the focus of this interesting book by Drs Jenicek and Hitchcock, and which are very important to each of us, including physicians.

Robert H. Ennis, PhD
Professor Emeritus of Educational Policy Studies
University of Illinois, Urbana-Champaign
President, Association for Informal Logic and Critical Thinking, 2001–2005
May 2004

Physician's Foreword

Few professions depend on thinking as much as modern medicine does. Medicine has long been described as "an art based on science." With the advancements in the last half of the 20th century, many would argue the scientific base of medicine is increasingly important. It is impossible to be scientifically based without thinking; as the science of medicine grows, so does the need to think clearly. More and more medical interventions are based on medical research—research that requires at least some ability to discern validity. As diagnostic tests and treatments multiply, clinicians and patients must choose the best course to follow from an ever-expanding list of possibilities. Good patient care requires careful and rational consideration of the alternatives.

For medical students entering the profession, at times medical "thinking" must seem comprised almost entirely of memorization. In truth, the science of medicine depends not so much on the ability to memorize (especially now with computers), as the ability to think logically. Pre-medical requirements in biology, chemistry, physics, and mathematics all are supposed to provide future physicians a foundation in scientific and logical thinking.

Ironically, medical schools do not require a pre-medical course in philosophy, particularly its branches of logic and epistemology. Neither I nor most physicians I know have ever taken such a course. So, our understanding of the relationship of logic in medicine to logic and epistemology in philosophy is hazy at best. We understand even less the philosophical concepts of *techne* (relating to the skills and art of a practitioner, in this case, a health care provider) and *phronesis* in medicine (combining art and science to make decisions in the care of the individual patient).

What we need is a textbook, one that lays out the fundamental concepts of logic in the field of philosophy, gives us a brief overview of the development of logic in human history, introduces us to its language, and demonstrates how logic is and is not used in medicine. We now have such a textbook in Jenicek and Hitchcock's *Evidence-Based Practice: Logic and Critical Thinking in Medicine.* With their succinct text, clinicians, as well as medical researchers and health planners, can understand better the worlds of "critical thinking" and "evidence-based medicine" and how they relate to classic philosophical thought. Readers learn how traditional activities of patient care and medical research intersect with logical thinking. They also see how medicine's approach to logic has contributed to philosophy, especially its concept of cause, with the development of ways to avoid bias in medical observations, the hierarchy of strength of evidence, and understanding of the role of chance. Finally, readers learn how medicine's logic is not always the same as that used by the rest of the world, especially in the legal profession, where the definitions of probability and cause are quite different from those in medicine.

This book provides a unique introduction to those who would enjoy discovering the history and concepts of logic as it relates to medicine. It combines the perspectives of a physician who has spent decades writing about how to make medicine more rational and a classical philosopher who has spent decades thinking about logic. Perhaps it is understandable that few physicians spend much time thinking about such a fundamental medical activity as thinking. Perhaps, too, it is time to change. Logic is as important to physicians as water is to fish—it surrounds us all and we swim in it every day.

Suzanne W. Fletcher, MD, MSc
Professor of Ambulatory Care and Prevention
Harvard Medical School and Harvard Pilgrim Medical Care
March 2004

Feel smart! Be smart!

Science in medicine *means questions, observations, measurement, analysis, and explanations.*

Philosophy in medicine *means thinking about medical thinking.*

Logic in medicine *means correct reasoning in research and practice.*

Critical thinking in medicine *means using logic to understand health problems and make reasonable decisions in patient and community care.*

If useful evidence in medicine is an egg yolk and the logical use of it is the white of the egg, this book is a scrambled egg made mostly of egg white. (The dieters will appreciate that!)

A Word From the Authors

Writing comes more easily
if you have something to say.
—Sholem Asch, 1955

Science in medicine provides us with the best possible evidence on human risks, on diagnostic methods to use, on the most effective treatment and other kinds of intervention, on the best or worst prognosis, and on the most rational ways to plan actions and make decisions. Science in medicine is about **producing the evidence**.

Logic and critical thinking is about rational **uses of evidence**. Complete and methodologically impeccable evidence about a health problem is not enough to make valid and valuable choices. If the interpretation of the evidence is not logically sound and if the evidence is used uncritically, the patient may be harmed. He or she may be equally harmed by a logically flawless use of poor or poorly evaluated evidence.

In any medical research paper, the introduction (formulation of a problem), the material and methods section, and the presentation of results summarize the scientific aspects of production of evidence. The discussion and conclusions sections review, analyze, and trace the meaning of evidence. They should provide us with a balanced view about our certainties and uncertainties pertaining to a health problem across presented findings and evidence. "Discussion" and "Conclusions" especially call for the mastery of rational thought and understanding as provided to us by logic and critical thinking.

We received from our teachers a remarkable wealth of facts, wisdom, and experience to produce valuable evidence. We need a similar enrichment of the proper uses of such evidence in daily practice and research. Why? Because our entire professional life is a wide world of arguments. Training in philosophy is already well anchored in the areas of probability and ethics. Mastery and uses of logic and critical thinking are equally important in our daily dealing with health problems and their solutions. These particular aspects of philosophy in medicine not only have an inherent value of "deep thought"; but also their practical implications and applications are immediate and essential for effective community and patient health care and for the solution of health problems. They still await an objective explanation and this book intends to prove it.

This book is not an essay, but a textbook that should guide its readers in choosing the objectives of teaching, what to teach, how to teach it, and what to retain from the whole message for better practice, for better research, and most important, for the benefit of the patient.

This book contains two parts. The first part offers the reader some basic and universally anchored principles and methods of logic and critical thinking. The second part applies these principles to various fields of medical endeavor: working with the patient, conducting research, handling health programs and policies in a community setting, interacting with society and the law, and, enhancing our own understanding as health professionals of what's going on and what to do.

The shaded sections of the text are meant to draw reader's attention to basic and important definitions when they appear for the first time in the text, key concepts, steps and stages of work to be followed, checklists to bear in mind, important conclusions, pitfalls to avoid, and recommendations for practice.

The Reader's Bookshelf, which appears at the end of this preface, is for beginners. It is intended to attract readers to additional readings without discouraging them by the complexity of the recommended references. We included encyclopedias and dictionaries where beginners usually start, as well as many introductory readings on logic "outside the medical world" and some basic medical readings focusing on reasoning in medical thinking and decision.

In fact, we do not want this book to produce some future full-fledged logicians in health sciences. Instead, we want to show the broadest possible array of readers how important it is to be better critical thinkers in their own professions (be it in daily practice, when reading and listening to medical information, or in conducting research, whether it is fundamental or oriented to bedside decision-making). Philosophy today may indeed be practical and down to earth!

One of our graduate students, an outstanding pediatric intensive care specialist, said at the end of his course, ". . . I don't know if I've got everything, but boy, I feel smart!" We wish the same and more for all our readers.

In many parts of the world, there is no space outside clinical epidemiology for teaching critical thinking, as outlined in this book, to medical and other health sciences students. We modestly hope that this outline will justify (and guide) future teachers to include logic and critical thinking in health sciences curricula as fully as other components of evidence-based medicine.

We cannot disagree with Simon Blackburn that the separation of philosophy as a discipline seems to be an artifact of academic administration rather than the reflection of a clear division between using a concept and thinking about it.

Although endeavors in critical thinking have developed rather independently in the arts and sciences and in medicine, their converging trend might best be introduced by listing some important references published on both sides of the academic barrier. Some of them are quoted at the end of this message and used in greater detail in the chapters that follow.

Joseph Wood Krutch once said teasingly that *logic is the art of going wrong with confidence*. His sting was even applied to evidence-based medicine, seen by Michael O'Donnell as *perpetuating other people's mistakes instead of your own*. It is our desire to help the reader feel and understand that **logic is the art of going right with confidence with meaningful evidence at hand.**

Some areas that have not been sufficiently tested are also quoted in this reading, such as fuzzy logic or chaos theory. We intend only to stimulate the curiosity of the reader and go beyond the established routine in this "unfinished symphony" of critical thinking in health sciences.

Curious where we have put our heart and soul (again)? Who has done what in this book? Today, editorial boards of medical journals wish more and more to have this point specified. Readers are curious, and academic administrators and bureaucrats insist on recording properly all endeavors of their flock. This book is a joint project. How did we do it? MJ conceived the idea and wrote the first draft. He started from Chapters 3 and 12 of his *Foundations of Evidence-Based Medicine* published in 2003 (see the Reader's Bookshelf). These chapters had been revised extensively before publication in light of comments by DH. Later on, DH revised the first draft of the present work, contributing in particular the bulk of the theoretical material in Chapters 2 and 4, and most of the Glossary. Each part of the book went back and forth several times until both authors approved every word. In this marriage made in heaven between a health professional and a philosopher, the more "cerebral" of us (DH) chiseled the precision of the written word while the more "visual" in the couple (MJ) worked hard on the artwork (figures) to make our thoughts as explicit as possible in today's cataract-ridden world of authors and readers as well.

We would like to express our appreciation for the advice, time, attention, and experience our colleagues provided in critically reading this endeavor and guiding it in the right direction.

Several prominent logicians and critical thinking specialists of our day looked at the pages that follow: Professors Jonathan E. Adler (City University of New York), J. Anthony Blair (University of Windsor), Robert H. Ennis (University of Illinois at Urbana-Champaign), Trudy Govier (independent scholar, Calgary), Nicholas Griffin (McMaster University), Ralph H. Johnson (FRSC, University of Windsor), Robert C. Pinto (University of Windsor), and Mark L. Weinstein (Montclair State University).

Several experienced academic physicians-practitioners-researchers-teachers offered us invaluable help by assessing medicine itself in this reading, and the relevance of this book for teaching: Professors Paul Grof (psychiatry, University of Ottawa), Madhu Natarajan (cardiology, McMaster University), Jeanne Teitelbaum (neurology, McGill's Montreal Neurological Institute and Université de Montréal's Maisonneuve-Rosemont Hospital), Karl Weiss (clinical microbiology, Université de Montréal and Maisonneuve-Rosemont Hospital), and Marianne Xhignesse (family medicine and Director of continuing medical education, University of Sherbrooke).

Mrs. Nicole Kinney (Linguamax Services Ltd.—text review) and Mr. Jacques Cadieux (Université de Montréal's Audiovisual Centre—infographics) smoothed out the message and made it pleasing for the eye as well as explicit and easy to understand for any inquisitive mind.

We are indebted to all of them not only for their time, energy, attention, and interest, but also for the significant improvements they have made to this book. The reader should be the foremost beneficiary of their contributions. We should of course make clear that we alone are responsible for any faults that remain. As the saying goes, "*the best way to be noticed is to make mistake(s)."*

Our final word of thanks goes to our foreword authors. One of them, Suzanne W. Fletcher, is an eminent physician, academic, and professional with a lifetime of experience in national and international health. The other, Robert H. Ennis, is the world's leading authority on the definition of the concept of critical thinking for purposes of education and assessment. Their "medical" and "philosophical" forewords reflect the distinctive character of our book—the bringing together again of medicine and philosophy (logic and critical thinking in particular).

So, here then, is an introduction to logic and critical thinking in health sciences. If we, readers and authors alike, succeed in infusing critical thinking into theory and practice in health sciences, all those in our care should benefit.

Milos Jenicek and David Hitchcock
June 2004

READER'S BOOKSHELF

Following is a health professional-friendly general bibliography by chronological order within each category.

Logic and Critical Thinking

1. Salmon WC. *Logic.* Englewood Cliffs, NJ: Prentice-Hall; 1963.

2. Thomas SN. *Practical Reasoning in Natural Language.* 2nd ed. Englewood Cliffs, NJ: Prentice-Hall; 1981.

3. Hitchcock D. *Critical Thinking. A Guide to Evaluating Information.* Toronto, Canada: Methuen; 1983.

4. Toulmin S, Rieke R, Janik A. *An Introduction to Reasoning.* 2nd ed. New York: Macmillan; 1984.

5. Moore BN, Parker R. *Critical Thinking. Evaluating Claims and Arguments in Everyday Life.* Palo Alto, Calif: Mayfield Publishing Company; 1986.

6. Copi IM. *Informal Logic.* New York, NY: Macmillan; 1986.

7. Michalos AC. *Improving Your Reasoning.* 2nd ed. Englewood Cliffs, NJ: Prentice-Hall; 1986.

8. Engel SM. *With Good Reason. Introduction to Informal Fallacies.* New York, NY: St. Martin Press; 1986.

9. Engel SM. *The Chain of Logic.* Englewood Cliffs, NJ: Prentice-Hall; 1987.

10. Damer TE. *Attacking Faulty Reasoning.* 2nd ed. Belmont, Calif: Wadsworth Publishing Company; 1987.

11. Weston A. *A Rulebook for Arguments.* An AVATAR book. Avatar Books of Cambridge. Indianapolis, Ind: Hackett Publishing Company; 1987.

12. Seech Z. *Logic in Everyday Life. Practical Reasoning Skills.* Belmont, Calif: Wadsworth Publishing Company; 1987.

13. Walton DN. *Informal Logic. A Handbook for Critical Argumentation.* Cambridge, England and New York, NY: Cambridge University Press; 1989.

14. Harrison FR III. *Logic and Rational Thought.* St. Paul, Minn: West Publishing Company; 1992.

15. Popkin RH, Stroll A. *Philosophy Made Simple.* 2nd ed rev. A Made Simple Book. New York, NY: Broadway Books; 1993.

16. Hansen HV, Pinto RC, eds. *Fallacies: Classical and Contemporary Readings.* University Park, Calif: The Pennsylvania State University Press; 1995.

17. Ennis RH. *Critical Thinking.* Upper Saddle River, NJ: Prentice-Hall; 1996.

18. Nolt J, Rohatyn D, Varzi A. *Schaum's Outline of Theory and Problems of Logic.* 2nd ed. Schaum's Outline Series. New York, NY: McGraw-Hill; 1998.

19. Hughes W. *Critical Thinking. An Introduction to the Basic Skills.* 3rd ed. Peterborough,Ontario: Broadview Press Ltd.; 2000.

20. Fisher A. *Critical Thinking. An Introduction.* Cambridge, England: Cambridge University Press; 2001.

21. Govier, T. *A Practical Study of Argument.* 5th ed. Belmont, Calif: Wadsworth; 2001.

22. Bowell T, Kemp G. *Critical Thinking. A Concise Guide.* London, England and New York, NY: Routledge; 2002.

23. Copi IM, Cohen C. *Introduction to Logic.* 11th ed. Upper Saddle River, NJ: Prentice-Hall; 2002.

Encyclopedias and Dictionaries of Philosophy

1. Hughes GE, Wang H, Roscher N. The History and Kinds of Logic. In: McHenry R, ed. *The New Encyclopaedia Britannica: Macropaedia/Knowledge In Depth.* Vol 23. Chicago, Ill: Encyclopaedia Britannica, Inc; 1992:226–282.

2. Blackburn S. *Oxford Dictionary of Philosophy.* Oxford, England and New York, NY: Oxford University Press; 1994.

3. Honderich T, ed. *The Oxford Companion to Philosophy.* Oxford, England and New York, NY: Oxford University Press; 1995.

4. Audi R, ed. *The Cambridge Dictionary of Philosophy.* 2nd ed. Cambridge, England: Cambridge University Press; 1999.

5. Bullock A, Trombley S, eds. *The New Fontana Dictionary of Modern Thought.* 3rd ed. London, England: HarperCollins Publishers; 1999.

6. Reese WL. *Dictionary of Philosophy and Religion: Eastern and Western Thought.* Expanded ed. Amherst, NY: Humanity Books; 1999.

7. Crofton I, ed. *Instant Reference Philosophy.* London, England: Hodder Headline; 2000.

8. Craig E, ed. *Concise Routledge Encyclopedia of Philosophy.* London, England and New York, NY: Routledge; 1999.

9. Martin RM. *The Philosopher's Dictionary.* 3rd ed. Peterborough, Ontario: Broadview Press; 2002.

10. Bunge M. *Philosophical Dictionary.* Enlarged ed. Amherst, NY: Prometheus Books; 2003.

Books in Epidemiology and Medicine Related to Philosophy, Logic, Reasoning, and Critical Thinking

1. Feinstein AR. *Clinical Judgment.* St. Louis, Mo: CV Mosby; 1967.

2. Susser M. *Causal Thinking in the Health Sciences: Concepts and Strategies of Epidemiology.* New York, NY: Oxford University Press; 1973.

3. Murphy EA. *The Logic of Medicine.* Baltimore, Md: The Johns Hopkins University Press; 1976.

4. King LS. *Medical Thinking: A Historical Preface.* Princeton, NY: Princeton University Press; 1982.

5. Cutler P. *Problem Solving in Clinical Medicine: From Data to Diagnosis.* 2nd ed. Baltimore, Md: Williams & Wilkins; 1985.

6. Wulff HR, Pedersen SA, Rosenberg R. *Philosophy of Medicine: An Introduction.* Oxford, England: Blackwell Scientific Publications; 1986.

7. Albert DA, Munson R, Resnik MD. *Reasoning in Medicine: An Introduction to Clinical Inference.* Baltimore, Md: The Johns Hopkins University Press; 1988.

8. C Buck, A Llopis, E Najera, M Terris, eds. *The Challenge of Epidemiology: Issues and Selected Readings.* PAHO Scientific Publication No. 505. Washington, DC: Pan American Health Organization; 1988.

9. Rothman KJ, ed. *Causal Inference.* Chestnut Hill, Mass: Epidemiology Resources Inc; 1988.

10. Elwood JM. *Causal Relationships in Medicine.* Oxford, England: Oxford University Press; 1988.

11. Evans AS. *Causation and Disease: A Chronological Journey.* New York, NY: Plenum; 1993.

12. Phillips CI, ed. *Logic in Medicine.* London, England: BMJ Publishing Group; 1995.

13. Jenicek M. *Epidemiology: The Logic of Modern Medicine.* Montreal, Canada: EPIMED International; 1995.

14. Sackett DL, Straus SE, Richardson WS, Rosenberg W, Haynes RB. *Evidence-Based Medicine: How to Practice and Teach EBM.* 2nd ed. New York, NY: Churchill Livingstone; 2000.

15. Last JM, ed. *A Dictionary of Epidemiology.* 4th ed. Oxford, England and New York, NY: Oxford University Press; 2001.

16. Guyatt G, Rennie D, eds. *Users' Guides to the Medical Literature: Essentials of Evidence-Based Clinical Practice.* Chicago, Ill: AMA Press; 2002.

17. Jenicek M. *Foundations of Evidence-Based Medicine.* New York, NY: Parthenon Publishing/CRC Press; 2003.

Other Professions and Domains

1. Gambrill E. *Critical Thinking in Clinical Practice: Improving Accuracy of Judgment and Decisions About Clients.* San Francisco, Calif: Jossey-Bass; 1990.

2. Aldisert RJ. *Logic for Lawyers: A Guide to Clear Logical Thinking.* 3rd ed. Notre Dame, Ind: National Institute for Trial Advocacy; 1997.

3. Waller RJ. *Critical Thinking: Consider the Verdict.* Englewood Cliffs, NJ: Prentice-Hall; 1988.

Part 1

Theory and Methodological Foundations

From Philosophy to Logic, From Logic to Medicine: Fundamental Definitions and Objectives of This Book

IN THIS CHAPTER

*In these days, we should be proclaiming the fact that uniformity
and dull conformity are a crime against intelligence
and are indeed the sad abortion of creation. At a time when science
both inside medicine and without is increasingly concerning itself
with practical affairs and is ceasing to be related in any way
to the fundamental problems of the meaning and purpose of life,
it is imperative that a place be found for philosophy
and its business of inquiring into the meaning of things.*

EARLE P. SCARLETT, 1972

Philosophy is not a theory but an activity.

LUDWIG WITTGENSTEIN, 1922

*Here is the beginning of philosophy: a recognition
of the conflicts between men, a search for their
cause, a condemnation of mere opinion . . .
and the discovery of a standard of judgment.*

EPICTETUS, CA FIRST CENTURY AD

*Science is what you know,
philosophy is what you don't know.*

BERTRAND RUSSELL, 1959

*The separation of philosophy as a discipline
can seem to be an artefact of academic
administration, rather than a reflexion
of a clear division between using
a concept and thinking about it.*

SIMON BLACKBURN, 1996

This book should help you reason logically and think critically in medicine and other health sciences. But where does critical thinking belong, what is needed to think critically, how and where should we apply critical thinking, and what can we expect as the result of such an application?

In this chapter, we discover through clinical and other scenarios the importance of logic and critical thinking in medical reasoning, in understanding health problems, and in making correct decisions about clinical cases and situations. We see how logic and critical thinking are as relevant to medicine as epidemiology or biostatistics.

The remainder of Part One presents some basic notions, methods, and techniques of logic and critical thinking for readers who wish to learn more about this field. Those who have already mastered and understand these concepts will find practical applications in Part Two.

1.1 WHY ARE LOGIC AND CRITICAL THINKING NEEDED IN OUR PRACTICE, RESEARCH, AND COMMUNICATION? WHY READ THIS BOOK?

To answer these questions, let us first consider the following scenarios.

Scenario 1: Communicating with your patient

In your practice, you see a sixty-year-old woman who has recently experienced fresh rectal bleeding. During this patient's colonoscopy, the surgeon finds a cancerous-looking lesion. This is confirmed by the pathologist through an exploratory biopsy analysis. Together with the surgeon, you suggest to this patient the surgical removal of her lesion by colon resection and adjuvant chemotherapy, if needed. This patient is a highly intelligent and experienced businesswoman. She wants answers to several questions: "How sure are you about your diagnosis? If you perform this surgery, how successful will it be? How would I specifically benefit from it? Are there any other alternatives to treat my problem? Will my prognosis, life expectancy, and quality of life improve? What about the chemotherapy? I've heard so much about its terrible side effects!"

Answers to any of these queries do not only involve knowledge of evidence, results of clinical trials, or clinical outcomes. The answers also involve a logical discourse (argument) with the patient, to whom we must explain all of our considerations and decisions in plain, understandable terms. If you say, "You are a good candidate for this treatment because your age, other characteristics, and your general medical history are comparable to those of the patients who participated in clinical trials proving the effectiveness of surgery/chemotherapy intervention," you base your recommendation on an argument by analogy. In past trials, the recommended intervention was effective for patients with a specified condition and specified characteristics. You have this condition and those characteristics. Hence (on the basis of such premises), the recommended intervention will likely be effective for you (conclusion). All of our answers to any of the previously mentioned questions must be logically sound. Knowledge and experience are not enough.

Scenario 2: Communicating with your peers

As a psychiatry resident, you discuss with your colleagues at morning floor rounds a patient you admitted overnight. The patient's relatives, who brought him to the hospital emergency department, reported that he had attempted suicide earlier that day. You might be asked, "Besides the suicide attempt and the patient's withdrawal, are there any other findings and considerations that led you to admit this patient? Given the patient's history and your clinical evaluation and findings, what is your working diagnosis? What were the risks if you decided not to admit this patient and instead to refer him to outpatient care? What do you suggest we do now with this patient? Should we keep him here or should we discharge him? When, where, and under what care?" Again, answers to all of these questions are conclusions of a logical discourse in a medical setting based on general and specific experience, knowledge, and evidence.

Scenario 3: Defending a health program in community medicine and public health

As a specialist in community medicine and as a public health officer, you have been informed by your epidemiologist about the high occurrence of home accidents and ensuing injuries in school-age children in your community, as seen in the emergency services of your regional hospitals. You may ask yourself, "How did the epidemiologist obtain such information? Is this a problem specific to our community and medical services? Do we know its causes? Do we have the resources to implement justifiable prevention programs?" Again, your experience, knowledge, epidemiological evidence, and good gut feeling and intuition are not enough. You must carry through a logical argument to convince all interested parties and stakeholders of the next steps to take. What injury prevention and medical care program, if any, should be implemented in the health services and the community? How should it be evaluated? Would it be cost-effective and cost-efficient? Justifying such a program as a priority and convincing other decision-makers to fund and participate in it requires more than current applicable legislation, experience from other comparable programs here and elsewhere, and an understanding of the epidemiology of injury. It requires an understanding of how all of these components fit together. A good logical argument is needed to solve the problem and questions raised.

Scenario 4: Medicine and health in the courts—communicating with and convincing men and women of law

As a physician and epidemiologist specializing in environmental medicine and occupational health, you are invited to be an expert witness. In a class action, a group of citizens blame a new type of home insulation for respiratory and allergy problems. The defendant's lawyer asks you to give your opinion on the following: How well-defined are the reported health problems? What do we know about the exposure? What do we know about the nature of the insulation material and its cause-effect relationship to the reported health problems? What can we conclude about the cause-effect relationship in the case of each individual plaintiff? How can the plaintiffs' exposure to the insulation material in their homes and workplaces be explained individually and collectively? Answers to all of these questions depend heavily on how "logically" you arrive at your opinion. Was the cause-effect relationship between the exposure to this insulation material and the health of individuals living in the insulated environment established and to what degree? If such convincing evidence exists in general, does it apply equally to each of the plaintiffs? A good argument must lead to and contribute to the making of the right decision of the court in this matter.

Scenario 5: Communicating with crowds

You are a well-known family physician in your community and you are invited by a local radio station to talk to its listeners and answer their questions about various health problems that concern them. Is the drinking water in the community well treated? Is drinking it a health hazard for a water-borne disease? Will eating organically grown fruits and vegetables improve one's health? And how risky is it to eat genetically modified foods? All of your recommendations or warnings are conclusions of your reasoning leading from premises to your recommendations. Having good evidence about the health value of the local drinking water or foods is fundamental. What is equally important is how you will use this evidence to arrive at your conclusions and convince your listeners.

Scenario 6: Writing a research article

As an academic physician specializing in internal medicine, you ran a successful clinical trial to evaluate the effectiveness of a new anti-hypertensive drug designed for patients of an advanced age who have been diagnosed with uncontrolled and extremely high blood pressure. The design of your trial was impeccable and all rules required by clinical epidemiology and biostatistics were respected. You realize that this new evidence and its uses will be accepted if you conceive your article as a flawless logical argument leading from what you have seen (premises) to your recommendation or rejection of this new drug for this type of patient.

All six of these scenarios show the equal importance of the best evidence available and its uses in an ideally impeccable process of thought. The communication of good evidence and of the ensuing conclusions and recommendations (in other words, explaining it and having it accepted by your listeners in the clinical and community setting) is a priceless and learned skill making treatment and prevention successful. Through the eyes of such scenarios, one might draw the following general picture of medical thought.

1.2 MEDICINE AS ART AND SCIENCE

Medicine as both art and science is seen as "evidence-based."[1] Careful observations are made. A sense is given to these observations in terms of diagnosis or prognosis. Causes are studied and identified in terms of risk and prognostic factors. Effective treatment is chosen and its beneficial or adverse effects are determined. This process is fact-driven; new findings are sought and used. This process also is evidence-generating and evidence-driven.

Another important aspect of evidence in medicine is how the evidence is used in the process of medical reasoning. Patients may be harmed because their diagnosis and treatment are based on poor evidence. They may also be harmed because the evidence, good or bad, is used inadequately. Hence, patients may benefit from good uses of good evidence, or they may be harmed by poor evidence or poor uses of evidence, good or bad. The **production of good evidence** in fundamental research oriented to clinical decision-making as well as its **uses through good reasoning and decision-making** are learned experiences. They must be. "You are intelligent enough to figure it out" is not sufficient to avoid harm. Neither is a memorized volume of information about health and disease.

Philosophy and its branches—in particular, logic and epistemology, which are the roots of critical thinking—are as vital for the good use of evidence as genetics, microbiology, physics, chemistry, biostatistics, and epidemiology are necessary for the production of evidence.

Medicine is

"the art and science of diagnosis, treatment, and prevention of disease, and the maintenance of good health."[2] We add: *in the care of individual patients and communities as well.*

The **art of medicine** includes

"sensory skills, and the systematic application of such skills and of knowledge in language, speech, reasoning, and motion, in order to obtain desired results."

The skills may be based on or reflect creative imagination, faithful imitation, innovation, or intuition. They bring gratification to the senses.

We tend to consider skills that are hard to define and quantify as part of the art (and not the science) of medicine. Things like serendipity or flair are thought to fall into the category of *either you have it or you don't*. Other skills such as memory, listening to the patient, advising the patient, empathy, insight, equipoise, conceptualization, observation, and inference are thought to be learned and/or improved by experience, according to the motto, *you will learn it somehow as you go along; just watch me!* Acquiring such expertise through experience is an essential part of becoming a good physician (or an expert of any other kind). These skills cannot be taught based only on rules. Having said this, one of the authors of this book had in his past experience at the Montreal General Hospital an extraordinary teacher of surgery who when working with patients, held a nonstop monologue describing what he was doing and why as an overview of debatable rules. One of his residents paid him the ultimate compliment by saying to us, "*Yes, he is a teacher!*"

Should these skills be learned more systematically, as surgeons already do with sensory and manual skills? For the moment, it seems that our training in the scientific aspects of medicine is better structured, better defined, and more uniform across the profession than is our training in the art of medicine.

In recent writings about the nature of medicine, some authors have proposed a third aspect that amalgamates both art and science. In terms of classical Aristotelian philosophy, the science of medicine is a kind of *episteme*, scientific, deductive knowledge. The art of medicine is a *techne*—a craft or productive skill of the practitioner. Making decisions in clinical practice requires adaptation of both *episteme* and *techne* to particular, ever-changing circumstances. Some authors have proposed naming the skill of adapting medical science and art to particular circumstances **medical "phronesis."** (We return to this concept in Chapter 6.) Paralleling this to music, *episteme* would mean writing and reading sheets of music, knowing notes, harmony, and so on. *Techne* would mean the technical mastery of a musical instrument. For Tyreman,[3] *phronesis* would mean musicianship: playing a sheet of music (using one's knowledge or *episteme* to read the score) on a musical instrument (using one's acquired *techne*), and conveying the soul of the music, whether to a gathering of family or friends, at a concert hall, or in a nightclub or stadium, is a phronetic endeavor. Phronesis, in this sense, plays an important role in the application of evidence to particular patients as a part of evidence-based medicine, or EBM. (See Chapter 6.) **Science** in general is

"the study of the material universe or physical reality in order to understand it."[4]

The **science of medicine** involves the

discovery, creation, evaluation, and application of new evidence and the evaluation of the impact of its practical uses.

Psychiatry also includes in such uses of evidence how the patient's mental functioning corresponds to physical reality in its broadest sense.

Historically, medicine went through four stages: from prevailing belief to increasing shared experience, then to understanding, and finally to organized reasoning, evaluation, and decision-making as we know it today. Philosophy applies to this fourth and last stage.

1.3 PHILOSOPHY IN MEDICINE OR PHILOSOPHY OF MEDICINE?

Philosophy is

the study of fundamental questions, that is, questions about concepts (What is health?) and principles (What fundamental ethical norms should govern medical practice?).

Among the topics philosophy studies are being, reality, thinking, perception, values, causes, principles of physical phenomena, and ethical principles.[5]

Four fundamental branches of philosophy are metaphysics, epistemology, logic, and ethics. **Metaphysics** involves exploring the nature of being and reality, **epistemology** studies knowledge, **logic** studies valid inference, and **ethics** studies values and conduct. Philosophy also has numerous fields of application: language, science (hence medicine), history, religion, politics, work, business, finances, military arts (war and peace) among others. Many of us have a fading memory, from high school or college, of philosophy as a dry and abstract discipline. As we see in this book, however, our mastery of its applications and uses in practical problem-solving and decision-making are vital, be it in medicine or elsewhere in the health sciences, and far more practical than we may think at first glance.

Figure 1-1 illustrates the components and domains of philosophy in medicine and society. The main branches of philosophy address the following basic questions:

FIGURE 1-1

Branches, trends, and applications of philosophy

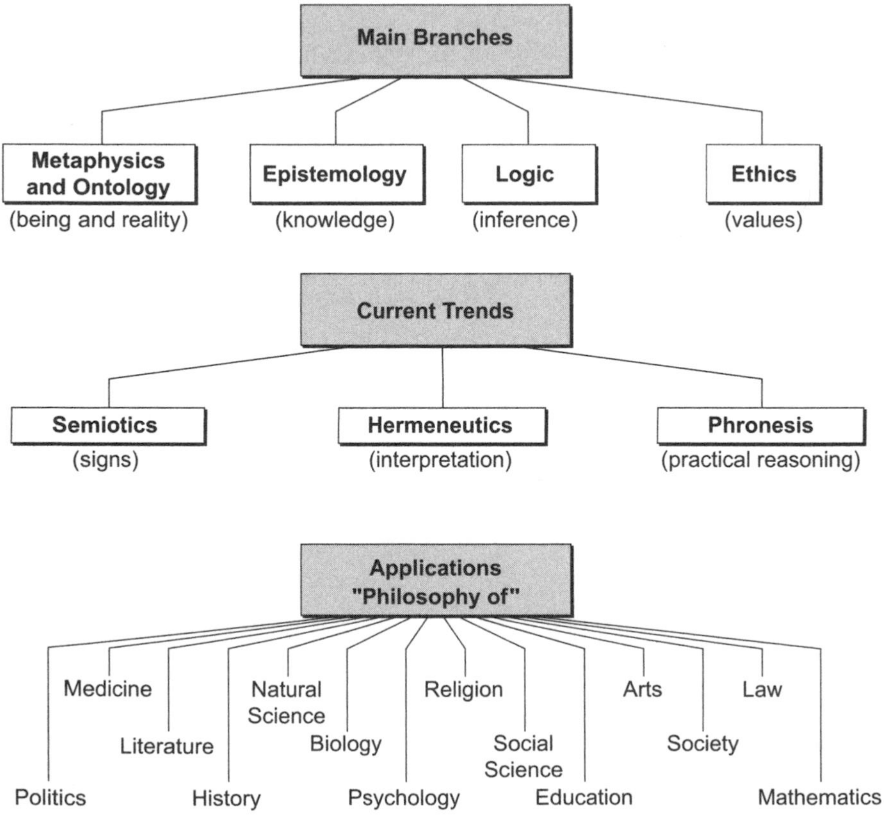

What is there? (Ontology and metaphysics.) How can we know? (Epistemology.) What follows? (Logic.) What are we to do? What is good, and what is bad? (Ethics.) These questions, and the answers to them, have a profound impact on decision-making, decisions themselves, and actions in various fields of human endeavor. From one endeavor to another, the magnitude of contribution of various branches of philosophy may vary. We may expect a lot of logic in the philosophy of science or the philosophy of economics, a lot of metaphysics in the philosophy of religion, and a lot of ethics in medical ethics.

Some turning points in the recent evolution and history of philosophy have important implications for medicine, such as the principle of verifiability of cause-effect relationships by experience as advanced in logical positivism by the Vienna Circle; increasingly flexible views of argumentation; expansions of the classical Aristotelian model of reasoning and argument; chaos theory; and fuzzy logic vs traditional yes-or-no thinking.

Physicians such as Murphy[6] and Wulff et al[7] see philosophy in medicine as *"a formal inquiry into the structure of medical thought."*

More precisely, from our perspective, **philosophy in medicine** means

> *the uses and application of philosophy to health, disease, and medical care. It is an activity whose aim is to study the general principles and ideas that lie behind our views, understanding, and decisions about health, disease, and care. Its objective is not a new or old finding (science follows this objective), but the understanding of the concepts and principles used to interpret phenomena that surround us and that concern us. Philosophically understanding our views of the physical world and of physical phenomena helps improve our biological understanding of health, disease, and care.*

In other words, philosophy in medicine not only examines our daily ways of doing things and making decisions. It also examines the methods used by medicine to formulate hypotheses and directions on the basis of evidence, as well as the grounds on which claims about patients and health problems may be justified.

For Schaffner and Engelhart Jr,[8] the philosophy of medicine is a kind of philosophy "... *encompassing those issues in epistemology, axiology, logic, methodology and metaphysics generated by or related to medicine. Issues have frequently focused on the nature of the practice of medicine, on concepts of health and disease, and on understanding the kind of knowledge that physicians employ in diagnosing and treating patients."* As we can see, their definition encompasses both **philosophy of medicine** (philosophical consideration of the nature of medicine's own additional contribution to philosophy in general, such as clinical trials as proof of cause-effect relationships) *and* **philosophy in medicine** (uses and applications of philosophy regarding various problems in medicine).

Across the medical literature, philosophy is scattered among various topics mainly covered by biostatisticians, epidemiologists, and a few clinicians. The latter shared their interest in these matters with "real" philosophers, logicians, and critical thinkers. In *Philosophy of Medicine: An Introduction*, Wulff et al[7] make connections between various branches of philosophy and topics in medicine; in *Reasoning in*

Medicine: An Introduction to Clinical Inference, Albert et al[9] focus essentially on clinical inference. In other terms, philosophy in medicine explores the methods used by medicine, the ways in which hypotheses and decision rules and decisions themselves are formulated from evidence, and the grounds on which medical claims about a health problem and its handling are justified. A career philosopher is increasingly becoming a kind of vital and valuable partner to health professionals,[10] as biostatisticians, economists, engineers, sociologists, economists, managers, and other specialists are already.

Traditionally, since the times of the Hippocratic oath, most philosophy in medicine was devoted to **medical ethics,** which focuses by definition on the **values** of health, disease, and care, and on the **morality** of our actions, behavior, and conduct. Surprisingly, the *Journal of Medical Philosophy* is devoted almost exclusively to medical ethics. We deal here instead with the less developed and less structured domain of medical thinking itself.

A neophyte may feel overwhelmed and puzzled by many terms: *thinking, reasoning, logic, critical thinking,* and others. Do these terms mean the same thing or not? They do not. Each term has its own significance and consequently its own *raison d'être.*

In clinical research and epidemiology, we are almost obsessed by definitions, not only conceptual ones (What is hypertension?) but also operational ones (What values [eg, blood pressure] separate normalcy from a disease on which the clinician must act, make a more profound diagnostic workup, or prescribe a conservative or radical treatment plan?). Let us devote our attention similarly to some basic, mostly conceptual definitions in the realm of philosophy in medicine, as we do in epidemiology, biostatistics, clinical pharmacology, psychiatry, medical sociology, and elsewhere. What is logic? What is critical thinking? What is reasoning? Defining these concepts will help further explain the topics of this book.

For whatever reason, many readers may not find this information in their basic training. Many curricula still do not tackle these topics, either directly in an organized manner or as an integrated and integral part of training a physician. The practical importance of philosophy in medicine is much greater than one might expect.

Pellegrino[11,12] stresses the difference and complementarity of *philosophy in medicine, philosophy of medicine, philosophy and medicine,* and *medical philosophy.* Currently all of these terms are used across the medical literature. For Pellegrino:

Philosophy *in* medicine means

> *"uses of the formal tools of philosophical inquiry to examine the matter of medicine itself as an object of study."*

Philosophy *of* medicine is

> *"a philosophical inquiry into the nature of medicine with a view to elaborating some general theory of medicine and medical activities."*

Philosophy and medicine remain totally independent disciplines. A philosopher may use empirical data from fundamental and clinical microbiology to advance the conceptualization of body-environment reaction and adaptation. A physician will use the tools of formal and informal logic to elaborate a system of diagnosis, treatment decision analysis, and action prescription in the form of clinical algorithms.

Consequently, this book is about philosophy *and* medicine, in particular about **both** logic and critical thinking **and** medicine.

1.4 PHILOSOPHY OF SCIENCE, SCIENTIFIC METHOD, EVIDENCE, AND EVIDENCE-BASED MEDICINE

Is there some relationship between philosophy of science, scientific method, and evidence? Definitely!

Philosophy of science means the systematic study[13(see also 27)] of

- *the inner workings and functioning of science, and*

- *the extent of its ability to gain access to the truth about the material world, and*

- *such concepts of scientific inquiry as laws of nature, causality, probability, and explanation.*

Scientific method includes as important components:

- *defining the domain and the problem of interest*

- *critical review of the available evidence*

- *formulating a hypothesis*

- *observation and/or experimentation involving data collection and implying some kind of measurement*

- *recording of the findings*

- *analysis and interpretation of the findings using both quantitative and qualitative methods*

- *confirmation or refutation of the hypothesis*

- *generation of a new hypothesis and/or of directions for further inquiry and practice.*

Evidence in medicine means

". . . any data or information, whether solid or weak, obtained through experience, observational research, or experimental work (trials). This [sic] data or information must be relevant to some degree (more is better) either to the understanding of the problem (case) or to the clinical decisions (diagnostic, therapeutic, or care-oriented) made about the case. . . ."[1]

"Evidence" is not automatically correct, complete, satisfactory, or useful. It must be evaluated, graded, and used according to its own merit.

What then is EBM?

Three closely related definitions of EBM have been formulated:

- *"The process of systematically finding, appraising, and using contemporaneous research findings as the basis of clinical decisions."*[14]

- *"The conscientious, explicit, and judicious use of current best evidence in making decisions about the care of individual patients."*[15]

- *"The integration of the best research evidence with clinical expertise and patient values."*[16]

In this sense, it is also applied closely to evidence-based public health.[17-19]

The steps for the practice of EBM closely reflect the above-mentioned scientific method as well as the steps of formulating, implementing, and evaluating any health program. These **EBM steps** are:

- Formulating the question concerning the patient that has to be answered (*identifying need for evidence*)

- Searching for the evidence (*producing the evidence*)

- Appraising the evidence (*evaluating the evidence*)

- Selecting the best evidence available for clinical decision-making (*using the evidence*)

- Linking the evidence with clinical knowledge, experience, and practice and with the patient's values and preferences (*integrated uses of evidence*)

- Using the evidence in clinical care to solve the patient's problem (*uses of evidence in specific settings*)

- Evaluating the effectiveness of the uses of the evidence in this case (*weighing the impact*)

- Teaching and expanding EBM practice and research (*going beyond what was already achieved*)

Hence, science is here to produce high-quality evidence. Philosophy should contribute to its soundness, logical acceptability, and good use by fitting it into the correct way of thought.

Philosophy has a much broader appeal for medicine than logic or ethics. Table 1-1 illustrates essential steps in EBM and some relevant domains of philosophy at each step. Logic is relevant at each EBM step (with epistemology, among others, helping us understand what is involved in the production of evidence), hermeneutics is relevant to understanding the patient, and ethics is relevant to the use of evidence.

In addition to the application of classical domains of philosophy to medicine, some authors recently attempted to see certain medical activities as a reflection of

TABLE 1-1

Relevance of philosophy to evidence-based medicine

World and cascade of evidence	Some relevant domains of philosophy
Building ground for evidence (clinical data acquisition)	*Logic, hermeneutics, semiology*
Producing evidence (carrying out medical research)	*Logic, epistemology, philosophy of science*
Evaluating evidence (evaluating results of research)	*Logic, hermeneutics, epistemology*
Using evidence (putting results of research to use in clinical and community medical practice)	*Logic, "phronesis," ethics*

other, still controversial trends such as **hermeneutics**,[20-22] which are for them *"the art of interpretation in its broadest sense"* or **semiotics**[23,24] as *"the study of interpretation of signs"* or **phronesis**,[3] which might be seen in medical terms as *"the best possible use of evidence in particular, concrete, and specific situations, patients, conditions, and settings."* We can expect further development and evaluation of these recent views in the medical literature.

Evidence-based medicine must make sense! To follow the objectives of EBM, medical science uses what philosophers call an **"object language"**—speaking directly about clinical (bedside) and paraclinical (laboratory) observations.

Philosophy in medicine uses a sort of **"metalanguage"** by focusing its attention on the meaning of what the object language provides. Does it accurately reflect the reality it is supposed to describe?

A psychiatrist may conclude that his or her patient produces only a "word (or verbal) salad"—a statement in an object language. What does this mean? What kind of mental health problem does verbal salad represent? A metalanguage is needed to clarify and find the answer to these questions. We still don't always know or agree on meanings in the world of medical communication.

Whereas the science of medicine bases its theories, understanding, and actions wholly on established facts, philosophy deals with conceptual issues and issues of principle that arise even where the facts have not been firmly established. In addition, philosophy also covers other areas of inquiry, where entirely satisfactory facts are not available.[25]

Tonelli[26] maintains that EBM should use philosophy to go beyond the empirical evidence at the core of EBM and investigate the complex variation of clinical judgment from one patient to another.

1.5 THINKING, LOGIC, REASONING, AND CRITICAL THINKING

Good medicine not only relies on good evidence but also on how evidence is interpreted, understood, and used. How is evidence integrated within our reasoning, and how do we convey our conclusions to their intended recipients? How do we think about it? Is what we say logical? Does the path of our reasoning reflect critical thinking?

When we ask such questions, the meaning of the terms *thinking, logic, reasoning,* and *critical thinking* may seem obvious. Let us, however, make explicit their distinct meaning and their relationship.

Thinking is a mental action, which, if verbalized, is a matter of combining words in propositions. For example, the premises and conclusion of a logical argument are propositions.

Definition making has its proper rules,[27] which are not always easy to follow. The more definitions we have of a given subject, the more we are uncertain about its exact context and demarcations. In fact, the term *logic* means different things to different people,[28-30] and definitions of logic abound. Some of them are worth quoting in our context:

- The normative science that investigates the principles of valid reasoning and correct inference,[28] dealing either with conclusions that follow necessarily from the reasons or premises (**deductive logic**) or with conclusions that follow with some degree of probability from the reasons or premises (**inductive logic**).

- The basic principles of reasoning developed by and applicable to any field of knowledge; the **logic of science**.[31]

- "*Logic is not the science of belief, but the science of proof, or evidence*" (John Stuart Mill).[32]

Logic then, is

". . .a normative discipline, one that lays down standards of correct reasoning to which we ought to adhere if we want to reason successfully."[29]

Logic focuses, as we will see in more detail in the next two chapters, on the strengths and weaknesses of arguments and on how arguments are linked in their drive to the conclusion that should result from them.

Logic as applied to medicine is then

". . .a system of thought and reasoning that governs understanding and decisions in clinical and community care. It defines valid reasoning, which helps us understand the meaning of medical phenomena and justifies clinical and paraclinical decisions on how to act in response to such phenomena."[1]

Reasoning itself is

". . .thinking directed towards reaching a conclusion. The reasons from which it begins are called 'premises'; what they lead to and support is called the 'conclusion'. . . ."[28]

Ideally, "*reasoning is thinking enlightened by logic. . . .*"[29]

Correct reasoning is

"the result of applying logical principles to particular cases. . . ."[29]

Fueled by satisfactory evidence, it produces **knowledge**.

Common knowledge may be defined as

shared knowledge between individuals.

For example, the realm of common knowledge in medicine includes, among others, human anatomy, allergy, human genetics, and intensive care. Understanding common knowledge is one of the fundamental conditions of effective communication and consequent action (care) in medicine.

Good decisions in practice and research require an organized combination of all the above, brought by modern philosophers under the umbrella of critical thinking. Hence, **critical thinking** means a broader framework that integrates and synthesizes all the above.

Critical thinking was best defined by Ennis[33] as

"reasonable reflective thinking that is focused on deciding what to believe or do."

Critical thinking in medicine is about ways of deciding and conveying well to others what we believe and what we are doing or intend to do, not for our personal intellectual satisfaction, but for the full benefit of the patient and the community.

Sounds too theoretical? Our first overview of basic definitions is more familiar to arts and pure science than to the health sciences. It should help us understand more clearly the practical implications and applications of logic and critical thinking as they will be briefly outlined in the following chapters.

1.6 WHERE IN MEDICINE MAY WE FIND PRACTICAL APPLICATIONS AND PRACTICAL USES OF PHILOSOPHY, LOGIC, AND CRITICAL THINKING AND THEIR EXPECTED BENEFITS?

The answer is in both medical practice and medical research. Information and skills are not enough. Medical practice and research also rely heavily on logic and critical thinking:[1]

- **In our research papers**, discussion of our findings relies not only on the "hard" evidence of the findings themselves, but more importantly on their critical analysis and sound interpretation. So do our recommendations.

- **At scientific gatherings and in medical journals**, we must convincingly explain our findings.

- **In the clinical management of individual patients** in daily hospital and family practice, we must "make ourselves understood and understand what the patient means and what he or she wants to say."

- **At clinical rounds**, we must find common ground with our peers for the clinical evaluation and care of our patients.

- **At business meetings on health programs and policies**, often involving stakeholders other than health professionals, we must justify health interventions "logically" as well as the commitment of human and material resources to the recommended actions.

- **In litigation and in societal discussions** involving occupational and environmental health issues for individual patients and whole communities, our arguments must be understood by not only health professionals but also the broader public.

- **At any other forum "outside the hospital or medical office" in civic, political, and public life** that focuses on decision-making carried out by other decision-makers and, last but not least, by concerned individuals, we should be able to muster good arguments for our position.

After two chapters covering some of the basics of logic and one chapter on critical thinking, we devote one chapter each to their applications in writing and reading reports of medical research, in clinical practice, and in interactions with the "outside world" of non-health professionals. As expected, different domains of philosophy will predominate in different fields of application. For example, in medical research, we may be predominantly concerned with the best ways of studying and interpreting cause-effect relationships. In working with patients, we may be very interested in **hermeneutics** (ie, what do they want to say, what message do they convey?), and **heuristics** ("rules of thumb" for discovery). Elsewhere (eg, in critical care, in genetic considerations, or in discussions of cloning humans), medical ethics may play an important and often decisive role. In the legal and quasilegal world, the domain of fallacies in argumentation is important. Not all interested parties necessarily search for absolute truth, but they all want to win the case! We need to be on the lookout for tricky maneuvers.

For Jaspers,[34] "*every doctor is a philosopher.*" There is a reason for this. If a physician does not adopt and apply philosophy in a practical manner in medical problem-solving, several difficulties may occur. In the specialty of psychiatry, for example, the Association for the Advancement of Philosophy and Psychiatry points out several important consequences of such neglect:

- the naïve empiricism of the most recent entries in the *Diagnostic and Statistical Manual of Mental Disorders* (*DSM-IV*) by the American Psychiatric Association,[35]

- confusion of the scientific and philosophical aspects of the mind-body problem,

- declining interest in a rigorously phenomenological discipline of psychopathology,

- virtual elimination of detailed idiographic or single-case studies, and

- insufficient attention to the interface of psychiatric theory and practice with sociopolitical and economic forces.[36]

Harper[37] considers the use of philosophy in medicine as a kind of "*philosophical climbing frame*," which makes better doctors. It "*. . . allows us to step out from underneath into a position where we have a better perspective. . . . We will also be in a position to look beyond the confines of our own little medical world and see that there are other stockpiles and climbing frames, the ascent of which might be useful, interesting, or both.*"

As we may now understand better, this book is not about EBM itself, but about how we see, read, interpret, use, and evaluate evidence in a larger context. Or rather, how we should do so. First, let us consider (in Chapters 2 and 3) some general remarks about logic, good reasoning, and good argument. Then (in Chapter 4), we can consider in a little more detail what critical thinking is and apply the process of critical thinking to the challenge posed to medicine by so-called *complementary and alternative medicine.* This general background will enable us to apply principles of good reasoning and good argument to reading and writing research reports (Chapter 5), to clinical practice (Chapter 6), and to our interactions with the outside world (Chapter 7).

Before moving any further, some readers may feel that they would benefit from a succinct background text about philosophy today. Popkin and Stroll's *Philosophy Made Simple*[38] is a good introduction for curious onlookers, including those in the health sciences.

References

1. Jenicek M. *Foundations of Evidence-Based Medicine.* New York, NY: The Parthenon Publishing Group; 2003.

2. *Mosby's Medical Dictionary.* 2nd ed rev. St.Louis, Mo: Mosby; 1987.

3. Tyreman S. Promoting critical thinking in health care: phronesis and criticality. *Med Health Care Philos.* 2000;3:117–124.

4. *On-line Medical Dictionary.* Available at: http://cancerweb.ncl.ac.uk/omd.

5. Thompson B. *Philosophy.* (Teach Yourself Books.) London, England and Lincolnwood, Ill: Hodder Headline PLC and NTC/Contemporary Publishing; 2000.

6. Murphy EA. *The Logic of Medicine.* 2nd ed. Baltimore, Md: The Johns Hopkins University Press; 1997.

7. Wulff HR, Pedersen SA, Rosenberg R. *Philosophy of Medicine: An Introduction.* Oxford, England: Blackwell Publishing; 1986.

8. Schaffner KF, Engelhardt HT Jr. Philosophy of medicine. In: *Conscise Routledge Encyclopedia of Philosophy.* London, England: Routledge; 2000:552.

9. Albert DA, Munson R, Resnik MD. *Reasoning in Medicine: An Introduction to Clinical Inference.* Baltimore, Md: The Johns Hopkins University Press; 1988.

10. Kamm FM. The philosopher as insider and outsider. *J Med Philos.* 1990;11:347–374.

11. Pellegrino ED. Philosophy of medicine: towards a definition. *J Med Philos.* 1986;11:9–16.

12. Pellegrino ED. What the philosophy of medicine is. *Theor Med Bioeth.* 1998;19:315–336.

13. Helicon Publishing Ltd, ed. *Instant Reference: Philosophy.* (Teach Yourself Books.) London, England and Lincolnwood, Ill: Hodder Headline PLC and NTC/Contemporary Publishing; 2000.

14. Rosenberg W, Donald A. Evidence-based medicine: an approach to clinical problem solving. *BMJ.* 1995;310:1122–1126.

15. Sackett DL, Rosenberg WM, Gray JA, Haynes RB, Richardson WS. Evidence-based medicine: what it is and what it isn't. *BMJ.* 1996;312:71–72.

16. Sackett DL, Straus S, Richardson WS, Rosenberg W, Haynes RB. *Evidence-based Medicine: How to Practice and Teach EBM.* 2nd ed. London, England: Churchill Livingstone; 2000.

17. Jenicek M. Epidemiology, evidence-based medicine, and evidence-based public health. *J Epidemiol.* 1997;7:187–197.

18. Jenicek M, Stachenko S. Evidence-based public health, community medicine, preventive care. *Med Sci Monit.* 2003;9(2):SR1–7.

19. Brownson RC, Baker EA, Leet TL, Gillespie KN. *Evidence-based Public Health.* Oxford, England: Oxford University Press; 2003.

20. Packer MJ, Addison RB, eds. *Entering the Circle: Hermeneutic Investigation in Psychology.* Albany, NY: State University of New York Press; 1989.

21. Cooper MW. Is medicine hermeneutics all the way down? *Theor Med.* 1994;15:149–180.

22. Svenaeus F. Hermeneutics of clinical practice: the question of textuality. *Theor Med Bioeth.* 2000;21:171–189.

23. Burnum JF. Medical diagnosis through semiotics. Giving meaning to the sign. *Ann Intern Med.* 1993;119:939–943.

24. Nessa J. About signs and symptoms: can semiotics expand the view of clinical medicine? *Theor Med.* 1996;17:363–377.

25. *The Columbia Encyclopedia* [online]. 6th ed. New York, NY: Columbia University Press; 2002. Available at: www.bartleby.com/65.

26. Tonelli MR. The philosophical limits of evidence-based medicine. *Acad Med*. 1998;73:1234–1240.

27. Audi R, ed. *The Cambridge Dictionary of Philosophy.* 2nd ed. Cambridge, England: Cambridge University Press; 1999:213–215.

28. Department of Philosophy, University of Guelph. *Logic Outline.* 7th ed, rev. Guelph, Ontario, Canada: University of Guelph; 2000.

29. Johnson DM. Reasoning and logic. In: Sills DL, ed. *International Encyclopedia of Social Sciences.* New York, NY: Macmillan Co and The Free Press; 1968:344–349.

30. Hughes GE, Wang H, Roscher N. The history and kinds of logic. In: McHenry R, ed. *The New Encyclopaedia Britannica: Macropedia/Knowledge in Depth.* Vol 23. Chicago, III: Encyclopaedia Britannica, Inc; 1992:226–282.

31. *New Illustrated Webster's Dictionary of the English Language.* New York, NY: PAMCO Publishing Company; 1992.

32. Cooper DE. *World Philosophies: An Historical Introduction.* 2nd ed. Oxford, England: Blackwell Publishing; 2003.

33. Ennis RH. *Critical Thinking.* Upper Saddle River, NJ: Prentice Hall; 1996.

34. Jaspers K. *General Psychopathology.* Chicago, III: University of Chicago Press; 1963.

35. Task Force on DSM-IV and the American Psychiatric Association. *Diagnostic and Statistical Manual of Mental Disorders.* 4th ed. Washington, DC: American Psychiatric Press; 2000.

36. Wallace E, Radden J, Sadler JZ. The philosophy of psychiatry: who needs it? *J Nerv Ment Dis*. 1997;185:67–73.

37. Harper CM. Philosophy for physicians. *J R Soc Med*. 2003;96:40–45.

38. Popkin RH, Stroll A. *Philosophy Made Simple.* 2nd ed, rev. New York, NY: Broadway Books; 2001.

CHAPTER 2

Logic in a Nutshell I: Reasoning and Underlying Concepts

What Is Required? Does It Make Sense?

IN THIS CHAPTER

Ye shall do no unrighteousness in judgment . . .
THE HOLY BIBLE, OLD TESTAMENT, LEVITICUS (UNDATED)

*Logic is not an enemy of feeling, emotion, and passion.
If it is true, as the philosopher Pascal said, that
"the heart has reasons of its own," logic can take
these reasons into account and work with them too.
So instead of opposing the heart's desires,
logic can help the heart to achieve them.*
STEPHEN S. THOMAS, 1981

Logic is the art of going wrong with confidence.
JOSEPH WOOD KRUTCH, QUOTED IN 1977,
S. W. MERRELL AND J. M. MCGREEVY, 1991
*(DEFINITELY, IF PREMISES ARE UNSUPPORTED
BY THE BEST EVIDENCE AVAILABLE!)*

*Without logic and critical thinking,
physicians risk quickly becoming simply
practitioners of medical technologies.*

In this chapter, we outline basic elements of logic and illustrate how they apply to medical problems:

- We need to know more than what the best evidence is for our clinical decisions.

- We also need to know how to use evidence in a logical way. It is our correct and critical thinking which guides our mind and hand toward a properly executed tracheal intubation or lumbar puncture or which leads us to do something else or to do nothing.

- We need to learn and understand how medical evidence should be used in our reasoning and decision-making.

In this chapter, we examine the classical paradigms of our thinking about medical problems in terms of classical logic and less traditional logic as well. It is essential for all physicians to learn more about medical reasoning and to understand its workings.

2.1 A BRIEF HISTORICAL NOTE

Logic as the theory of correct reasoning has always been one of the cornerstones of philosophy and human thinking. The roots of our modern understanding of reasoning are surprisingly ancient. In **Western philosophy and logic,**[1-3] Aristotle of Stagira (384–322 BC) in ancient Greece developed a sound and complete theory of what has come to be known as *categorical syllogisms*. Chrysippus of Soli (ca 280–207 BC) developed a sound system of *propositional logic*—the logic of the words *not, both . . . and, either . . . or,* and *if . . . then,* which govern propositions. Medieval logic developed theories about *sophismata* (puzzling cases) and *supposition* (different references of terms in different contexts), among others. In the 17th and 18th centuries, Gottfried Wilhelm Leibnitz made substantial contributions to the development of formal logical calculi. The 19th century was one of the most prolific periods of advances in modern logic. George Boole, Gottlob Frege, and Charles Sanders Peirce developed symbolic logic and blurred demarcations between logic and mathematics. In the 20th century, Bertrand Russell considered pure mathematics as part of logic, but Kurt Gödel's theorems showed that a sound formal theory of arithmetic was necessarily incomplete. More recently, *informal logic* has emerged in reaction to the mathematization of formal logic as a kind of logic in natural conditions, setting, and speech. This new trend is reflected in the text of this book.

In **Eastern philosophies,**[1-3] Aristotelian logic is related to language in Islamic philosophy (Al-Farabi) and in the ancient Chinese philosophy originating from the same period as logic in ancient Greece (Hu Shi, Gongsun Lung, Mohists). Logic in India was related rather closely to religion. India's Nyaya school of philosophy developed its own way of argumentation (illustrated further in this chapter) from the third century BC to the second century AD. Since the 19th century, Japanese philosophers (Nishida Kitaro, Tanabe Hajime) focused on dialectical logic or *ronri* (principles of discourse and argument). Logic in medicine is the fruit of such rich historical endeavors and of experience acquired by generations across time and continents.

In the health sciences and other sciences, modern philosophers, epidemiologists, and biostatisticians, by virtue of their specialties and domains of interest, examined problems of probability and uncertainty, cause-effect relationships, the deductive and inductive nature of medical research, and observational or experimental studies in disease etiology and therapeutics.[4-12] (More information about them may be found in Chapter 5.) Their views have been extensively reviewed and synthesized,[13-15] and some elements of logic have appeared in several more recent monographs.[16-18]

Theoretical studies of the uses of logic in medicine have been rather scarce and fragmented. In 1976, Murphy published *The Logic of Medicine*,[11] which focuses mostly on various aspects of probability and uncertainty in medical understanding and decisions. King's *Medical Thinking: A Historical Perspective*[19] followed in 1982. In the eighties, epidemiologists tackled many important philosophical issues in the study of cause-effect relationships.[7-15] In 1987, Slaney[20,21] presented in two articles a short outline of formal logic and its applications in medicine. Finally, in 1995, Phillips[22] brought together a set of publications devoted to various aspects of logic in medicine.

This chapter is intended to be a basic companion and starting point in the fundamental workings of logic as it applies to various clinical problems and settings.

2.2 LOGIC IN GENERAL AND LOGIC IN MEDICINE

We want medicine to be logical in order to better understand it and to use it effectively to the benefit of the patient. But are things that are "logical" more easily understood than things that "make sense"? Is logic part of our understanding of health and disease? The answer to these questions is a definite "yes," since logic heavily underlies our epidemiologic and biological thinking, interpretations, and practical decisions.

Let us now focus on the basic principles and applications of logic.

Many of us left school with the idea that philosophy is too abstract and theoretical, especially for our medical minds that are driven to the resolution of concrete and practical problems in patient health. At the beginning of the 20th century a group of philosophers known as the Vienna Circle[2,3,23] proposed that the object of philosophy is a logical clarification of thought; it is not a theory, but an activity. These first proponents of *logical positivism* advocated that logic, mathematics, and experience could reduce the content of scientific theories to truth.[24] Their *verification (or verifiability) principle* claims that a proposition (statement) is meaningful if, and only if, some experience acquired through the senses would suffice to determine that it is true or false.[24,25] This principle has proved impossible to articulate and defend in a form that would achieve the positivists' goal of stigmatizing metaphysical and value claims as nonsensical or nonfactual while at the same time making scientific claims meaningful. Nevertheless, logical positivists built bridges between speculative logic and experimental considerations in health sciences.

For medicine, in light of the focus on evidence that experimental research provides, several views of logical positivists are worth stating:

- There are two sources of knowledge: logical reasoning and sense perception.

- Logical reasoning includes mathematics, which is reducible to formal logic.

- Empirical knowledge obtained through a combination of sense perception and logical reasoning includes physics, biology, [and] psychology.

- Experience (sense perception) is the only judge of scientific theories. However, scientific knowledge does not exclusively arise from experience: scientific theories are genuine hypotheses that go beyond experience.

- There is a distinction between observational and theoretical terms.

- There is a distinction between synthetic and analytic statements.

- There is a distinction between theoretical axioms and rules of correspondence.

- Scientific theories are of a deductive nature.

In this approach, experience and experimental work join pure thinking as part of scientific theorizing. More recent developments in the philosophy of science[6,26-29] have challenged every one of the views just mentioned. Science now tends to be regarded by philosophers as a historically situated activity in which techniques, apparatus, and assumptions play as large a role as sense perception and logic in constituting what is accepted at any given time.

Logic itself is part of a broader framework of **critical thinking**: *"reasonable reflective thinking that is focused on deciding what to believe or do."*[30]

Reasoning is *thinking directed toward reaching a conclusion*. Ideally, it is structured and objectified by logic, as defined earlier.

Logic itself is the *"normative science, which investigates the principles of valid reasoning and correct inference."*[31] It deals with conclusions that either follow necessarily from the reasons or premises (**deductive logic**) or follow with some degree of probability from the reasons or premises (**inductive logic**). Logic investigates, systematizes, and demonstrates rules of correct reasoning.[32]

If the principles of logic are applicable to any field of science, medicine should also be subjected to its general rules. The *logic of medicine* is **a system of thought and reasoning that governs understanding and decisions in clinical and community care. It defines valid reasoning, which helps us understand the meaning of medical phenomena and leads us to the justification of the choice of clinical and paraclinical decisions about how to act on such phenomena.**

Logic focuses primarily on strengths and weaknesses of the links in reasoning and arguments between premise (or premises) and conclusion.

Arguments are studied in two ways by formal and informal logic. **Symbolic** or **formal logic** builds a *formalized system of reasoning, using abstract symbols for the various aspects of natural language.* Artificial intelligence is based on formal logic. Formal logic abstracts from the content propositions, statements, or deductive argument structures or logical forms they embody. A symbolic notation is used to express these structures, and the list of such symbols must be found elsewhere.[1,23,33]

Informal logic[31,34,35] uses *methods and techniques to analyze and interpret seemingly informal reasoning as it happens in the context of natural language used in everyday life.* Examples of such reasoning occur in an exchange of information between physicians on clinical rounds; in professional, administrative, or judiciary medical reports; or in scientific papers.

Let us first explain some basic elements and principles of logic. (Their application to specific problems and challenges in medicine may be found in subsequent chapters.)

For those readers whose knowledge of the basic principles of logic has faded with time, Part One briefly deals with the application of informal logic to medicine.

2.3 REASONING AND ARGUMENTS

In Western culture, we owe the fundamentals of logic to ancient Greek philosophers such as Aristotle and Chrysippus of Soli and to such later thinkers as Gottfried Wilhelm Leibniz, George Boole, John Stuart Mill, Gottlob Frege, Charles Sanders Peirce, and Bertrand Russell. Formally, logic concerns **inferences**, which may occur in solo **reasoning** or in **arguments** addressed to others. **Reasoning** is *thinking leading to a conclusion.* For example, one may say to oneself, "This 70-year-old patient of mine has lung cancer, so he should stop smoking," thus inferring the conclusion that the patient should stop smoking from the diagnosis of lung cancer. (As we see in Chapter 6, this is bad reasoning.) An **argument** is *a set of statements, some of which—the premises—are offered as reasons for another statement, the conclusion.* For example, one may say to the patient, "You have lung cancer, so you should stop smoking," thus presenting one's reasoning to the patient in an attempt to convince him to stop smoking. Definitions of "argument" in logic textbooks vary.[34,36,37] An argument in this sense is generally expected to show that its conclusion should be accepted. It is therefore not about quarreling or fighting. It is about **explaining and defending our beliefs with good evidence and having them endorsed by others**.

We call *back-and-forth discussion in which at least one person advances arguments* "**argumentation**." Arguments and argumentation are ubiquitous in daily medical practice and in fundamental and bedside decision-oriented research. Examples of such arguments and argumentation can be found during **clinical rounds; in patients' charts; in public health, community medicine,** and **health policies; in medical and research articles; in our quest for grants in medical research; and in tort litigations.** Last but not least, we need logic and arguments supporting our recommendations when **we talk to the patient.**

In fact, ". . . *the critical standards of logic have application in any subject which employs inference and argument—in any field in which conclusions are supported by evidence.*"[38]

The basic model of medical reasoning and argument is **reasoning from one or more premises to a conclusion**. For example, our assessment of risk or diagnosis or our decision to treat is a product of reasoning, which can be addressed to others as an argument. Each piece of reasoning and each argument must be formulated as clearly as possible to give the correct meaning to whatever we do. Each of our premises must be the best possible piece of sustainable evidence.

When discussing clinical cases during floor rounds, we are advancing arguments (sometimes even arguing), providing reasons for some conclusion about the case. During clinical rounds, several colleagues may propose their sometimes contradictory, sometimes convergent views about the case (premises). Based on one, two, or more than two such premises, physicians attending rounds reach some conclusion about the diagnosis, treatment, or prognosis of the patient. Often, more than one argument is needed to solve a clinical problem.

To better understand argumentation used on rounds or anywhere in medical practice and medical research, we must know (1) how arguments are constructed (*What is required?*) and (2) how to evaluate them (*Does it make sense?*). Sections 2.4 and 2.5 help us with this.

2.4 COMPONENTS AND ARCHITECTURE OF REASONING AND ARGUMENTS: *WHAT IS REQUIRED?*

Since the time of Aristotle, reasoning and arguments have been thought to consist solely of one or more premises and a conclusion. In fact, the ancient Stoics defined an argument as "a system composed of premises and a conclusion."[39] Recently Toulmin[40,41] extended this analysis to allow for other components. We start with the traditional analysis and then expand it with Toulmin's model.

2.4.1 Classical Layout of Arguments: Premises and Conclusions

As mentioned, reasoning means directing thinking toward a conclusion. Reasons are called "premises," and they support a "conclusion." When addressed to someone else, the reasons and their pathway to a conclusion (included) form an argument.

An example of reasons leading to a conclusion is the classical categorical syllogism of Aristotle. The **categorical syllogism** is *a form of reasoning or argument consisting of two premises and a conclusion.* For example, we can state:

Premise A (p1): *All surgeons are physicians.*

Premise B (p2): *Peter is a surgeon.*

Conclusion (C): *Therefore, Peter is a physician.*

Figure 2-1 illustrates the architecture and building blocks of a classical categorical syllogism.

- **Premises** are statements of evidence.

- A **conclusion** is a statement that is supported by evidence.

- **Inference** is the "path from premises to conclusion."

Within premises and conclusions, in a categorical syllogism, three terms are used:[35]

- The **major term** (symbolized by the letter *P*, ie, **predicate**) is the predicate of the conclusion. It appears in the **major** premise. (In our example, **P** = physician.)

- The **minor term** (symbolized by the letter *S*, ie, **subject**) is the subject of the conclusion. It also appears in the **minor** premise. (In our example, **S** = Peter.)

- The **middle term** (symbolized by the letter *M*) appears in each premise but **not** in the conclusion. (In our example, **M** = surgeon.)

For a logician, a categorical syllogism is deductively valid (defined in Section 2.5.3) if **S, P,** and **M** are correctly combined. (See Chapter 3 for methods of testing for such correct combinations.)

In everyday life, premises are presented in any order. Often only the minor premise (B) is presented, and the major premise (A) is tacit. For example:

Premise A (major): *Anyone with a streptococcal infection of the throat present for less than 10 days* **(M)** *must be treated with antibiotics* **(P)**. *

FIGURE 2-1
_____

Architecture and building blocks of a classical categorical syllogism

MAJOR PREMISE	MINOR PREMISE	CONCLUSION

MIDDLE TERM

SUBJECT

All pediatricians **(M)** are physicians **(P)**	Mary **(S)** is a pediatrician **(M)**	Mary **(S)** must be a physician **(P)**

PREDICATE

Another example:

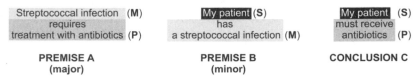

Streptococcal infection **(M)** requires treatment with antibiotics **(P)**	My patient **(S)** has a streptococcal infection **(M)**	My patient **(S)** must receive antibiotics **(P)**
PREMISE A (major)	**PREMISE B** (minor)	**CONCLUSION C**

Premise B (minor): *My patient* **(S)** *has a streptococcal infection of the throat present for less than 10 days* **(M)**.

Conclusion C: *My patient* **(S)** *must be treated with antibiotics* **(P)**.

* *If the infection has been present more than 10 days, the benefit of treatment by antibiotics may be questionable.*

In practice, a clinician is likely to think only of premise B (my patient has an infection) before making his or her therapeutic decision (conclusion C).

Such syllogisms follow the pattern:

A $(\alpha, p1)$; **B** $(\beta, p2)$; **therefore C** (γ, c).

Logicians recognize many other forms of reasoning and argument besides categorical syllogisms. (Chapter 3 outlines them in greater detail.) Traditionally, all syllogisms were analyzed and categorized into premises and conclusion. **The number of premises can be any finite number greater than or equal to one.**

2.4.2 Toulmin's Modern Scheme for Layout of Arguments

Stephen Toulmin[40,41] proposed four additional components for the layout of arguments. Although nontraditional, his scheme for the "layout of arguments" closely ties into our project of combining evidence-based medicine (EBM) with good reasoning and good argument. We will refer to it throughout the rest of this text.

Toulmin's scheme has six components:

- **claim** (conclusion)

- **grounds** (premise [or premises])

- **warrant**

- **qualifier**

- **rebuttals**

- **backing**

Take the following example: *A female patient has streptococcal pharyngitis, so presumably she should be treated with penicillin, unless she has a known allergy to penicillin. According to the best evidence available from clinical trials and other analytical studies, a 10-day course of penicillin is the treatment of choice for streptococcal pharyngitis.*

Figure 2-2 (theoretical model) and Figure 2-3 (practical application) illustrate the six components with reference to this example.

The claim

The **claim** or conclusion is *the proposition at which we arrive as a result of our reasoning, or which we defend in argument by citing our supporting grounds.*

FIGURE 2-2

Toulmin's modern layout of arguments and its six components: theoretical model*

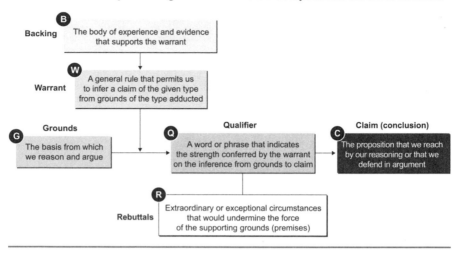

* Principles adapted from Figures 22-8 and 22-9 in Toulmin S, Rieke R, Janik A.[41]

Often the claim is an answer to a question at issue in the context. In our example, the claim (conclusion) is the proposition "*This patient should be treated with penicillin.*" It is an answer to the question, "*What treatment is appropriate for this patient?*"

Hence, the claim can be seen as the equivalent of the conclusion in more traditional terminology. In cultures with a European heritage, the claim is usually explicit, whether in reasoning, argument, or argumentation. In some Asian cultures, however, participants in "argumentative" discussions tend to leave their claims unstated, so as not to disrupt the harmony of the group, which is highly valued. In such discussions, the claim will emerge only at the end of the discussion, once participants have communicated to each other the reasons (grounds) relevant to the question at issue and have converged on an agreed answer.

The grounds

The **grounds** are *the basis from which we reason or argue.* They are *the specific facts relied on to support a given claim or conclusion.*

The grounds are the answer we give if someone challenges our claim by asking, "*What do you have to base yourself on?*" They are always explicitly stated. More traditionally, they are known as the premise or premises of the reasoning or argument. The grounds in our example are the single premise "*This patient has streptococcal pharyngitis.*"

We may consider the grounds as the equivalent of the premises in more traditional terminology.

FIGURE 2-3

Toulmin's modern layout of arguments and its six components: practical application

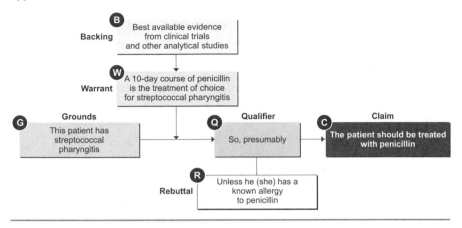

The warrant

The **warrant** is a *general rule that permits us to infer a claim of the given type from grounds of the type we have adduced.*

If we compare reasoning or arguing to baking a cake, the grounds or premises are the ingredients, the conclusion is the finished cake, and the warrant is the recipe for combining the ingredients to produce the cake. Warrants are **general** and are **usually unstated**; we reason and argue **in accordance with them**, rather than from them. They are general principles that are part of our background information in the field in which we reason or argue (in this case, medicine) and that can act as **licenses** permitting us to infer a conclusion of a certain sort from corresponding grounds or premises. In our example, we are inferring a recommendation about treatment of a particular patient from a diagnosis of streptococcal pharyngitis. The warrant for such an inference is: "*Given a diagnosis of streptococcal pharyngitis, a patient should be treated with penicillin.*" More colloquially, we can express warrants as general statements ("*Patients with streptococcal pharyngitis should be treated with penicillin.*") or as conditional statements ("*If a patient has streptococcal pharyngitis, that patient should be treated with penicillin.*").

Warrants can be highly general. A patient diagnosed with lung cancer may take into account the probabilities of the possible outcomes of surgery and/or chemotherapy and of some other more conservative treatment. The patient may consider the costs and benefits of each option-outcome combination in light of her or his values, preferences, and wishes and then decide on the treatment that promises to be most beneficial. The warrant for this reasoning might be the rule for decision making under probability: if the probabilities of each outcome of each option are known, choose that option with the greatest expected value. Most patients would use a more qualitative but highly general warrant, for example, choose an option whose worst possible outcome you can tolerate.

We may consider the warrant as the equivalent of an unstated (tacit) major premise in a classical Aristotelian categorical syllogism.

The qualifier

The **qualifier** is a *word or phrase that indicates the strength conferred by the warrant on the inference from grounds to claim, and thus the strength of support given to our conclusion by the grounds we offer* (assuming those grounds are true).

If the warrant can be applied without hesitation in all cases, without exception, we could qualify our conclusion by such words as "necessarily" or "certainly," or insert the word "must." For example: *The new emergency room patient has just gone into cardiac arrest; you **must** call the resuscitation team.* In this book, such warrants are called *universal warrants.* If the warrant is not definitively established or holds only in most cases, we may qualify our conclusion by a word such as "probably"; for example, the warrant that angina pectoris generally attacks men who are (in old-fashioned terminology from 1799) "*inclined to corpulency*"[42] would license the inference "*This new patient I am about to see reportedly suffers from angina pectoris, so he is **probably** a man inclined to corpulency.*" If the warrant is poorly established or holds only in some cases, we may qualify our conclusion by the word "possibly" or insert the word "may." For example, a pulsating abdominal mass is only sometimes an aneurysm of the abdominal aorta, so one should conclude from feeling such a mass only that the patient *may* have an aneurysm of the abdominal aorta. If the warrant has known exceptions or contraindications, the conclusion can be qualified by a word such as *presumably.* The word *presumably* in our example is such a qualifier. Qualifiers are not always expressed; one could simply argue, "*This patient has streptococcal pharyngitis, so she should be treated with penicillin.*" However, even well-established warrants such as the rule of treating streptococcal pharyngitis with penicillin have exceptions. **Good reasoning about the diagnosis, treatment, and prognosis of individual patients requires attention to such possible exceptions** as well as to how well established (evidence-based) the warrant is and whether it holds only in most or some cases.

The rebuttals

Rebuttals are *extraordinary or exceptional circumstances that would undermine the force of the supporting grounds* (premises).

To offer a rebuttal of an inference is to point to some circumstance in the particular case that makes the warrant inapplicable. In our example, information from the patient that she is allergic to penicillin would rebut the inference. Potential rebuttals can be made explicit in one's reasoning or argument through an "unless" clause, which may be open-ended ("*unless there is some contraindication in the particular case*"). In our example, there is one known exception-making condition, an allergy to penicillin, so the rebuttal can be quite specific: "*unless the patient has a known allergy to penicillin.*"

The backing

Backing is *the body of experience and evidence that supports the warrant.*

Just as we do not usually make our warrants explicit in our reasoning and arguments, so we do not usually make explicit the evidence on which these warrants are based. But, if we supply our warrant, someone may challenge us by asking, "*Why do you think that?*" An answer to that challenge will cite the evidence that backs up the general rule we are using. In EBM, that is the best available evidence, which should support the warrants we use to draw inferences. Somewhat unusually, our example alludes to such evidence (although it does not actually produce it in the form of citations of peer-reviewed papers in good medical journals): "*According to the best evidence available from clinical trials and other analytical studies, a 10-day course of penicillin is the treatment of choice for streptococcal pharyngitis.*" Here the phrase *the best evidence available from clinical trials and other analytical studies* alludes to evidence that could be cited to back up our warrant: "*A 10-day course of penicillin is the treatment of choice for streptococcal pharyngitis.*"

Sometimes warrants are backed by theoretical arguments rather than by evidence. Consider, for example, an inference from the positive results of a well-designed and well-executed randomized clinical trial to a conclusion that the treatment tested is more effective than the treatment received by the control group. (Headache sufferers receiving analgesic A were significantly more likely to feel relief after 30 minutes than were headache sufferers receiving analgesic B. Hence analgesic A is more effective for headache than analgesic B.) Here the warrant is that positive results of well-designed and well-executed randomized clinical trials prove causal effectiveness. If asked to justify this assumption, which lies at the heart of EBM, we would not appeal to the best available evidence. Rather, we would appeal to our conception of causation and to highly general features of our universe (things don't just happen, they are caused). In Chapter 5, where we focus on the

---

Implicit character of some components of Toulmin's model

It is important to realize that some elements of Toulmin's scheme are usually implicit. The warrant is almost never stated, nor are we conscious of it in our mental reasoning. We reason and argue **in accordance with** warrants, not from them; they are not premises, but rules of inference. The evidence that backs up our warrants (in EBM the best available evidence) tends to be stated only when we are called on to justify drawing our conclusion from the data. Rebuttals are often left unstated, for example, when the contraindications to a recommended treatment are well known. Even the qualifier is often implicit, although clarity demands that we specify whether we take our conclusion to follow strictly or only with some probability or subject to exceptions. The only components that are always explicit are the traditionally recognized components: claim (conclusion) and grounds (reasons, premises).

discussion and conclusions section of articles in medical journals, the theoretical character of the backing for such warrants shows up in the absence of a box for backing in our "Toulmin diagrams." The warrant will be taken to be self-evident, or at least not requiring backing by the best available evidence.

2.4.3 Reconstructing Arguments from the Natural Language of Daily Life

Arguments in everyday medical communication are mostly "hidden" in the flow of the message, which only rarely has an obvious structure. Discussion and conclusions of research findings do not always necessarily follow the order of Toulmin's scheme, or the classical Aristotelian syllogism. In everyday life and communication and even in medical literature, building blocks and architecture of arguments, as illustrated by Figure 2-1 and Figure 2-2, may be buried by the natural language of argumentation. For example: *We have found in the literature only one case report of such an unusual neurological deficit after stroke.* (Premise A?) *Our case series of five patients shows a comparable clinical picture to the above-mentioned index-case.* (Premise B?) *We may conclude that this clinical presentation of this type of stroke represents a broader and more representative pattern of manifestations of this particular clinical entity.* (Conclusion C?)

If the components of an argument are already clear, it may be submitted to direct evaluation by the criteria of the next section focusing on structure and content. If they are not, a standardized argument must be "deciphered, extracted, unearthed" from the flow of words and messages, or "reconstructed," as logicians say.

The reconstruction of an argument takes place in two phases:

1. Premises and conclusions are identified and reformulated (if necessary) from the natural language.

2. The structure of the argument is displayed in a tree diagram based on such identification and reformulation of premises and conclusions (ie, point 1).

Reconstruction of arguments[43] is covered in more detail in Chapter 6.

Identification and reformulation of premises and conclusions

To get a better understanding of argumentation in natural language, it is necessary, mostly in the world of research and teaching, to reconstruct syllogisms and other types of arguments, that is, to reorganize and reword them in a workable ensemble for analysis and improvement according to one of our structured models of reasoning. Important aids in such a reconstruction are words indicating relationships between propositions, especially **premise indicators** and **conclusion indicators** (defined in the shaded section that follows). Unfortunately, many of these words are ambiguous. The word "since", for example, can be used as a premise indicator, that is, to introduce a premise. (*"Since the patient is dehydrated, he must be given fluids."*) However, it can also be used **causally** to introduce a cause. (*"Since he smoked three packs of cigarettes a day for 40 years, he ended up developing lung cancer."*) It can also be used **temporally** to introduce an event at the beginning of some ongoing state or process. ("*Since I started running three times a week, I have never felt better.*") Here, *since* means "after this" and not "because of this," which requires an inference.

Premise indicators are words such as *for, since, because, assuming that, seeing that, granted that, in view of, given that,* and *in as much as.*[42] If they are used inferentially (as opposed to causally or temporally), they indicate that what immediately follows them is a premise.

Conclusion indicators are words such as *therefore, thus, hence, so, for this reason, accordingly, consequently, which proves that, which means that, as a result,* and *in conclusion.*[42] If they are used inferentially (as opposed to causally or temporally), they indicate that what immediately follows them is a conclusion.

Table 2-1 offers a more complete list of premise and conclusion indicators as tip-offs for more or less hidden reasoning or arguments.[43-48]

Sometimes, missing premises and conclusions must be completed on the basis of the context of the argument. In particular, arguments may be accompanied by statements of specific conditions under which the argument applies. For example, an argument about the risks of nosocomial (hospital) infections and their control may be made more specific by defining these infections, types of hospitals, and means available to control them.

Let us consider an example of everyday communication in medicine, and how it can be reconstructed:

An internal medicine resident may inform the clinical microbiology fellow of the following: "*The nurse on call told me that the elderly immunocompromised patient in Room 20 is distressed and disoriented, and has chills and fever. It looks to me like he may have sepsis. After ordering blood cultures, we started treatment with a combination of antibiotics, given that a delay in treatment might be hazardous for the patient. As soon as we get the results of the blood cultures, we will adjust treatment accordingly. . . .*"

We may reconstruct the above-mentioned resident's message as a report of the following reasoning:

- Premise A: *The elderly patient in Room 20 is immunocompromised.*

- Premise B: *He is distressed and disoriented.*

- Premise C: *He has chills and fever.*

- Conclusion D: *He may have sepsis.* (From A, B, C)

- Conclusion E: *Order blood cultures/Blood cultures are ordered.* (From D)

- Conclusion F: *A delay in treatment may be hazardous for him.* (From D)

- Conclusion G: *Start treatment with antibiotics/Treatment with antibiotics is started.* (From F)

- Conclusion H: *As soon as we get the results of the blood cultures, we will adjust treatment accordingly.* (From D, E, G)

Our reconstruction was aided by one inference indicator, the premise indicator "*given that*" used to introduce the premise "*A delay in treatment might be hazardous*

TABLE 2-1

Inference indicators (premise indicators and conclusion indicators) in reasoning and arguments in natural language*

Premise indicators	Conclusion indicators
As	Accordingly
Assuming that	Allows us to infer that
As indicated by	As a result
As shown by the fact that	Bears the point that
Being as	Consequently
Being that	Demonstrates that
Because	Establish(es) that
Firstly (or first)	For this reason
Follows for (from) the fact that	From which we can infer that
For	From which we may conclude that
For the reason that	Hence
Given that	I conclude that
Granted that	Implies that
Inasmuch as	In conclusion
In the first place	Indicates that
In the second place	In this way, one sees that
In view of the fact that	It follows that
It is established that	Justifies the view (belief) that
It is a fact that	Leads me to believe that
May be deduced from	Let us
May be derived from	Must
May be inferred from	Points to the conclusion that
One cannot doubt that	Proves that
On the correct supposition that	Shows that
Secondly (second)	So
Seeing that	Suggests that
Since	The moral is
The reason is that	Then (without preceding if)
This is true because	Therefore
Whereas	Thus
	We have proved that
	We may conclude that
	We may establish that
	We must
	We propose that
	Which means that
	Which proves that
	Which shows that
	You see that

* Compiled and modified from references 43–48.

for the patient," from which the resident inferred that it was appropriate to start treatment with a combination of antibiotics. The resident's communication contains no conclusion indicators; to indicate the structure of his reasoning more clearly, the resident could have said, "*So before getting results of blood cultures, we started treatment with antibiotics,*" thus indicating by the conclusion indicator "so" that the decision to start treatment was drawn as a conclusion from the suspicion that the patient was becoming septic.

The first inference, from premises A, B, and C to conclusion D, follows in virtue of several warrants: a compromised immune system is a risk factor for sepsis, and symptoms of sepsis include confusion, chills, and fever. The warrant for the second inference, from D to E (first part), is that blood cultures are needed to confirm a tentative diagnosis of sepsis. The warrant for the third inference, from D to F, is that a delay in treatment is hazardous for patients with sepsis. The warrant for the fourth inference, from F to G (first part), is that antibiotics are the treatment of choice for sepsis. The warrant for the fifth inference, from D, E (second part) and G (second part) to the final conclusion H, is that the results of blood cultures used to test for sepsis may indicate a need to use treatment other than a combination of antibiotics. (See the section that follows for a display of the resident's reasoning in a tree diagram.)

Here is another example of everyday medical communication with more or less hidden reasoning and arguments. Before leaving the hospital, we may say to a colleague on call, "*Do not forget to check this patient who has a fever of unknown origin. Results from the laboratory workup should arrive at any moment. I'm very concerned about him. All patients with a ruptured abscess have a fever. His condition may worsen quickly. Because this patient is febrile, and given his other clinical manifestations, he may have a ruptured abscess. If incoming laboratory and other paraclinical test results confirm the diagnosis, we should treat him with antibiotics as soon as possible and contact the surgeon on call for additional assessment and surgical care if indicated.*" Identifying the premises and conclusions in this communication and reconstructing the argument in a tree diagram is left as an exercise for the reader.

Sometimes, a reconstruction of argumentation may lead to more than one chain of premises (**branching of syllogisms**) and their fusion into a final conclusion. This type of reconstruction is, however, beyond the scope of this introductory text.

Detailed information on ways of reconstructing arguments may be found elsewhere.[43]

Displaying the structure in a tree diagram

The structure of an argument may be better understood by outlining it in the form of a **tree diagram**,[17,48] a schematic representation of links between premises (P_1, P_2, ... P_n) and conclusion or conclusions (C).

This structure may be as simple as linking one single premise to one conclusion:

After Harry contracted chlamydial urethritis, he was successfully treated with antibiotics.

Hence, Harry will not be able to transmit Chlamydia to his spouse.

In other instances, arguments may be more complex. Premises may lead to other premises, which are joined by some additional premises and merged toward a single conclusion:

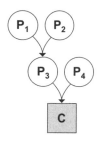

P₁: *When we proposed a disease prevention program focusing on passive smoking in public places, we had the support of all politicians at the local level in our region.*

P₂: *Even municipalities with strong opponents to the program ratified it.*

P₃: *So, the representatives of all municipalities support our program.*

P₄: *However, a considerable majority of residents outside the regional capital and a nonnegligible minority within the capital itself strongly opposed our program.*

C: *Therefore, municipal decision-makers approved the program based on medical arguments but at the expense of a good number of people in the target population of our health program whose views were not accommodated.*

In expanding our reasoning about a problem, such linking or chaining of ideas in a **sequence of arguments** occurs. For example, the following is the tree diagram of the resident's reasoning about the elderly patient with suspected sepsis:

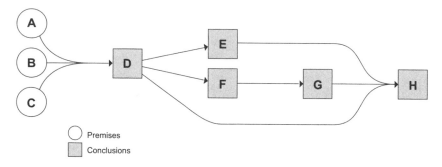

A: *The elderly patient in Room 20 is immunocompromised.*

B: *He is distressed and disoriented.*

C: *He has chills and fever.*

D: *He may have sepsis.*

E: *Order blood cultures/Blood cultures are ordered.*

F: *A delay in treatment may be hazardous for him.*

G: *Start treatment with antibiotics/Treatment with antibiotics is started.*

H: *As soon as we get the results of the blood cultures, we should adjust treatment accordingly.*

Completing arguments and compensating for ambiguity and vagueness may be, in some cases, a considerable challenge even for an experienced person.

2.5 EVALUATION OF REASONING AND ARGUMENT: DOES IT MAKE SENSE?

What is good reasoning? What is a good argument? What is good argumentation? Goodness is relative to function. We will identify one common function of reasoning, argument, and argumentation, and we will provide criteria of evaluation relative to that function.

2.5.1 Criteria for Good Reasoning

Reasoning is *thinking leading to a conclusion.* A common function of such thinking is to produce a correct answer to a question whose answer is not immediately obvious to the reasoner but may be inferred from information at the reasoner's disposal. What is the correct diagnosis of this patient's condition? What tests are appropriate to order as part of this patient's regular checkup? What is the best treatment for this patient's diagnosed condition? What is this patient's prognosis? Sometimes the answers to these questions are obvious, but when they are not, we must reason. Naturally we want to arrive through this reasoning at a correct answer.

Unfortunately, there is no instant test or gold standard for correctness of conclusions. We cannot write the conclusion on a piece of paper, dip it in a liquid, and determine from the color of the paper whether the conclusion is correct or incorrect. We are not infallible visionaries, but human beings, working with incomplete information of less than perfect quality. Instead of correctness or truth, we must make do with the next best alternative: justification by the best obtainable evidence. This is why many warrants hold in most or some cases rather than in all cases, why we qualify our conclusions with such words as "probably" or "possibly," and why we acknowledge potential rebuttals of our conclusions.

Our goal, then, is to reach the answer that the best relevant obtainable evidence justifies us in accepting. To reach this goal:

- we must be *justified in accepting the premises*; that is, they must be evidence-based. Further,

- our premises *must include all the relevant justified obtainable information.* Further,

- the conclusion must follow in virtue of a *justified general warrant.* And,

- if the warrant is not universal, we must be justified in assuming that in the particular case there are *no known contraindications (rebuttals) that rule out application of the warrant.*

These four conditions—**justified premise (or premises), complete informa-tion, justified warrant, no known contraindications**—are individually necessary and jointly sufficient for arriving at a justified conclusion.

Let us consider each of them in more detail.

Justified premises

There are many sources of justified premises. Examples are direct observation, writ-ten records of direct observation, memory of what one has previously observed or experienced, personal testimony, previous good reasoning or argument, expert opinion, appeal to an authoritative reference source, popular belief, value commit-ments, and intuitive hunches. (There is more on these sources later in this chapter.)

No matter how one's premises are justified, it should be kept in mind that *being justified is not the same as being correct.* A premise justified by direct observation, or a written record of a direct observation, or an authoritative reference source, may later turn out to be false. The flushed and slightly sweaty face of your patient may be the temporary effect of having run to your office to avoid being late for his or her appointment, rather than a more permanent condition. The laboratory result may turn out to be the result from another patient's blood sample. At one time, author-itative reference sources identified spicy food, acid, and stress as the major causes of gastric and duodenal peptic ulcers. It is now recognized (since 1982) that more than 90% of ulcers are caused by a bacterial infection with *Helicobacter pylori*. The moral is: *Always be prepared to revise your opinion in light of compelling new evidence to the contrary.*

Premises may thus be based either on mere belief or on knowledge, which affects their truthfulness. As Bowell and Kemp[43] point out, a **belief** is not necessarily the truth. **Truth** is a property of propositions. It is defined as the attribute of asserting what is really the case.[44] Its opposite is falsity, the attribute of asserting what is not really the case. The better the evidence for a belief, the more likely it is to be true. Ideally, in medicine, truth should be supported by the best evidence as defined by clinical epidemiologists. Most often, evidence is imperfect and so less likely to give us the truth. Hence, EBM contributes to the building of an elusive ideal of truthful propositions. **Knowledge** can be defined as *justified true belief.*[49] Even the best of our knowledge ("scientific knowledge"), however, depends on the dominating par-adigms of the time and evidence occurring within the framework of such a para-digm.[34] Beliefs sometimes accepted as true may change within new paradigms. For example, the paradigm of a peptic ulcer as a disease related to stress, diet, and other noninfectious factors is replaced by the paradigm of a peptic ulcer as an infectious disease related to exposure to *Helicobacter pylori*. **We must recognize our fallibility as human beings and be prepared to change our opinion.**

Complete information

If you are trying to answer a question correctly on the basis of obtainable informa-tion, you need to take into account all the good relevant information that is practi-cally obtainable. Relevant information is information that could make a difference to the answer you reach. That is, a justified warrant links it to a possible answer to your question; authoritative recent clinical guidelines are one source of such justified warrants. If you consider only information that supports one answer, and ignore information that points to a different answer, you are more likely to reach an incorrect conclusion than if you consider everything. **Do not forget to listen carefully to what your patient is telling you.** A common human failing is to close prematurely on a particular answer, then seek supporting evidence for this answer, while failing to seek (or even ignoring) evidence that points in a different direction. In recent years, several convictions for murder have been reversed on the basis of DNA evidence that proved conclusively that the convicted person could not have committed the murder; in these cases, detectives, prosecutors, and juries were successively led to the wrong conclusion, often because the detectives were trying to get the evidence to convict their prime suspect and ignoring evidence that pointed away from him or her. In some of these cases, the detectives even pressured witnesses to change key details of their testimony. The tendency to suppress unwanted evidence also occurs in intelligence work. It can even be seen in the context of scholarly and scientific writing (including reports of medical research), and it certainly is present in medical practice. **Do not ignore a sign, symptom, or test result that points in a different direction from your *impression*, or tentative diagnosis.**

In diagnosis, it is often necessary to seek additional information by further examination or by ordering tests. In general, seeking additional information is advisable where it is relevant, needed, and obtainable. A good example is obtaining a test result needed for a differential diagnosis, where a positive result on the test is the gold standard for confirming a suspected condition.

In making treatment decisions, obtaining and using complete information involves attending to the broader context, to the whole patient. If the patient will have trouble complying with a complicated recommendation, that fact is relevant in deciding what to recommend; a simple recommendation that the patient will actually follow may be better than a more complicated recommendation that is theoretically ideal. If a treatment for condition X may have adverse effects on conditions Y and Z, the treatment decision should take into account whether the patient has all three conditions.

Justified warrant

If your reasoning is to justify your conclusion, that conclusion must follow from your premises in accordance with a justified general warrant. The warrant should actually apply to the inference. This means that it should be **equivalent to some generalization of the so-called *associated conditional*: If the premises are true, then the conclusion is true.** No conclusion follows in just one particular case; if it follows in one case, it follows in parallel cases. An applicable warrant picks out a class of such cases. Suppose you reason as follows:

Premise A: *The patient in whom we have transplanted a new kidney has a fever.*

Premise B: *Clinical and paraclinical (laboratory) workup for infection and organ rejection has ruled out infection.*

Conclusion C: *Adjusting the dosage of the patient's antirejection drugs would probably be the best choice.*

Any warrant by virtue of which this conclusion follows from the premise will be some generalization of the associated conditional:

Associated conditional: *If the patient in whom we have transplanted a new kidney has a fever, and clinical and paraclinical (laboratory) workup for infection and organ rejection has ruled out infection, then adjusting the dosage of the patient's antirejection drugs would be the best choice.*

The obvious generalization of this conditional proposition is the warrant:

Warrant: *Adjusting the dosage of antirejection drugs is generally the best choice for kidney transplant recipients with a fever if clinical and paraclinical (laboratory) workup for infection and organ rejection rules out infection.*

In forming an associated conditional to discover applicable warrants, qualifiers and rebuttals are removed from the conclusion, for example, the word "probably" in the earlier example. The generalization may hold mainly or only sometimes rather than always and may be subject to provisos (ie, conditions of exception or rebuttals). For example, we inserted the word "generally" in the above warrant to reflect the fact that the conclusion was qualified by the word "probably."

Additionally, the warrant should be **justified**. Since warrants are general, the evidence that justifies them tends to take the form of clinical trials and other analytical studies, the conclusions from which are incorporated into authoritative clinical guidelines and references. (More information on such reasoning and argument may be found in Chapter 5.) Well-established explanatory models, such as the explanation of many ulcers as caused by bacterial infection, are also justified warrants.

No known contraindications

As indicated earlier, many warrants come with rebuttals, or exceptional conditions under which the conclusion is incorrect. We use the term *contraindications* for such rebuttals, to link up with the term commonly used in relation to drugs. For reasoning to be good, we must be justified in assuming that no contraindication in the particular case rules out application of the warrant. We must know of no such contraindication. If a possible contraindication has serious consequences (eg, infection as a contraindication to prescribing antirejection drugs for a febrile kidney transplant recipient), we must find out whether the exceptional condition is present. Otherwise, we can act as if there is no contraindication, simply on the basis that we know of none, but we should be alert to the possibility of discovering some exceptional circumstance pertaining to the particular case. In our example of the patient with streptococcal pharyngitis, we must be justified in assuming that the patient has no allergy to penicillin. If the patient had received penicillin before with no hypersensitivity reaction, that is good evidence. If the patient had not previously had penicillin or does not remember if she had a hypersensitivity reaction, more caution is indicated. We may proceed *as if* we know that the patient is not allergic to penicillin, but it would be prudent to advise the patient what to do in the case of possible adverse reactions.

Figure 2-4 represents in the form of a flowchart an algorithm of steps (decisions, actions) for the evaluation of reasoning to a single conclusion.

The four conditions—justified premises, complete information, justified applicable warrant, no known contraindications—are individually necessary and jointly sufficient for good reasoning. If any one of the four conditions is absent, the reasoning

FIGURE 2-4

Algorithm for evaluation of reasoning

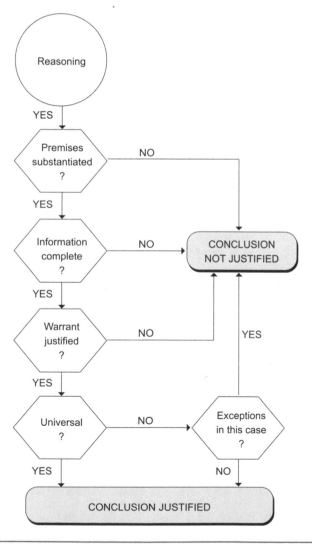

is not good; it does not justify the conclusion. If they are all present, the reasoning is good; it does justify the conclusion. **Justification is not the same as truth.** Even bad reasoning can, by a lucky chance, arrive at a correct conclusion. And even good reasoning can, by an unlucky chance, arrive at an incorrect conclusion. The reason for preferring good reasoning to bad reasoning is that, on the whole, one is *more likely* to arrive at the correct answer to one's question through good reasoning than through bad reasoning.

Here is a short example of good reasoning: *This patient has a pulsating abdominal mass, so she may have an aneurysm of the abdominal aorta.* In calling it good reasoning, we assume that the reasoner has felt the pulsating abdominal mass, thus justifying the premise by direct observation. We assume, a little artificially, that the pulsating abdominal mass is all the obtainable justified information relevant to whether the patient has an aneurysm of the abdominal aorta. More likely, other relevant signs and symptoms would present themselves and would need to be included in the premises. The warrant is that a pulsating abdominal mass is sometimes an aneurysm of the abdominal aorta. Since the warrant holds only in some cases, the conclusion is qualified by the word *may.* There are no rebuttals for such a modest claim. Further investigation is needed to arrive at a definite diagnosis.

2.5.2 Sources of Justified Premises

A number of possible sources of justified premises were mentioned earlier. Here are some details.

Direct observation

In general, the most basic source of justified premises is through **direct observation**. An experienced physician is trained to notice such things as complexion, affect, and posture. The stethoscope and the sphygmomanometer allow the physician to collect additional observations. These signs of the patient's medical condition are the first basis of diagnosis. In general, an observation is justified when:

- The sense being used (eg, sight or hearing) is in good condition.

- The conditions for observation are adequate (eg, not too dark or too noisy).

- Any instruments used (eg, a sphygmomanometer or stethoscope) are in good condition and functioning properly.

- The observer is close enough to what he or she is observing and takes care to notice accurately (rather than just taking a hurried glance while preoccupied with something else).

- The observer has whatever expert knowledge is required to use any instruments involved (eg, a stethoscope) and to interpret what is observed.

- No other justified information contradicts the observation.

A physician examining a patient generally meets these conditions.

Written records of direct observation

A second source is **written records of direct observation**. This is one function of medical charts; they make it possible to restore previous observations without depending on the vagaries of memory, which is notoriously plastic and unreliable.[50] The sooner we write it down, the more likely it is to be accurate. Waiting allows our memory to play tricks on us. Care in record taking is important.

Memory

A third source is **memory** of what one has previously observed or experienced. Memories decline in accuracy with the passage of time, with retelling to others, and with exposure to discussions by others of the "remembered" events. Memories are also less accurate about peripheral or unimportant details than about emotionally salient and central facts. In the laboratory setting, psychologists have been able to create vivid and detailed "memories" of supposed personal experiences that their subject never had.[50] Let us be careful about relying on memory alone. Put it in the patient's chart!

Personal testimony

A fourth source is **personal testimony** of what has been directly observed or experienced. Such testimony is no better than the observation or experience on which it is based. It must be scrutinized in terms of the criteria mentioned earlier for observation, written records, and memory; for example, testimony based on distant memories is suspect if unsupported by written records made at or near the time of the observation. The patient's symptoms, as reported to the physician, are an example of personal testimony, which must be evaluated for accuracy. It is important to listen carefully to what the patient is saying and to probe if necessary for further clarification; the physician cannot simply ignore or dismiss the patient's reports. Interpretation is often required. An example of generally credible testimony of what has been directly observed is a laboratory report of a test ordered on a patient; this report is a written (or electronic) record, produced at the same time as the observation, which usually meets the conditions mentioned earlier for a justified observation report. It is particularly important in evaluating testimony to be on guard against second-hand, third-hand, or more distant testimony. As the game of "telephone" dramatically shows, the quality of messages passed from one person to another tends to deteriorate with each transmission. Patients' verbal reports of their blood pressure on their last visit, for example, are generally not as trustworthy as the written record in the chart or computer file, provided the record has been entered carefully. An additional complication in evaluating testimony is the possibility that its author may distort the truth through a careless or intentionally deceptive formulation. Patients' reports of their symptoms are rarely lies, but they are often vaguely formulated, and probing may be needed to determine exactly what the patient has been experiencing.

Previous reasoning or argument

A fifth source is **previous good reasoning or argument**. The patient's entire complex of signs, symptoms, and test results may lead the physician by means of a justified warrant to a specific diagnosis. This diagnosis, in turn, becomes the premise of a new piece of reasoning, leading to a decision about how to treat the patient. If the diagnosis was justified by the earlier reasoning, it becomes a justified premise of the new reasoning about how to treat the patient.

Expert opinion

A sixth source is **expert opinion**. The verdict of a specialist called in for a consultation on a difficult case is an example of such an expert opinion. In some cases, it is possible and desirable to scrutinize the reasoning by which the expert arrived at the opinion in question. In other cases, however, it is either impossible or undesirable to undertake such scrutiny, and the acceptability of the expert's opinion must be judged indirectly.

There are seven criteria for a good expert opinion:

1. The opinion in question must belong to some subject matter in which there is expertise. Whether a patient has an obstruction of the vessels that lead to the brain is a question that expert knowledge must settle. Whether it is in the patient's best interest to have an operation immediately to surgically correct (with bypass or otherwise) this section is not entirely a question of expertise; it depends partly on the patient's values, wishes, and preferences. Expertise can only determine the risks and consequences of the options of operating immediately or waiting for some time. An opinion can belong to an area of expertise even if the expertise is not based on formal education; there are experts on baseball history and on stamps, for example.

2. The person expressing the opinion must have the relevant expertise; for instance, expertise in psychiatry does not enhance one's ability to interpret X-ray films. The requirement of relevant expertise is violated routinely in advertisements in the mass media when celebrities give testimonials to the merits of some product for which their celebrated accomplishments are irrelevant.

3. The author must use the expertise in arriving at the opinion. The relevant data must have been collected, interpreted, and processed using professional knowledge and skills.

4. The author must exercise care in applying the expertise and in formulating the expert opinion.

5. The author ideally should not have a conflict of interest that could influence, consciously or unconsciously, the formulated opinion. For example, an expert opinion as to the drug of choice for a certain condition is less trustworthy if its author is a major shareholder in the company that holds the patent on the drug. Even the acceptance of gifts from the sales representative of a pharmaceutical company can make a physician's prescription of that company's drug more suspect; both medical research and medical practice need clear conflict-of-interest guidelines for such situations.

6. The opinion should not conflict with the opinion of other qualified experts; if experts disagree, further probing is required.

7. The opinion should not conflict with other justified information; if an expert opinion does not fit with what you otherwise know, scrutinize its credentials carefully and perhaps get a second opinion.

Sometimes, we do not know directly whether these seven conditions are met, and we must judge by inference. Your patients may not know how up-to-date your knowledge is in your field of expertise, but they will make inferences about it on the basis of their experience of whether the side effects they experienced were ones you warned them were possible, whether the prognosis you gave them turned out to be accurate, and so on. You make similar inferences about the quality of your colleagues' expertise and about their care in applying it, on the basis of your experience of the quality of their expert opinions.

Authoritative reference source (best evidence)
A seventh source is **an authoritative reference source**. This is the appropriate source for general information relevant to risks, diagnosis, treatment decisions, and prognosis. Ideally, authoritative references in medicine embody the best available evidence at the time they are composed. They are primarily a source of warrants in accordance with which physicians reason and argue, but general information obtained from them may sometimes function as a premise.

The seven sources of justified premises just mentioned (direct observation, written records of direct observation, memory of what one has previously observed or experienced, personal testimony, previous good reasoning or argument, expert opinion, and appeal to an authoritative reference source) are the most common ones. We use other sources for our premises, for example, commonly accepted opinions, value judgments, or intuitive hunches. Sometimes propositions derived from these sources are justified; sometimes they are not. Judgment is required to decide whether a proposition derived from such a source is justified.

2.5.3 Criteria for Good Arguments and Good Argumentation

As defined earlier, an **argument** is *a set of statements, some of which—the premises—are offered as reasons for another statement, the conclusion*. Thus, arguments have the same premise-conclusion inferential structure as does reasoning. However, arguments are expressed in statements, which are typically addressed to one or more other people. Individuals who advance arguments are typically trying to justify or prove the conclusion to one or more other people. We will call an argument that actually justifies or proves its conclusion to its intended audience a **cogent argument**, the word "cogent" coming from a Latin term meaning compelling. (We are talking about arguments that **ought to** convince members of the intended audience, not necessarily about arguments that actually succeed in convincing them; some people remain unpersuaded by conclusive arguments based on indisputable evidence. It is another question, not discussed in this text, which features of arguments make them persuasive.) Generally speaking, a cogent argument must be **good reasoning as far as its author is concerned**. But it must also be **good**

reasoning as far as its intended audience is concerned. That is, both the author and the intended audience must be justified in accepting the premises, the premises must include all good relevant information obtainable by both, and the conclusion must follow by virtue of a warrant that each is justified in using. Finally, if the warrant is not universal, each must be justified in assuming that in the particular case there are no exceptional circumstances (rebuttals) that rule out application of the warrant. Quite often, the audience's justification is different from that of the author of the argument; for example, the arguer may have justified a premise by direct observation, but the audience's justification will be the personal testimony of the arguer. Hence, the argument must be tailored to the intended audience. It must be logical for the audience to whom it is addressed. Also, it must be stated in a language that the audience can understand.

Ethics as well as logic requires that a good argument be good reasoning for its author. Perhaps the intended audience justifiably believes a proposition that the arguer knows is false. Can the arguer use it as a premise? The resulting argument might be convincing. But it would be devious to use it.

For an example of a cogent argument, consider the following situation: *In an emergency room, the attending pediatrician examines a 5-year-old boy who is choking and unable to vocalize or cough. His parents explain that the boy often runs with food in his mouth and that his 14-year-old sister gives him whatever she eats when she baby-sits him. Our pediatrician succeeds in dislodging a foreign body from the boy's airways. He suggests to the parents that they should teach him good eating habits and explain to the boy's sister that she should give him food appropriate for his age.*

The pediatrician might argue as follows: "*Your son was choking because some food was trapped in his airway. From what you tell me, this could have happened either because he was eating when he was running or because he was eating food inappropriate for his age. You should therefore teach him good eating habits, and your daughter should give him food appropriate for his age.*" The premise that the trapped food caused the choking is justified by the pediatrician's extraction of it from the boy's airway, the fact that the choking immediately stopped, and background knowledge of the mechanism of breathing. For the pediatrician, the extraction is a matter of personal experience; for the parents, the extraction is a matter of personal testimony by the pediatrician. The premise as to the possible causes of food being trapped in the boy's airways is justified partly by the parents' personal testimony and partly by background knowledge of causal mechanisms that can cause food to lodge in a young child's airways; the pediatrician has the knowledge, but the parents may have to trust the pediatrician's expert opinion. These two premises include all the information relevant to this particular recommendation. The warrant is that one should eliminate possible sufficient causes of a traumatic and life-threatening experience for one's child; this warrant is justified by the concern of parents for their child's well-being. (Because the pediatrician is recommending elimination of sufficient causes, rather than of necessary causes, there is no guarantee that the recommended actions will prevent a recurrence; see Chapter 5 for the difference between sufficient and necessary causes.) The pediatrician assumes, and the parents would presumably agree, that there is no contraindication in this case to the recommended action; there is no reason to suspect that there are overriding reasons as to why the boy should eat while running or why the boy's sister should give him what she eats. Thus, the four conditions for good reasoning—justified premise, complete information, justified warrant, and no known contraindication—are met by both the arguer and the addressee.

What is good argumentation? **Argumentation**, as defined earlier, is *back-and-forth discussion in which at least one person advances arguments*. Such discussion can have many purposes. Argumentation in discussions with patients, in clinical rounds, and in exchanges in medical journals typically has the function of arriving through the discussion at a justified position on some question at issue. Should the patient begin to take a daily low dosage of aspirin as a prophylaxis against coronary artery disease? What is the correct diagnosis of the patient who presents the following signs and symptoms? What are the risks and benefits of combined (estrogen and progestin) hormone replacement therapy? If the function of argumentation is to arrive at a mutually agreed-on justified position on such a question, the contributions to the discussion must be **relevant to the question**. Going off on an irrelevant side issue makes the argumentation bad; in particular, it is usually irrelevant to personally attack a participant in the discussion. In addition, any arguments advanced must be **cogent** in the sense defined earlier.

Competing criteria of good argument and good reasoning

Competing criteria, not adopted in this book, can be found in logic textbooks. According to the **truth-validity-strength criteria,**[44] for example, reasoning and argument are good if (and only if) they are based on true premises and the inference from the premises to the conclusion is either deductively valid or inductively strong.

Truth is a property of propositions. It is defined as the attribute of asserting what is really the case.[44] Its opposite is falsity, the attribute of asserting what is not really the case. This book adopts the competing criterion of justified belief, which is all we, as fallible humans, can claim.

The terms "**deductively valid**" and "**inductive strength**" have a specific meaning:[44]

- **Deductive validity** is a property of the inference from premises to conclusion. As mentioned earlier, in a **deductively valid inference it is impossible for the premises to be true while the conclusion is false, because of their meaning.** This is a rarely attained ideal, both in general and for medical decisions, given the nature of the biological phenomena with which medicine deals.

- **Inductive strength** is also a property of the inference from premises to conclusion. We can define **inductive strength** as *the probability that the conclusion of an inference is true given that the premises are true*. An inductively strong argument is defined as follows: *Given that the premises are true, the conclusion is probably also true* (ie, to some extent).

Allowing inductive strength as well as deductive validity is more realistic for medical decision making, which often takes place under uncertainty with ill-defined probabilities. It is important to realize that the inductive strength of an inference is relative to the information in the premises. If further relevant information turns up, the conclusion may become more probable or less probable. Also, the probability in question is merely qualitative; there is no probability calculation for the inductive strength of inferences. Consequently, this book adopts Toulmin's concept of qualifiers[40,41] such as "presumably" and "probably" in preference to the vague concept of inductive strength.

2.6 FALLACIES: DEFINITION, CLASSIFICATION, AND EXAMPLES

Having defined good reasoning and good argument, let us now turn to bad reasoning and bad argument. Errors in reasoning and argument, or *fallacies* as we call them, are ubiquitous. The challenge is to avoid them in our own reasoning and arguments and to recognize and respond appropriately to them in the reasoning and arguments of others, for the sake of arriving at good solutions to health problems.

2.6.1 Definition of a Fallacy

A **fallacy** is *"any mistaken idea or false belief, or error in reasoning or in argument."*[51] A fallacy is also generally defined as a *"flaw in reasoning; anything that diverts the mind or eye; or any reasoning, exposition, argument, etc, contravening the canons of logic."*[37]

Hence, another way to evaluate reasoning and arguments is to understand whether they are free of fallacies or not.

The application of general logic is necessary to purge medicine from numerous fallacies threatening reasoning and decisions. Avoiding fallacies is necessary not so much to please formal logicians, but rather to put the best available evidence to the best use for the benefit of the patient.

A **fallacy** is a term used in logic to characterize some mistake in reasoning or argument, for example, in the transition from premises to conclusion. By contrast, a **falsity** refers to a single statement.[2] Our reasoning may then be **fallacious** because our arguments do not respect the rules of formal validity. Moreover, our propositions, interpretations, and decisions may be **false**, because of uses of inappropriate evidence. Hence, good medicine means correctly using good evidence.

A fallacy in logical discourse does not necessarily mean that the conclusion is false. It simply means that better evidence is needed to show that the conclusion is true. Fallacies may be based on illicit assumptions, ambiguity, irrelevance, or faulty causal reasoning. Some fallacies, such as the **ecological fallacy**[52] (where some associations applicable to groups are inappropriately applied to individuals), are already known to epidemiologists. However, logical thinking in medicine is still poorly taught.

Biases are defined as *any systematic deviation of results or inferences from the truth.*[52] (**Errors**, in contrast, are **not systematic**.) Their extent is now better known to epidemiologists. In fact, the list of biases in medicine[53] is ever-expanding.[54] As in any endeavour, proper reasoning to avoid fallacies should be the subject of more formal and structured training for every health professional, not only for those directly involved in medical research.

Formal fallacies, from which logicians protect us so well, do not arise out of the specific matter of the argument. Physicians must be on guard against them. They arise *from a structural pattern of reasoning that is generically incorrect.*[31]

2.6.2 Classification of Fallacies

The classification of fallacies across the literature is not uniform, and the list of fallacies is perhaps still not complete. It probably will never be complete, since there is no end to the number of ways in which one can go wrong—in logic or in life. The following classification gives some sense of the range of possible mistakes:[31]

Material fallacies (or **nonlogical fallacies**) are also called *fallacies of presumption* because the premises "presume" too much.[31] They covertly assume the conclusion or avoid the issue of interest. Uses of poor evidence for premises also fall into this category. Facts are misstated.

Formal fallacies (or **logical fallacies**) occur when the fault is in the very process of reasoning. An improper process of inference is at the root of formal fallacies.[31] They represent wrong connections between premises and conclusions, hence, deficiencies in the process of logical thinking.[44]

Verbal fallacies occur in arguments whose ambiguous words shift their meaning within the course of an argument.[51] The incorrect use of terms is a culprit.[51]

In medical decision making, one other category must be also considered: substantive fallacies.[44] **Substantive fallacies** (we also call them **content fallacies**) arise from *overly general premises leading to inappropriate conclusions.* Inadequate evidence supporting premises results in conclusions as new poor evidence. We may also call substantive fallacies **evidence-bound fallacies.** The evidence used in premises makes them truthful or not.

Theoretically, any fallacy in reasoning, argument, or argumentation is a violation of some criterion of good reasoning, good argument, or good argumentation. It would be possible to classify the fallacies we discuss in Section 2.6.3 according to the criteria given earlier for good reasoning, good argument, and good argumentation. However, such a classification may not be particularly helpful in practice.

In this book, we quote some of these fallacies, particularly those occurring in research (Chapter 5), in daily practice (Chapter 6), and when dealing with civic bodies outside the hospital or medical office environment (Chapter 7). Table 2-2 lists by name the fallacies important in these aspects of medical practice. (We explain, give practical medical examples, and comment on them in more detail in Chapters 5, 6, and 7.)

In this book, we generally do not bother to classify the fallacies according to any particular classification scheme. Occasionally, we use the simplest classification of fallacies, based on two categories, to assign them to one of two groups: fallacies dependent on form and those related to content (informal fallacies, evidence-bound, content-dependent). For the sake of immediate illustration and understanding, some of these fallacies are worthy of quotation now.

TABLE 2-2

Some fallacies in research, clinical practice, and communication with the outside world*

Fallacies in research (mainly causal reasoning and argument; see Section 5.4)

- Inferring cause from correlation
- *Post hoc, ergo propter hoc* or *after this, therefore because of this*
- Confounding necessary and sufficient cause
- *Argumentum ad ignorantiam* or *arguing from ignorance*
- Fallacy of division (community/individual fallacy, Rose's fallacy)
- Fallacy of accident
- Fallacy of composition

- Confusion of cause and effect
- "Domino" or "slippery slope" fallacy
- Perfectionist fallacy
- Irrelevant conclusion (irrelevant thesis, fallacy of diversion, "red herring")
- False dilemma
- *Ad populum* (or *appealing to the people*)
- Hypostatization
- Objectionable vagueness
- Equivocation

Fallacies in clinical practice

Making a diagnosis (see Section 6.2.2)
- Faulty evidence about the patient
- False dilemma
- *Argumentum ad verecundiam* (or *argument from authority*)
- Ockham's razor
- The "is-ought" fallacy

Treatment (see Section 6.2.3.2)
- Ignoring the qualification
- Suppressing evidence
- *Post hoc, ergo propter hoc* or *after this, therefore because of this*
- Slippery slope

Prognosis (see Section 6.2.4.2)
- Division and composition
- Oversimplification
- Misleading use of statistics

- Confusion of controllable with uncontrollable patient characteristics
- Confusion of risk factors with prognostic factors
- Gambler's fallacy
- Red herring

Understanding patients (see Section 6.3.2)
- Complex question

Medical communication (see Section 6.4.3)
- Accent
- Question-begging epithets
- False analogy
- *Ad misericordiam* (or *appeal to pity*)
- Sweeping explanation
- Equivocation
- Straw man

Fallacies and rhetorical ploys in communicating with outside world (see Section 7.5)

- Rhetorical ploys
- Appeal to novelty
- Appeal to popularity
- *Ad ignorantiam* (or *argument from ignorance*)

- Fallacy of ambiguity
- *Argumentum ad verecundiam* (or *argument from authority*)
- Statistical or clinical-epidemiologic fallacy (dangling relative)

* Some fallacies mentioned in one context also occur in other contexts where they are not specifically mentioned.

2.6.3 Examples of Fallacies

To avoid fallacious practice and research in medicine, we must be aware of several traps. A few fallacies from a much wider spectrum will be quoted here together with alternative titles that we might give them if related to reasoning, argument, and argumentation in the field of health:

1. A **fallacy of circular argument** ("begging the question") occurs when premises presume, openly or covertly, the very conclusion that has to be demonstrated.[31] Example: Patient Newbury always follows the treatments prescribed. How do we know? The patient always takes a nonsteroidal anti-inflammatory drug (NSAID) according to the physician's orders.

2. A *post hoc* **fallacy** (or fallacy of false cause) occurs when mere sequence or correlation is taken to prove a causal connection. This situation is already known to epidemiologists and other scientists as *post hoc, ergo propter hoc* reasoning, that is, "*after which, hence by which*" (or event B is due to event A just because B happens after A). A simple temporal sequence becomes a cause-effect sequence. For example, hyperacidity was caused by the meal, which preceded its occurrence; an embolism was caused by a transoceanic flight, because the victim was well on boarding the plane; epilepsy or autism are due to immunization, because they occurred after the child was immunized; and so on.

3. A **fallacy of many questions** occurs when a single answer is required for a question that might have several possible answers, such as: "Are the two patients in Room 212 sick? One appears to be so, but not the other." In this situation, any answer goes.

4. A **fallacy of** *non sequitur* ("*it does not follow*") occurs when there is not even a deceptively plausible appearance of valid reasoning because there is almost a complete lack of connection between the given premises and the conclusion drawn from them. For example:

   Premise A: *The computed axial tomography of the patient's right kidney shows a suspicious lesion.*

   Premise B: *This hospital and its department of surgery have outstanding reputations in the field of abdominal surgery.*

   Conclusion C: *This patient should have his right kidney removed.*

5. In an **"if ... then" form of reasoning**, formal fallacies may occur because of an improper handling of the **antecedent** (the phrase that follows "*if* . . .") or the **consequent** (the phrase that follows "*then* . . ."). A *fallacy of affirming the consequent*[45] asserts that because the consequent is true, the antecedent is also true:

   Premise A: *If this patient has diabetes, his blood sugar will be high.*

   Premise B: *His blood sugar is high.*

   Conclusion C: *Then (therefore), this patient has diabetes.*

In this kind of reasoning, the web of causes of high blood sugar is simply ignored. In reality, diabetes is not the only cause of high blood sugar.

6. A **fallacy of denying the antecedent**[45] occurs when arguing that, because the antecedent is false, the consequent must necessarily be false, too:

> Premise A: *If this patient has diabetes, his blood sugar will be abnormally high.*
>
> Premise B: *But this patient does not have diabetes.*
>
> Conclusion C: *Then (therefore) his blood sugar should be normal.*

A more complete compilation of a numerically open-ended list of fallacies in medical reasoning must still be worked up. The fallacies and their practical examples listed in the final sections of Chapters 5, 6, and 7 can serve as the starting points for such a compilation.

2.7 Conclusions

Reasoning is *thinking enlightened by logic.*[55] Rules of practice, basic and experimental research, and epidemiology, clinical epidemiology, and EBM are based on such reasoning. In return, all these disciplines help better structure our reasoning for the benefit of the patient. Mastering them, therefore, becomes a necessity. Obtaining good evidence is not enough. Its use must be logical, too. To be purposeful, **evidence must be used logically, and logic must be backed by evidence. The joint use of evidence and logic is a must. A patient can be harmed as much by the illogical use of evidence as by the use of a logical decision unsupported by evidence and even more by the use of faulty logic without evidence.**

The chapters that follow outline the fundamentals of the expanded uses of logic, critical thinking, and evidence and their practical applications in various domains of medical activity. They show how important it is to support logical reasoning through evidence in order to make it relevant for interpretations and decisions in health sciences. More central to this book, they outline basic principles governing the use of medical evidence in a structured, focused, and logical way within different facets of clinical and community medicine.

References

1. Craig E. *Concise Routledge Encyclopedia of Philosophy.* London, England: Routledge; 2000.

2. Cooper DE. *World Philosophies: An Historical Introduction.* 2nd ed. Oxford, England: Blackwell Publishing; 2003.

3. Reese WL. *Dictionary of Philosophy and Religion: Eastern and Western Thought.* Amherst, NY: Humanity Books; 1996.

4. Bernard C. *An Introduction to the Study of Experimental Medicine.* New York, NY: Macmillan Publishing Co Inc; 1927.

5. Zalta EN. *Stanford Encyclopedia of Philosophy.* Stanford, Calif: Metaphysics Research Lab at Stanford University; 2000. Available at: http//plato.Stanford.edu.

6. Kuhn TS. *The Structure of Scientific Revolutions.* 3rd ed. Chicago, Ill: University of Chicago Press; 1996.

7. Hill AB. Observation and experiment. *N Engl J Med*. 1953:248:995–1001.

8. Hill AB. The environment and disease: association or causation? *Proc R Soc Med*. 1965;58:295–300.

9. Surgeon General's Advisory Committee on Smoking and Health. *Smoking and Health.* Washington, DC: US Public Health Service; 1969. Publication No. 1103.

10. Evans AS. *Causation and Disease: A Chronological Journey*. New York, NY: Plenum Medical Book Co; 1993.

11. Murphy EA. *The Logic of Medicine*. 2nd ed. Baltimore, Md: The Johns Hopkins University Press; 1997.

12. Susser M. *Causal Thinking in Health Sciences: Concepts and Strategies of Epidemiology.* New York, NY: Oxford University Press; 1973.

13. Greenland S, ed. *Evolution of Epidemiologic Ideas: Annotated Reading on Concepts and Methods.* Chestnut Hill, Pa: Epidemiology Resources Inc; 1987.

14. Buck C, Llopis A. *The Challenge of Epidemiology: Issues and Selected Readings.* Washington, DC: Pan American Health Organization; 1988.

15. Rothman KJ, ed. *Causal Inference.* Chestnut Hill, Pa: Epidemiology Resources, Inc; 1988.

16. Sox HC Jr, Blatt MA, Higgins MC, Marton KI. *Medical Decision Making.* Boston, Mass: Butterworth-Heinemann Medical; 1988.

17. Albert DA, Munson R, Resnik MD. *Reasoning in Medicine: An Introduction to Clinical Inference.* Baltimore, Md: The Johns Hopkins University Press; 1988.

18. Wulff HR, Pedersen SA, Rosenberg R. *Philosophy of Medicine: An Introduction.* Oxford, England: Blackwell Publishing; 1986.

19. King LS. *Medical Thinking: A Historical Preface.* Princeton, NJ: Princeton University Press; 1982.

20. Slaney JK. An outline of formal logic and its applications to medicine—I. *Br Med J*. 1987;295:1195–1197.

21. Slaney JK. An outline of formal logic and its applications to medicine—II. *Br Med J*. 1987;295:1261–1263.

22. Tomassi P. Logic and medicine (1–29) and Logic and scientific method (30–58). In: Phillips CI, ed. *Logic in Medicine.* London, England: BMJ Publishing Group; 1995.

23. Audi R, ed. *The Cambridge Dictionary of Philosophy.* 2nd ed. Cambridge, England: Cambridge University Press; 1999.

24. *The Columbia Encyclopaedia* [online]. 6th ed. New York, NY: Columbia University Press; 2002. Available at: www.bartleby.com/65.

25. Murzi M. Logical positivism. In: Fieser J, Dowden B, eds. *The Internet Encyclopedia of Philosophy*; 2004. Available at: www.iep.utm.edu.

26. Popper KR. *The Logic of Scientific Discovery*. New York, NY: Basic Books; 1959.

27. Lakatos I, Musgrave A, eds. *Criticism and the Growth of Knowledge*. Cambridge, England: Cambridge University Press; 1970.

28. Feyerabend P. *Against Method: Outline of an Anarchistic Theory of Knowledge*. London, England: Verso Books; 1978.

29. Salmon M, Earman J, Glymour C, et al, (eds). *Introduction to the Philosophy of Science*. Englewood Cliffs, NJ: Prentice Hall; 1992.

30. Ennis RH. *Critical Thinking*. Upper Saddle River, NJ: Prentice Hall; 1996.

31. Hughes GE, Wang H, Roscher N. The history and kinds of logic. In: McHenry R, ed. *The New Encyclopaedia Britannica*. Vol 23. Chicago, Ill: Encyclopaedia Britannica Inc; 1992:226–282.

32. Engel SM. *With Good Reason: An Introduction to Informal Fallacies*. 3rd ed. New York, NY: St. Martin Press; 1986.

33. Blackburn S. *Oxford Dictionary of Philosophy*. Oxford, England: Oxford University Press; 1996.

34. Copi IM. *Informal Logic*. New York, NY: Macmillan Publishing Co Inc; 1986.

35. Engel SM. *The Chain of Logic*. Englewood Cliffs, NJ: Prentice Hall; 1987.

36. Weston A. *A Rulebook for Arguments*. Indianapolis, Ind: Hackett Publishing Co; 1987.

37. Michalos AC. *Improving Your Reasoning*. 2nd ed. Englewood Cliffs, NJ: Prentice Hall; 1986.

38. Salmon WC. *Logic*. Englewood Cliffs, NJ: Prentice Hall; 1963.

39. Diogenes Laertius. *Lives of Eminent Philosophers*. Vols 1 and 2. Loeb Classical Library 184 and 185. Cambridge, Mass: Harvard University Press; 1925.

40. Toulmin S. *The Uses of Argument*. Cambridge, England: Cambridge University Press; 1958:94–145.

41. Toulmin S, Rieke R, Janik A. *An Introduction to Reasoning*. 2nd ed. New York, NY: Collier Macmillan Publishers; 1984.

42. Parry, CH. *An Inquiry into the Symptoms and Causes of the Syncope Anginosa, Commonly Called Angina Pectoris; Illustrated by Dissections*. London, England: Cadell & Davis; 1799.

43. Bowell T, Kemp G. *Critical Thinking: A Concise Guide*. London, England: Routledge; 2002:155–205.

44. Copi IM, Cohen C. *Introduction to Logic*. 11th ed. Upper Saddle River, NJ: Prentice-Hall; 2002.

45. Popkin RH, Stroll A. *Philosophy Made Simple*. 2nd ed rev. New York, NY: Broadway Books; 2001.

46. Hitchcock D. *Critical Thinking: A Guide to Evaluating Information.* Toronto, Ontario: Methuen Publishing; 1983.

47. Nolt J, Rohatyn D, Varzi A. *Schaum's Outline of Theory and Problems of Logic.* 2nd ed. New York, NY: McGraw-Hill; 1998.

48. Hughes W. *Critical Thinking: An Introduction to the Basic Skills.* 3rd ed. Peterborough, Ontario: Broadview Press; 2000.

49. Gettier EL. Is justified true belief knowledge? *Analysis.* 1963;23:121–124.

50. Schacter DL. *Memory Distortion: How Minds, Brains, and Societies Reconstruct the Past.* Cambridge, Mass: Harvard University Press; 1995.

51. Harrison FR III. *Logic and Rational Thought.* St. Paul, Minn: West Publishing Co; 1992.

52. Last JM, ed. *A Dictionary of Epidemiology.* 4th ed. Oxford, England: Oxford University Press; 2001.

53. Sackett DL. Bias in analytical research. *J Chronic Dis.* 1979;32:51–63.

54. Jenicek M, Cléroux R. *Épidémiologie: Principes, techniques, applications [Epidemiology: Principles, Techniques, Applications].* Paris, France: EDISEM and Maloine Éditeurs; 1982.

55. Johnson DM. Reasoning and logic. In: Stills DL, ed. *International Encyclopedia of the Social Sciences.* New York, NY: Macmillan Company and The Free Press; 1968.

CHAPTER 3

Logic in a Nutshell II: Types of Reasoning and Arguments

How Can We Reason and Argue Better?

IN THIS CHAPTER

Good evidence is not everything.
It's also essential to know how you use it.
Good uses of good evidence are everything.

Using good evidence poorly is nothing.
Using poor evidence illogically is malpractice.

Nobody practices perfect medicine.
My colleagues are of the opinion that I am nobody.
Therefore, I practice perfect medicine.
What's wrong with my logic, you say?

To make medicine successful, we must know how to find the best available arguments and their conclusions, how to build them properly, how to evaluate them critically, and how to use them in practice and research.

In this chapter, we learn more about the inner workings of logic as applied to medicine. Classical Aristotelian logic is not the only option available. Old and new trends as outlined in Sections 3.2 to 3.7 can also enrich our ways of thinking and reasoning, although some still await wide application.

3.1 DEDUCTION, INDUCTION, AND ABDUCTION

In the evaluation of reasoning and arguments, logicians are interested in two characteristics:

1. **Deductive validity.** The conclusion *necessarily* (without exception) follows from the premises. It is impossible, just because of the meaning of the statements, for the premises to be true while the conclusion is false. Deductive validity is an either-or, yes-or-no property. Any inference is either *deductively valid* or *deductively invalid.*

2. **Inductive strength.** The conclusion *only probably* follows from its premises. It is improbable, in the absence of other relevant information, for the premises to be true while the conclusion is false. Inductive strength is a matter of degree. Hence, an inference may be either *inductively weak* or *inductively strong.* (In either case, it is deductively invalid.)

Although deductive validity guarantees the truth of the conclusion **if** the premises are true, by itself it is neither sufficient nor necessary for the truth of the conclusion.

Two situations can arise:

- **One or more of the premises are false (untrue), and the conclusion of a deductively valid argument is false**: "*All physicians wear white coats* (not necessarily true). *All psychiatrists are physicians* (true). *Therefore, all psychiatrists wear white coats.*" (They don't.)

- **A deductively invalid argument may by chance have a correct (truthful) conclusion**: "*Some people who wear white coats are physicians* (true). *All psychiatrists wear white coats* (false; not all psychiatrists wear a white coat). *Therefore, all psychiatrists are physicians.*" (True, even though one premise is false and the inference is deductively invalid.)

Formal deductive validity depends on the form of the argument,[1] not on its content.

"All physicians are health professionals; George is a physician; therefore, George is a health professional" is a **formally valid inference based** (we suppose) **on truthful premises**. Its conclusion is therefore true.

"All physicians are health professionals; George is a health professional; therefore, George is a physician" is a **deductively invalid inference,** despite the (supposed) fact that George is a health professional. He may be a pharmacist, microbiologist, laboratory technician, or physiotherapist. It is also possible that he is a physician, but this argument does not prove it, because the inference is deductively invalid.

As indicated in Chapter 2, requirements for good reasoning and good arguments target both structure and content. The inference from the premises and the stripped-down warrant to the conclusion must be formally deductively valid; that requirement is a structural one. The premises and warrant must be justified, the premises must be complete, and there must be justification for assuming that no exceptional circumstances apply; those are content requirements.

Thus, all good arguments rely on their content and form. The content is largely given by the quality of evidence supporting the premises and warrants. Our sister book is devoted mainly to the production and evaluation of the best evidence.[2] Here, let us continue to focus instead on its evaluation and uses.

Logic and medicine, in general, have assigned slightly different meanings to deduction and induction. In **formal logic,** as we have seen, inferences may be **deductively valid** (given that the premises are true, the conclusion is definitely true) or **inductively strong** (given that the premises are true, the conclusion is probable, in the absence of further information). Deductive logic applies when premises can be secured from which a desired conclusion follows necessarily. Since certainty, however rare, is highly desirable in medicine, deductive logic is of interest for decisions in this field. Nonetheless, many conclusions may follow only inductively because of the nature of the problem under scrutiny. Figure 3-1 illustrates this classification of inferences.

In **medicine, in general,** the terms *deduction* and *induction* are applied, not to the product of reasoning or argument, but rather to the **process** of reasoning.

FIGURE 3-1

Classification of inferences in logic

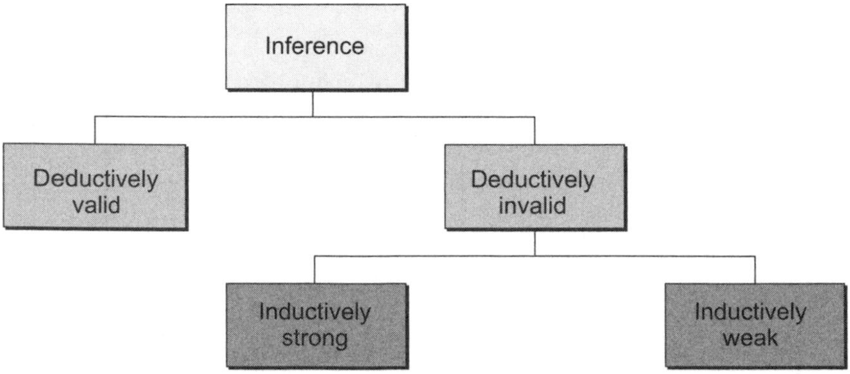

For Cutler,[3] **deduction** means going from established facts and general statements to an individual case. A conclusion is only as good as the propositions (established facts and general statements) from which it is deduced. In fact, there are other types of deductively valid inferences. For example, the deductively valid inference from the proposition that "no virus responds to an antibiotic" to the conclusion that "anything that responds to an antibiotic is not a virus" goes from a single general proposition to another general proposition.

Inductive reasoning often involves inference from a study of individual cases to a general principle. Once established by such studies, the principle can then be applied deductively to other cases.

In epidemiology, **deductive reasoning** often involves using a general principle (or hypothesis) as a starting point for the collection, analysis, and interpretation of data to confirm or refute this principle. **Inductive reasoning** typically involves the use of established facts (existing data and information) to draw a general conclusion or to confirm a hypothesis. Deductive reasoning and inductive reasoning go in opposite directions. Deductive reasoning goes from previously formulated hypotheses to the gathering of data whose analysis and interpretation leads to their acceptance or rejection, whereas inductive reasoning goes from data to hypothesis formulation and either acceptance or rejection. Debates continue on whether deduction or induction is preferable. However, most research in this area is an iterative process that moves back and forth between induction and deduction.

As clinicians, we reason more or less successfully by induction (Francis Bacon, 1561–1626), rather than by deduction (René Descartes, 1596–1650). Let us look at an example of both inductive and deductive approaches to a clinical question.

By **induction**, that is, drawing a probable conclusion:

- This alcoholic patient who vomits fresh blood is known to have ruptured esophageal varices. *(Individual)*

- That alcoholic patient who vomits fresh blood is known to have ruptured esophageal varices. *(Individual)*

- Alcoholic patients who vomit fresh blood have ruptured esophageal varices. *(General)*

Often, clinicians try, successfully or not, to generalize beyond the basic argument: Alcoholic patients who vomit fresh blood bleed from ruptured esophageal varices. (Or, patients bleeding from ruptured esophageal varices are alcoholics.) Such generalizations are not always legitimate in the eyes of logicians. In an inference from individual cases to a general conclusion, the applicable warrant is that generally all members of a certain kind have any characteristic observed in all examined members of that kind. In our example, the observed characteristic is ruptured esophageal varices, not bleeding from ruptured esophageal varices. And the kind whose members were examined is alcoholic patients vomiting fresh blood, not people bleeding from ruptured esophageal varices.

Generalizing from examined instances does not always produce a correct conclusion; for example, in many people's experience all examined swans are white, but in fact not all swans are white—some are black. Hence, generalizing from examined instances is inductive rather than deductive reasoning.

Historically, most practical clinical experience was gained by inductive generalization from examined instances.

Another example of induction in medicine follows.

- This delusional patient is schizophrenic. *(Individual)*

- That delusional patient is schizophrenic. *(Individual)*

- Delusional patients have schizophrenia. *(General)*

By **deduction**, that is, drawing a necessary conclusion:

- Alcoholic patients who vomit fresh blood have ruptured esophageal varices. *(General)*

- This patient who vomits fresh blood is an alcoholic. *(Individual)*

- Therefore, he has ruptured esophageal varices. *(Individual)*

Or:

- Delusional patients are schizophrenic. *(General)*

- This patient is delusional. *(Individual)*

- Therefore, he (or she) must have schizophrenia. *(Individual)* Let's check this out!

The justification of our concluding statements depends on the strength of evidence that *all* alcoholic patients who vomit fresh blood have ruptured esophageal varices or, in the case of the second example, that *all* delusional patients have schizophrenia. Everything depends on the question asked.

Let us return now to **induction and deduction in logic** and to their specific meaning in this domain. For some, deduction ("leading forth," "evolutionary," "unfolding") means that once a set of axioms (uncontested facts) has been established, all their logical consequences are already fixed.[4] On the other hand, we can make other predictions, which follow inductively (with probability) from our basis, as in clinical prognosis at the hospital or weather forecasting outside.

Formal logic focuses on deductive validity, and it abstracts from the content of our inferences. In fact, it is an a priori study. In this respect, it contrasts with the natural sciences and all other disciplines that depend on observation for their data.

Both deduction and induction are equally important for medicine. For example, we may particularly need deductively valid inferences in making crucial therapeutic decisions and handling critical cases and situations in medicine and surgery. On the other hand, there is no meaningful prognosis without inferences that are not deductively valid but are inductively strong.

Besides induction and deduction, abduction appears of interest and useful in the health sciences' "evidence-based era."

TABLE 3-1

Deduction, induction, and abduction in daily life and medicine

Deduction

Daily life

P$_1$: All fish in this lake are trout.	P$_2$: This fish is from this lake.	C: Therefore, **necessarily**, this fish is a trout.

Medicine

P$_1$: All premature babies have low birth weight.	P$_2$: This baby is premature.	C: Therefore, **necessarily**, this baby has low birth weight.

Induction

Daily life

P$_1$: This fish is from this lake.	P$_2$: This fish is a trout.	C: Therefore, **probably**, all fish in this lake are trout.

Medicine

P$_1$: These babies are premature.	P$_2$: These babies have low birth weight.	C: Therefore, **probably**, all premature babies have low birth weight.

Abduction

Daily life

P$_1$: These fish are trout.	P$_2$: The fish in this lake are trout.	C: **Perhaps**, these fish are from this lake.

Medicine

P$_1$: These babies have low birth weight.	P$_2$: Premature babies have low birth weight.	C: **Perhaps**, these babies are premature.

P$_1$ and P$_2$ indicate premises; C, conclusion.

The examples in Table 3-1 drawn from daily life and medicine may further clarify the deduction/induction/abduction concept.

Abduction is defined in several ways:

- **"The process of generating a hypothesis"**[5] (from C. S. Peirce)

- **A mode of probable inference**[6] (from C. S. Peirce)

- **"A tentative acceptance of an explanatory hypothesis which, if true, would make the phenomenon under investigation intelligible."**[7] In other terms: Some phenomenon (fact) of interest is observed. If some hypothesis related to it were true, this phenomenon (fact) would be commonplace. Therefore, the hypothesis may be true (modified from Reese[6]).

Thus, abduction is a specific kind of induction. When induction is contrasted with abduction, the contrast is between generalizing from instances (induction) and generating a hypothesis from observed data and information (abduction).

Abduction is of increasing interest in medicine given various degrees of uncertainty in most medical observations, analyses, interpretations, and decisions. For one author[8,9] medicine must deal with uncertainty related to parts of the problem that are not provable, whatever the reason might be. Does this uncertainty speak against evidence-based medicine (EBM)?[10] Certainly not. Abduction is attractive in thinking under uncertainty while taking into account medical information coming continuously from open dynamic systems and individual-specific settings. Models are just partially capturing this situation. In the framework of C. S. Peirce's philosophy, Upshur[11] considers clinical encounters and inferences in clinical medicine as characteristically abductive: "*. . . They should be regarded as tentative statements that the inference holds, is provisionally the case, or pragmatically justifies action. . . .*"[11] In the terminology of Toulmin,[12,13] the warrant for an abductive inference is merely provisional or presumptive.

Abductive reasoning is an open-ended system allowing us to adjust premises, inference, and conclusions according to the changing picture of research, clinical experience, and setting of practice with individual patients. For Upshur,[11] abductive reasoning is both rigorous and probabilistic, yet able to recognize the uncertainties and particularities of day-to-day practice.

3.2 CLASSICAL ARISTOTELIAN LOGIC

The most well-known form of deductively valid inference is a classical Aristotelian categorical syllogism. Many inferences can be construed as categorical syllogisms once the warrant is made explicit and added as a premise.

The **categorical syllogism** is *a form of argument consisting of two premises and a conclusion, each of which is a categorical statement.*

For example, we can state:

Premise A (P$_1$): *All sciences contain logic.*

Premise B (P$_2$): *Medicine is a science. (Note: It is also an art.)*

Conclusion (C): *Medicine contains logic.*

Such syllogisms follow the pattern:

A (α, P$_1$); B (β, P$_2$); therefore C (γ, C).

They are **categorical syllogisms** because they are composed entirely of **categorical statements**. Each categorical statement contains a **subject term** and a **predicate term**. For example, in premise A, the subject term is "science" and the predicate term is "contains logic." A categorical statement either **affirms** or **denies** that some predicate belongs to either **all** or **some** members of some subject class.

Simple affirmative or negative statements about an individual ("Mrs Fitzpatrick is critically ill") can also be regarded as categorical statements by treating them as statements about all members of the class consisting of just that individual.

Thus, there are four types of categorical statements:

- **Universal affirmative** or **A** statement (*affirmo*): "All patients in our intensive care unit require continuous monitoring of their vital signs." "Mrs Fitzpatrick requires continuous monitoring of her vital signs."

- **Universal negative** or **E** statement (*nego*): "None of the patients in our intensive care unit should be transferred to another ward without a thorough assessment of their needs, risks, and prognosis." "Mrs Jones does not require continuous monitoring of her vital signs."

- **Particular affirmative** or **I** statement (*affirmo*): "Some patients in the coronary care unit can be transferred to other wards without a thorough assessment of their prognosis and needs."

- **Particular negative** or **O** statement (*nego*): "Some patients with respiratory distress syndrome cannot be transferred to other wards without a thorough assessment of their care needs and prognosis."

Three such categorical propositions (two premises and one conclusion) form a categorical syllogism. The propositions are linked by common terms in such a way that, although each proposition contains two terms (its subject term and predicate term), the whole categorical syllogism contains only three terms. As already mentioned in Chapter 2, the three terms in such a syllogism[14] are labeled as follows:

- The **major term** (symbolized by the letter *P*, ie, **predicate**) is the predicate of the conclusion. It appears in one of the two premises, which is thus called the **major premise**.

- The **minor term** (symbolized by the letter *S*, ie, **subject**) is the subject of the conclusion. It also appears in the other premise, which is thus called the **minor premise**.

- The **middle term** (symbolized by the letter *M*) appears in each premise, but not in the conclusion.

In everyday life, premises are presented in any order. Very often, one premise is presented (B), and the other (A) is tacit. Usually, the major premise is tacit; in Toulmin's[12,13] terminology, this tacit proposition is a warrant that licenses the inference from the minor premise to the conclusion. For example:

Premise A (major): *No otherwise healthy person with a viral infection of her upper respiratory tract (M) needs antibiotics (P).*

Premise B (minor): *My patient (S) has a viral infection of her upper respiratory tract but is otherwise healthy (M).*

Conclusion C: *My patient (S) does not need antibiotics (P).*

In practice, a clinician is likely to consider only premise B (*my patient has a viral infection of her upper respiratory tract, but is otherwise healthy*), then infer his or her therapeutic decision (conclusion C) in accordance with tacit premise A, which warrants the inference from B to C. (Conclusion C is not the only therapeutic decision the clinician should make. The clinician will advise the patient to stay warm and comfortable, rest, drink plenty of fluids, and take over-the-counter medication to control fever and pain.)

Figure 3-2 illustrates the architecture and building blocks of a categorical syllogism through this example.

3.2.1 Testing Categorical Syllogisms by Diagramming

Not all categorical syllogisms are deductively valid. There are various ways to test them for deductive validity. One of these is to use so-called Venn diagrams in which circles represent the sets **P**, **S**, and **M** and the arrangement of the circles represents relationships between **P**, **S**, and **M**. These diagrams were actually invented by the Swiss mathematician Leonhard Euler in the 1700s. About a century later,[15] the English mathematician, John Venn, developed an alternative method of diagramming categorical statements, which he argued was more suitable for testing the validity of categorical syllogisms. Here, we will use Euler's diagrams rather than Venn's, because they are better known, especially in medicine. Following common practice, we will nevertheless refer to them, incorrectly, as *Venn diagrams.*

Clinicians are already familiar with Venn diagrams from the field of diagnosis. Sports fans see them visually as "Olympic circles." They can serve as a pictorial representation of the extent to which various entities (sets) of interest like diagnoses are mutually inclusive or exclusive.[16] A **Venn diagram** is a diagram of circles. Each area displayed by these circles represents a distinct class. It is used to picture all possible relations holding between those classes.[17] Practical examples may be found in rheumatology,[18] psychiatry,[19,20] and elsewhere.

FIGURE 3-2

"Architecture" and "building blocks" of a categorical syllogism: clinical example

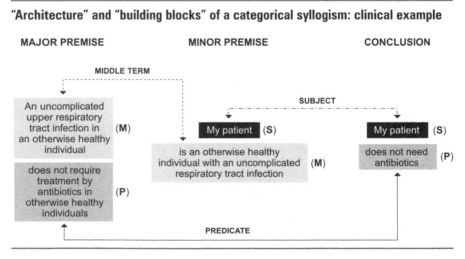

Figure 3-3 illustrates uses of circle diagrams in psychiatry. It shows relationships between four subtypes of depression using their proportional representation and overlapping of the circles (subtypes of depression). Absolute numbers of depressed patients under study are used in this graphical expression.

Figure 3-4 shows a circle diagram representing proportional relationships between three entities: affective disorder, suicide attempts, and suicide. It shows that an affective disorder plays a more important role in suicide than in suicide attempts.

In medicine, both the proportional overlapping of signs or symptoms of competing diseases in a differential diagnosis and the probabilities of various outcomes in prognostic studies are often represented in the form of Venn diagrams.

In logic, the subjects and predicates of the premises and conclusion of a categorical syllogism are also pictured as overlapping or disjoint circles, but they are used and analyzed in a different way. A categorical statement does not tell us the proportion of overlap between the sets referred to by its subject and predicate term, only whether the subject is included in the predicate (universal affirmative), is excluded from it (universal negative), at least partially overlaps with it (particular

FIGURE 3-3

Circle diagram* of subtypes of depression in psychiatry†

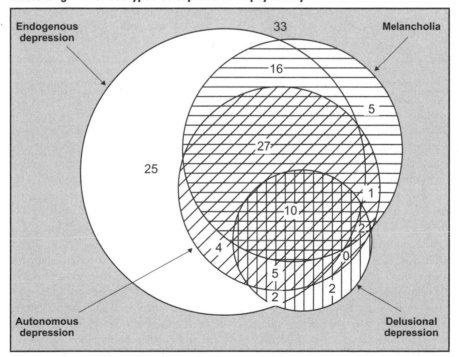

FIGURE 3-4

Circle diagram of relationships in psychiatry between affective disorders, suicide attempts, and suicide*

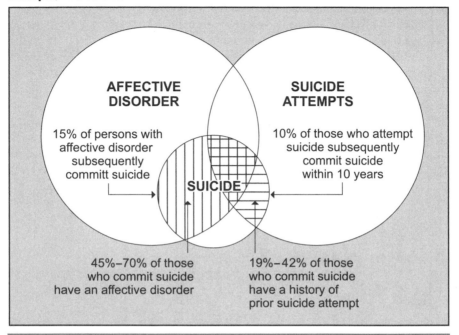

* Adapted with permission from the American Medical Association. (Avery D, Winokur G. Suicide, attempted suicide, and relapse rates in depression: occurrence after ECT and antidepressant therapy. *Arch Gen Psychiatry.* 1978;35:749–753). Copyright © 1978, American Medical Association. All rights reserved.

affirmative), or at least partially does not overlap with it (particular negative). Figure 3-5 shows the relationships between a subject (S) and a predicate (P) in categorical statements according to Venn's own method of diagramming, as well as according to Euler's method. Euler's diagrams, the so-called "Venn diagrams," actually contain more information than the statements they depict. For example, the diagram for a universal affirmative statement of the form "All S are P" shows S as a proper subset of P—that is, it shows that there are individuals in class P, but not in class S. But S may be coextensive with P. For example, the statement *"Every person whose leg veins show blood clots with the use of venous duplex ultrasonography has deep venous thrombosis"* is true. However, the class of people who show thrombi (blood clots and their effect) with the use of venous duplex ultrasonography (S) is coextensive with the class of people with deep venous thrombosis (P), since venous duplex ultrasonography is the gold standard (at the time of this writing) for evaluation of deep venous thrombosis. Strictly speaking, then, to depict a categorical statement with Euler's "Venn diagrams," you may need several alternative diagrams.

Use of Venn diagrams to test a categorical syllogism for deductive validity requires that one try to diagram the premises in a single diagram so as to depict the conclusion as false. In other words, one works against the conclusion. If this **cannot** be done, the syllogism is valid; the information in the premises forces one to represent

FIGURE 3-5

Venn's and Euler's diagram representation of various relationships between subjects and predicates in categorical statements

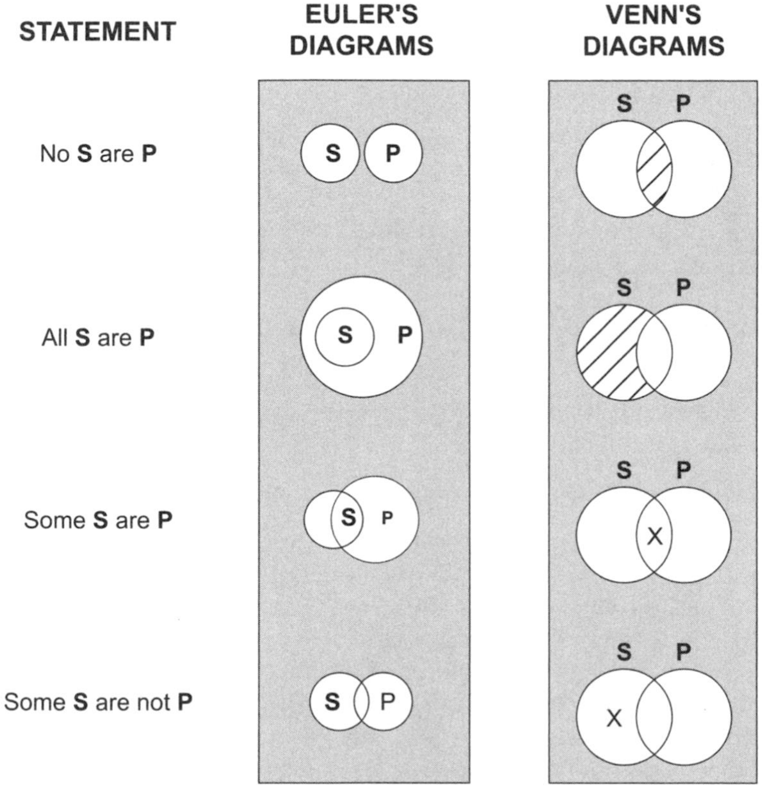

STATEMENT	EULER'S DIAGRAMS	VENN'S DIAGRAMS

S indicates subject; P, predicate.

the conclusion as true. If this **can** be done, the syllogism is invalid; it is possible for the premises to be true and the conclusion is false. Details of this method are given by Ennis.[21,22] Examples follow.

Many logic texts use circle diagrams to test categorical syllogisms for validity. Most of these use the diagrams introduced by Venn, the real Venn diagrams. Detailed instructions on how to construct and use the real Venn diagrams are given by Seech[16] and many others. It is also possible to test categorical syllogisms by seeing whether several rules apply.

A physician must also ensure that the premises are correct. Let us consider the following syllogism:

Premise A: *All sore throats are streptococcal infections.* (Incorrect)

Premise B: *Streptococcal infections respond well to antibiotics.* (Correct)

Conclusion C: *All sore throats should be treated with antibiotics.* (Incorrect)

FIGURE 3-6

Testing the validity of categorical syllogisms by using Venn diagrams*

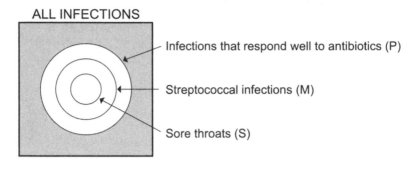

ALL INFECTIONS

Infections that respond well to antibiotics (P)

Streptococcal infections (M)

Sore throats (S)

* The syllogism is deductively valid, because diagramming the information in the premises forces us to diagram the conclusion as true.

No competent logician would regard this argument as formally correct. Instead, what follows formally from the premises is this:

Conclusion C: *All sore throats respond well to antibiotics.* (Incorrect)

Let us use this example to illustrate the Venn diagram test of deductive validity. First, we check that it is a categorical syllogism: two categorical premises and a categorical conclusion (all universal affirmative or **A** statements), with three terms (minor term **S** "sore throats," major term **P** "[infections that] respond well to antibiotics," middle term **M** "streptococcal infections") each used in the same sense throughout. If we diagram the premises in a single Venn diagram, we must put the circle for sore throats inside the circle for streptococcal infections and the circle for streptococcal infections inside the circle for infections that respond well to antibiotics. But, if we do that, we **must** put the circle for sore throats inside the circle for infections that respond well to antibiotics. In other words, we are forced to diagram the conclusion as true. So our Venn diagram test proves the deductive validity of our argument. (See Figure 3-6.)

But the conclusion is incorrect! Hence, in some situations, although **S, P,** and **M** may be correctly combined, they can lead to incorrect conclusions. That can happen only when at least one premise is incorrect, in this case the premise that all sore throats are streptococcal infections (premise A). In fact, not all sore throats are streptococcal infections. The conclusion might be true (although it is not), but the syllogism above does not prove it.

Let us apply our Venn diagram test to an example of deductively invalid reasoning in surgery:

Premise A: *The patient has a tender abdomen.*

Premise B: *Some patients with a tender abdomen have appendicitis.*

Conclusion C: *The patient must have his appendix removed right away.* (No other considerations are taken into account.)

FIGURE 3-7

Testing the validity of categorical syllogisms by using Venn diagrams*

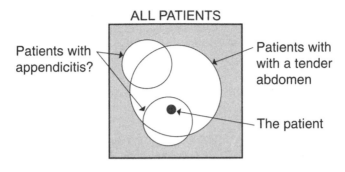

ALL PATIENTS

Patients with appendicitis?

Patients with with a tender abdomen

The patient

---

* The syllogism is deductively invalid, because diagramming the information in the premises does not force us to diagram the conclusion as true.

This is obviously jumping too quickly to a conclusion! The surgeon who is so anxious to operate has implicitly drawn a prior conclusion:

Conclusion C: *The patient has appendicitis.*

With this conclusion, the argument is a categorical syllogism: two categorical premises and a categorical conclusion (one premise a particular affirmative or **I** statement, the other premise and the conclusion universal affirmative or **A** statements), with three terms (minor term **S** "the patient," major term **P** "has appendicitis," middle term **M** "patients with a tender abdomen") each used in the same sense throughout. But is it deductively valid?

Let us test it with a Venn diagram. We put the circle for the patient inside the circle for patients with a tender abdomen (premise A). Then, we try to make the circle for patients with a tender abdomen intersect the circle for patients with appendicitis (premise B) without making the circle for the patient intersect with it (conclusion C, false). Can we do this? Yes. (See Figure 3-7.) As far as our premises are concerned, the patient might have appendicitis or might not. Since we can make a Venn diagram of the premises in which the conclusion is shown as false, the argument is deductively invalid. The conclusion does not follow necessarily from the premises.

Elsewhere, both premises may be untrue and the conclusion may be incorrect.

Premise A: *All sore throats are streptococcal infections.*

Premise B: *No streptococcal infections should be treated with antibiotics.*

Conclusion C: *No sore throat should be treated with antibiotics.*

It is left as an exercise to the reader to determine if the above categorical syllogism is deductively valid, using a Venn diagram.

Finally, if a categorical syllogism is formally valid and its premises are true, then the conclusion must be true:

Premise A: *Some sore throats are streptococcal infections.*

Premise B: *Streptococcal infections must be treated with antibiotics.*

Conclusion C: *Some sore throats must be treated with antibiotics.*

To determine that our premises are true, we must base them on solid evidence. Streptococcal infections, for example, should be confirmed by laboratory testing. Premise B is justified by solid evidence that antibiotic treatment of streptococcal infections prevents potentially serious late complications.

It is left as an exercise to the reader to use a Venn diagram to show that the above argument is deductively valid.

Thus, clinical reasoning must use the most appropriate evidence as a basis for each premise. Also, the premises as a group must be linked in a way that makes the argument logically valid. This is a necessary part of the art of medicine as defined in Chapter 1. Correct premises based on good evidence are driven by deductively valid inference to equally correct conclusions, which themselves become new evidence in the next argument (syllogism) and so on, in our chain of reasoning and problem solving. Errors sometimes cause an unexpected snowball effect.

The above picture of good clinical reasoning must be qualified by recognizing that our warrants (major premises) sometimes hold only generally or provisionally. There are exceptions. In such cases, the inference from the premises and the warrant with the qualifiers and rebuttals removed will be deductively valid. But the qualifiers and rebuttals mean that our conclusion does not follow necessarily from our premises. Even if we are certain of the premises, we need more evidence to be certain that our conclusion is true.

3.2.2 Syllogisms in Everyday Communication

Let us recall this example from Chapter 2:

Before leaving the hospital, we may say to a colleague on call: "*Do not forget to check this patient who has a fever of unknown origin. Results from the laboratory workup should arrive at any moment. I'm very concerned about him. All patients with a ruptured abscess have a fever. His condition may worsen quickly. Because this patient is febrile, and given his other clinical manifestations, he may have a ruptured abscess. . . . If confirmed by incoming laboratory and other paraclinical tests results, we should treat him with antibiotics as soon as possible and call the surgeon on call for additional assessment and surgical care if indicated. . . .*"

As we may see from this example, our natural language in everyday life is not a sequence of syllogisms whose purpose it is to please a logician's inquisitive mind. To understand if our "natural" argumentation is good or bad, we may need to reconstruct arguments from our natural language. We have already discussed such reconstruction in Chapter 2.[23-27]

In everyday clinical life, in fact, we do not usually communicate in the form of classical syllogisms. We may use **only one or more than two categorical premises** supporting and leading to some categorical conclusion. In the natural language of daily life, the conclusion may be presented first ("my patient must get antibiotics") and premises follow ("because he or she has a bacterial infection proven sensitive to antibiotics") in the **reverse order of a classical syllogism.**

In medical practice, **syllogisms** may look **truncated** by keeping one of the premises tacit: "my patient must be given antibiotics" because "he has a bacterial infection." This tacitly assumes that patients with bacterial infections must be given antibiotics. Traditionally, such an assumption is regarded as an unstated premise, and an argument with such an unstated premise is called an **enthymeme.**[28] For Hitchcock[29,30] however, *"[S]uch arguments generally do not have tacit premises. Rather, they should be evaluated as they stand to see whether there is a justified general principle (universal or probabilistic—'most,' 'usually'; presumptive—'presumably'; or possibilistic—'sometimes') in accordance with which the conclusion follows non-trivially from the premises."* Such a general principle is what Toulmin[12,13] calls a **warrant.** In this example, only a nonuniversal warrant *"most patients with a bacterial infection must receive antibiotics"* is justified, since there are known exceptions: some agents may be resistant to antibiotics.

As in other domains of logic, the solidity and value of an argument in medical decision making rely equally on:

- the best evidence supporting each premise

- the premises leading to the proposed conclusion

- freedom from fallacies

For example, a randomized, double-blind, controlled trial may be the best evidence for the effectiveness of drug control of arthritis in elderly patients. In our office, we have to decide how to treat an elderly person with arthritis who is seeking some relief from pain and dysfunction. We can reason in the following way:

Premise A: *The results of many controlled clinical trials, as well as their systematic review, prove that drug M is effective in controlling the symptoms of chronic degenerative arthritis diagnosed according to a set of inclusion and exclusion criteria.*

Premise B: *My patient is elderly and arthritis was diagnosed by the same set of inclusion and exclusion criteria.*

Conclusion C:
   1. Drug M will be effective in controlling the symptoms in my patient.
   2. My patient is a good candidate for treatment with drug M.
   3. I should prescribe drug M to my patient.

It should be noted that although the inference to conclusion C1 is formally valid, neither the inference to conclusion C2 nor the inference to conclusion C3 is formally valid. In each case, they follow only presumptively. There might be exceptions to conclusion C2: contraindications, or cheaper and equally effective drugs to choose from. Conclusion C3 is right provided that my patient complies well with the treatment regimen; the patient might comply better with other treatments. These considerations are in addition to those found in premises A and B, from which conclusions C2 and C3 follow only presumptively. C2 and C3 follow neither formally from premises A and B nor in accordance with a universal warrant. Formal logic can take us only so far in medicine.

As we can see from the previous-mentioned examples of syllogisms and their uses, correct reasoning and argument are vital to all decisions in prevention and care. The application of logic is necessary to purge medicine of numerous flaws of reasoning that threaten decisions, not so much to please formal logicians, but rather to **put to the best use the best available evidence for the best benefit to the patient**.

3.3 CONTEMPORARY LOGIC

Not all deductively valid reasoning and argument consists of Aristotelian syllogisms. In this section, we mention some other types.

Logical operators and **connectives**[31] such as *if. . . then, if and only if, it is not the case that . . ., both . . . and*, and *either . . . or* form the basis of **propositional logic**. Good introductions to classical propositional logic can be found in a number of elementary textbooks in mathematical logic.[32-34]

The logic of the **quantifiers** *all* and *some* extends beyond Aristotelian syllogisms. Contemporary logic adds its logic to propositional logic to create a more advanced system called **predicate logic**. (References 32 to 34 also provide an introduction to predicate logic.) One can then add rules for identity or equality, symbolized by an equal sign. Predicate logic with identity is called **first-order logic** if the quantifiers quantify only over individuals and not over their properties and relations.

In the study of risk, treatment, prognosis, or disease outcome, we may be interested in knowing whether ensuing conclusions, given the premises that lead to them, are necessary, possible, or impossible. Such properties are called *modal notions* and the logic associated with them is termed **modal logic**.[35] More advanced introductions to symbolic logic, such as those by Nolt[32] and Forbes,[33] include a section on modal logic.

Modal logic is an add-on, or extension, to some underlying logic. The underlying logic in elementary textbooks of symbolic logic is classical first-order logic. The key assumption of classical logic is that every statement is either definitely true or definitely false (although we may not know which). In Section 3.7 we examine an alternative to classical logic, namely, fuzzy logic.

3.4 HISTORICAL NOTE ON INDIAN LOGIC

Historically, Aristotelian (Western) logic is not the only type of logic. For example, in Eastern philosophy, the Nyaya school in India (third century BC to second century AD) developed methodological reasoning called Tarka, which operates using five stages rather than the three stages of an Aristotelian categorical syllogism.[36,37] Table 3-2 illustrates such a five-stage process of reasoning.

TABLE 3-2

Tarka methodological reasoning in Indian philosophy

Stages (steps)	Down-to-earth example[36]	Medical example
1. **Primary hypothesis** (Proposition)	There is a cow on the road somewhere.	My patient is worried that he may have cancer somewhere in his digestive tract given the fresh blood he has seen in his stools.
2. **Principal reasoning** (Reason)	There is cow dung on the road.	Colonoscopy shows a bleeding lesion in the colon of this patient.
3. **Major theory** (Must have concrete examples. Premise also includes relationship between classes of things such as cancer and bleeding lesions; see example.)	Where there is dung, there is an animal.	Where there is a bleeding lesion, there may be a cancer.
4. **Application** (Premise-supporting examples are applied to the particular case.)	This is cow dung, therefore . . .	Biopsy confirms that this lesion is malignant.
5. **Conclusion is asserted**	There is no dung without a cow. Therefore, there is a cow on the road.	There are no lesions of this kind without cancer. Therefore, my patient has colon cancer.

This formal method of reasoning also implies causality. Later, however, Tarka reasoning was reduced to three stages, which in our example might be:

- *Bleeding lesions of the colon indicate colon cancer* (P_1).

- *I found a bleeding lesion in the colon of my patient* (P_2).

- *As confirmed by biopsy, my patient has colon cancer* (C).

Thus, Tarka reasoning was brought closer to Aristotelian logic, which continues to be a part of Western thought and logic today.

3.5 UNCERTAINTY AND PROBABILITY IN MEDICINE

Statements and conclusions in our logical discourses may be made either with certainty or with some lesser degree of probability. Essentially, there are three possible "operating systems" in medicine for reasoning with less than perfect certainty:

- probability theory and its applications (well established),

- chaos theory and its uses in clinical research (emerging), or

- fuzzy logic and fuzzy set theory in handling imperfect or hard to interpret data (also emerging and increasingly attractive for many).

Are these tools contradictory or complementary?

Past generations of physicians tried to make medicine "as scientific as possible" by adopting a **deterministic paradigm of medicine**. This was accomplished by sending medicine to the laboratory and operating rooms. As examples, Pasteur's postulates defined infection, and a surgeon could see, touch, and repair a ruptured organ. Certainty was the ideal goal.

What is certainty? We can explain it from three different perspectives: psychological, statistical, and logical.

1. Certainty may be purely psychological: a simple state of mind; a spontaneous, intuitive, and unsubstantiated conviction. At best, we base it on some grounds of past personal or collective experience. "I'm sure of it. I'm telling you, I've seen it!"

2. A conviction of certainty (or uncertainty) may be based on probabilistic assessment and quantification of events. "Fifty percent of persons of some advanced age have some degree of atherosclerosis. My patient belongs to this age group. I may be 50% certain [or uncertain] that he has some degree of atherosclerosis. Let us do a more detailed clinical work-up to see if this particular patient really has some degree of atherosclerosis and if this degree is clinically important enough to warrant medical care."

3. Our certainty is the product of a deductively valid inference from premises known to be true. The premises are true (evidence-based), and from them there follows necessarily a conclusion, which becomes new solid evidence itself. Mr. Spock's "It's logical, Captain" in the *Star Trek* television series reminds us of this type of certainty.

Modern medicine should increasingly be based on the probabilistic and logical paradigms of certainty and uncertainty. In fact, in the last century, medicine has shifted toward a **probabilistic paradigm of medicine**.

In daily practice, most observations and decisions in health sciences are made under various degrees of uncertainty. **Probability is the quantification of such uncertainty**.

In medicine, we refer to probability more than we think. For example, a surgical resident admits a patient with an acute abdomen and concludes his or her report not by a definitive diagnosis, but by an "impression" (in the clinical jargon of medical charts): peritonitis, possibly ruptured appendix. Such a formulation can ideally be quantified in terms of probability.

This is just one example of the importance of probability in the daily life of clinicians. The management of clinical problems by different physicians and their success may reflect meanings attributed to words used to reflect probability.

What are the causes of our uncertainty in medicine?

- Our poor knowledge of the problem under study (etiology of essential hypertension or many cancers).

- Missing data for the complete understanding of a problem if all data are needed to solve the problem. However, "there are never enough data."

- Not all available data are correct, because of poor measurement.

- Findings are poorly interpreted.

- Time, place, and patients' demographic and clinical characteristics may vary.

- Conclusions are erroneously put into practice.

- The effectiveness of implemented decisions is not realistically determined.

- Poor distinctions are made between causes of disease cases and disease as an entity as well as between causes of disease itself (risk) and those of disease course and outcomes (prognosis).

This applies to research as well as to practice.

Most of our conclusions have a certain degree of **randomness**. We are not always absolutely sure that the patient has the disease we diagnose. For example, we might be uncertain about the recurrence of cancer after the surgical removal of its primary lesion. Our conclusions are more or less **educated guesses**, based on our experience and our knowledge of uncontested facts, causes, gauging uncertainty, and uses of probability.

A **stochastic process** is a process that incorporates some degree of randomness.[38] An example is the decay of a radioactive isotope, where the rate of decay (as measured by the half-life of the isotope) can be known, but not the time at which an individual atom will decay. Those who use the technical term *stochastic* want to circumvent the ambiguities of the term *random*[39] (governed by chance).

Bayes' theorem,[40] formulated in the18th century, was revolutionary for its probabilistic considerations that, in medicine, are mainly concentrated in the area of diagnosis. (For more information about diagnosis see Section 6.2.2.) However, it also applies to other kinds of evidence. For Murphy,[39] two important conclusions can be drawn from Bayes' views:

1. In all but trivial cases, there is uncertainty. There are therefore always at least two conjectures or explanations under consideration.

2. The most rational assessment of new evidence is that which combines the probability of our hypothesis on the basis of previous evidence (the prior, or *a priori*, probability) with the likelihood of the new evidence according to our hypothesis and according to its competing hypotheses (the posterior and prior likelihoods of the evidence) to produce a revised estimate of the probability that our hypothesis is true (posterior probability).

Another important characteristic of our observations within the framework of probability theory is our "black or white" (binary) categorization of events. Subjects are male or female, young or old, healthy or sick (with a disease of interest). They are treated or not; they are exposed or not to noxious factors such as carcinogens or poor diet.

Hence, such characteristics and events, as well as their associations, may be the subject of studies based on a probabilistic view of events.

Goodman's[41] view aptly concludes this section: "... *Making clinical sense of a case means explaining its logic: why the patient exhibits certain symptoms, how this patient is similar to others, how various findings relate, and the mechanism by which interventions will affect the future outcome. In groups, individual details are averaged out, but these details may be critical to the causal explanation for an individual patient. Inevitably, however, a gap exists between what we understand in a given patient and what we are able to predict: this is where probability fits in. ...*"

More information about the fundamentals of probability theory[42,43] and its applications to medicine[41,44,45] can be found in the literature.

3.6 Chaos Theory in Medicine

Until recently, we were accustomed to perceive the human body as a stable, well-organized biological system. Physiological functions often have their predetermined and fixed frequencies, amplitudes, rhythm, and levels of functioning. Exposed to various factors, the organism tends to maintain a predetermined balance (Claude Bernard's *milieu intérieur stable*), a process named **homeostasis** in the thirties by Walter B. Cannon. In this traditional concept, bodily functions tend to be regular and stable: heartbeat, electrolyte balance, body temperature, and the periodic rhythm of functions. In the interpretation of human physiology and pathology, deviations were interpreted in relation to these reference points.

Since the 1960s, in the framework of chaos theory, human functions as well as the workings of medicine have come to be considered not as "regular" but as "chaotic." In human biology, chaotic behavior was defined as "*an aperiodic, seemingly random behavior in a deterministic system that exhibits sensitive dependence on initial conditions*"[46] or "*apparently random or unpredictable behavior in systems governed by deterministic laws.*"[47] Small causes may lead to more important consequences, there is not necessarily a linear relationship between cause and effect, and the biological universe is unpredictable. "Chaotic" behavior is seen rather than normalcy. Becoming "regular" is a sign of a health problem in some cases. An absolutely regular heart rhythm is considered a prelude to myocardial infarction. Besides physiologic functions, health services may also be seen as "chaotic," such as emergency hospital services (They are already perceived as such, without any need for logic, by any medical student starting his or her experience in the emergency department!). More information about this may be found in our other writings.[2]

For logic and critical thinking, accepting "chaos" means that we will be obliged to review what premises are correct, what is an acceptable inference, and whether our conclusions are acceptable in terms of "chaos" as a reference point.

Our long-term predictions (prognosis) may prove difficult, if not impossible. Our interpretations will be based not only on fragmented problems and questions about them but also on the evaluation of a given problem as a whole. We must be alert to the possibility that a small unnoticed factor in our patient might make a clinically important difference in the correct diagnosis, treatment decision, or prognosis.

3.7 FUZZY SETS AND FUZZY LOGIC

Fuzzy set theory and fuzzy logic complete and sometimes oppose probabilistic thinking in medicine. We may expect these new ways of looking at medical phenomena to be followed by methodological adjustments and developments, as well as by their wider application, evaluation, and growing use in medical practice and medical research.

We discuss three topics in this section: the distinction between fuzzy logic and fuzzy set theory, the paradigm of fuzziness in medicine, and the essentials of fuzzy reasoning in fuzzy logic.

3.7.1 Distinction Between Fuzzy Logic and Fuzzy Set Theory

The terms "fuzzy logic" and "fuzzy theory" are often used interchangeably in the current literature. Let us reserve **fuzzy theory** for the view that the phenomena around us are not necessarily dichotomous (black or white, sick or healthy), but that many things are a matter of degree and should be analyzed and understood as such. **Fuzzy logic** should be reserved more narrowly for the domain of reasoning and argument based on fuzzy theory. Readers must often "read between the lines" to understand the exact meanings of some authors.

Our observations are subject to random and systematic errors in measurement and interpretation as well. Different combinations of clinical and paraclinical manifestations occur in different patients and throughout the clinical course of disease. In addition, the biological nature of our observations and data in medicine makes them not only imperfect and incomplete but also hard to interpret and explain. In daily life, we can remove sugar grain by grain from a spoon. However, when do the contents of the spoon cease to be a spoonful of sugar? In medicine, our evaluation of low or high blood glucose can be difficult if values are assessed in small increments. Theoretically, a fasting blood glucose level of 3.7 mmol/L (668 mg/L), which is at the lower limit of the 95% normal range for adults, can be considered low, as well as that of 3.4 and so on. At 5.18 mmol/L and above, we might consider the blood glucose level still normal but a bit high, then high, then definitely high, and finally we might assign it a diagnostic value as it becomes an indication for treatment. As the blood glucose level increases, the degree of fit of its interpretation as a "normal" blood glucose level decreases and vice versa.

For Steinmann[48] or Asbury and Tzabar,[49] these "sets of observations" are the subject of symbolic reasoning as a model of human thinking. Data are symbols to which we assign some meaning. Our meaning is imperfect because hypoglycemia or hyperglycemia, hypertension or hypotension can mean several values whose sets (or ensembles) are imprecise, overlapping, or "fuzzy." Such vague concepts are the subject of **fuzzy set theory**.

In probability theory and applications, we simplify demarcations and limits of **sets** (ie, collections of defined or distinct items). We clearly define who is healthy and who is ill, who smokes and who does not, who is treated and who is not. In fuzzy set theory, such a binary system (yes or no, black or white, 0 or 1) is replaced by a scale of values from 0 to 1, "yes, perhaps, probably, definitely no," and different shades of gray between white and black. **Fuzzy sets** infuse the notion of continuity in both deductive and inductive thinking.

Probabilities assume that something will occur or not. Fuzziness measures the degree to which something occurs or some conditions exist. It fills up Aristotle's "excluded middle."

If diagnostic, therapeutic, or prognostic reasoning is based on the assessment of several variables that might be considered "fuzzy sets," it requires some kind of logic to deal effectively with such multidimensional spaces of vagueness; it needs **fuzzy logic**. This logic is not fuzzy in itself since it is based on solid mathematical foundations. However, the data to which it is applied are fuzzy.

Different fuzzy sets can belong to other sets as well.

3.7.2 Paradigm of Fuzziness in Medicine

Proponents of fuzzy theory and fuzzy logic argue that classical logic in daily reasoning may be further away from the reality of overall human thinking and communication.[44] Classical logic works with an "excluded middle." One has a disease or one does not; one smokes or one does not. Protagonists of fuzzy logic point out that a patient is not simply sick or not but also might be "a little sick," "moderately sick," or "severely sick." However, we cannot say that a woman is "a little pregnant," "moderately pregnant," or "very pregnant." This might be possible from the point of view of fuzzy theory, but it is not supported by the biological reality of pregnancy. We have convincing evidence that there is no "excluded middle"—a future mother cannot be "a little," "moderately," or "very" pregnant. So do we first need some additional and perhaps special evidence for the excluded middle to accept its reality and to take it into account in our reasoning? Should we know how to apply it as correctly as we already use evidence in classical reasoning and argument?

For the sake of explicitness, Figure 3-8 illustrates in a visual manner a fuzzy transition between healthy weight and obesity. Subjectively, a layperson may consider an individual obese anywhere within a chosen range of appearance. Based on an excluded middle, one might categorize people only as either obese or not obese, in accordance with local values and acceptance of paradigms of beauty ranging from today's fashion models to the models for the paintings of Petrus Paulus Rubens. The fuzzy picture fits better the way we use the term *obese*.

Despite all our attention to clinimetrically valid and well-defined observations, our daily life and communication is full of "excluded middles" and fuzzy terms. We might hear on the radio that "it will be *partly* cloudy tomorrow, with *occasional* showers and *some heavy* rain by the end of the day." Similarly, an intern may report,

FIGURE 3-8

"Excluded middle" concepts of classical logic vs fuzzy concepts

Excluded Middle

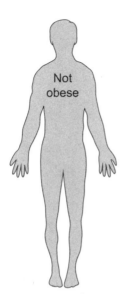
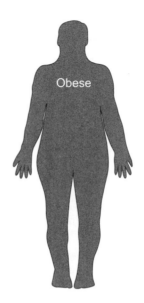

Fuzzy Concept

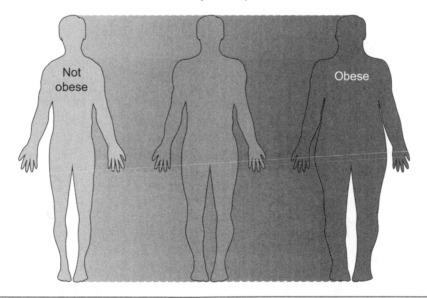

"We have admitted a diabetic, insulin-dependent patient with a history of *recent* surgery, showing a *worrisome* hyperglycemia and *advanced* decompensation of his (her) acid-basic balance, and appearing *considerably* confused." (All fuzzy terms are in italics.) Such a message may mean either of the following:

- that our intern does not know exactly what is he or she talking about, or

- that we have at hand (and that we know and understand all) stringent operational clinimetric criteria defining which hyperglycemia is *worrisome*, which metabolic decompensation is *advanced* (ketoacidosis requiring insulin, fluid, electrolyte and mineral replacement?) and what degree of mental confusion is *considerable*. (Is the patient belligerent? Does he or she not know the day or year?)

A staff member may suggest to the intern: "Your treatment and follow-up orders are *fine, watch* the patient *closely*, and do not forget to *give him (her) some* potassium! It is *unlikely* that we will need to do *more* than that." (Presumably, the intern will not consider such orders as "fuzzy" and will correctly calculate potassium requirements for this patient and choose the right manner by which potassium should be given while also knowing about the full array of diagnostic and therapeutic options in this case.) Another good example of fuzzy communication is given by Asbury and Tzabar:[49] "If the arterial pressure is *slightly* above the *desired* range, increase the infusion rate *a little*. If the arterial pressure falls *catastrophically*, stop the infusion *temporarily*." Zadeh[50] calls the highlighted words such as *slightly* and *desired* **fuzzy predicates**, **fuzzy quantifiers**, and **fuzzy probabilities**. He concludes that classical probability theory and classical logic do not well represent common-sense knowledge and usage. Fuzzy logic focuses on such kinds of uncertainty and lexical imprecision. Values of observations (statements, evidence) are directional and progressive between the existent and the nonexistent.

Propositions from Sadegh-Zadeh[51] stating that nosology, diagnosis, and treatment are fuzzy, specific to the available information and its context, or that somebody may be ill or not,[52] do not facilitate practical decision making in clinical life. For the moment, clinicians have two ways of dealing with such uncertainty:

- they may attempt some kind of **hardening of soft data**[2] and use this "sharper" information for sharp conclusions and decisions, or

- they may leave fuzzy terms as they are and submit them to the process of fuzzy logic.

The concept of fuzzy health, illness, and disease is still debated. Applications of fuzzy theory in medicine may focus on differential diagnosis, mixed diagnosis integrating Western and Eastern medicines, optimal selection of treatment, or real-time monitoring of patient data.[45] Fuzzy theory may prove particularly useful, however, in the case of health problems having multiple causes, a wide spectrum of clinical manifestations, or multiple therapeutic choices.[49,50]

3.7.3 Essentials of Fuzzy Reasoning in Fuzzy Logic

In contrast to sharp Aristotelian logic, fuzzy logic means approximate reasoning where everything is a matter of degree:[50]

- While appreciating **truth** of information, things may not only be true or false but also *very true* or *not quite true.*

- **Predicates** (properties stated about subjects) are not sharp either. The patient *feels ill;* the uterus of an expectant mother is *much larger than usual.*

- A single **predicate modifier** in classical systems, negation or *not,* is introduced into a larger set, including such modifiers as *very, more or less, quite, rather,* and *extremely.*

- **Quantifiers** are also more numerous than just *all* and *some: few, several, usually, most, almost always, frequently, approximately 10 cm.*

- Numerical or interval-valued **probabilities** are replaced by entities qualified as *likely, unlikely, very likely, by the end of the day,* and so on.

- Bivalent **possibilities** such as *possible* or *impossible* are expanded by degrees such as *quite possible, almost impossible,* and others.

Fuzzy logic is used in four kinds of reasoning:[51]

- In **reasoning from simple propositions about specific individuals**, there are no fuzzy quantifiers and/or probabilities in the premises. However, if the premises are fuzzy, the conclusion is also fuzzy: This patient has anemia; this patient is malnourished; hence, this patient is anemic and malnourished. (The conclusion is a conjunction of the premises here.)

- In **syllogistic reasoning**, the inference may be made from premises containing fuzzy quantifiers: *Most* patients with ketoacidosis have poorly controlled insulin-dependent diabetes; *Most* patients with ketoacidosis have recently undergone a pathologically and physiologically challenging event such as myocardial infarction or extensive surgery; Hence, *some* patients with ketoacidosis have poorly controlled insulin-dependent diabetes and have recently had a serious acute and radical clinical condition.

- The classical categorical syllogism is replaced by a **fuzzy syllogism** based on one or more fuzzy premises. Its conclusion will necessarily be fuzzy. It may be deductively invalid:

Premise A: *Many* North Americans are becoming *increasingly obese.*

Premise B: *Many* North Americans are not *physically active enough.*

Conclusion C: *Many* North Americans are both *increasingly obese* and not *physically active enough.*

- In **dispositional reasoning**, propositions are not necessarily always true. *Heavy* drinking of alcohol is a *leading cause* of liver cirrhosis. To avoid liver cirrhosis, avoid *heavy* drinking of alcohol.

- In **qualitative reasoning**, the input-output is expressed as a collection of fuzzy if-then rules in which the antecedents (premises) and consequents (conclusions) involve linguistic variables. This kind of reasoning bears some similarity to if-then reasoning in the field of artificial intelligence.[25]

For the moment, routine or "scientific" clinical reasoning is still not studied and understood enough from the point of view of fuzzy logic and fuzzy theory. Let us remember, however, that classical logic has been studied, understood, and applied for many centuries and that fuzzy logic is only a few decades old.

Providing a logical structure and rules for logical reasoning in daily life and using daily-life terms and information (evidence) properly are both necessary. They are a reality of everyday clinical practice. So far, some foundations of evidence and its uses have been traced, mainly in logic itself and in medical research. Their integrated uses in daily clinical practice will certainly not be quickly forgotten.

An additional challenge emerges. The use of fuzzy logic requires the availability of good "fuzzy" evidence, which fits "fuzzy" premises (antecedents) and "fuzzy" conclusions (consequents). For the moment, our understanding of "not-fuzzy" evidence appears better and more complete than our mastery of evidence of the fuzzy kind.

Let us see if logic can be brought to the individual patient's bedside. Patients, in fact, should all benefit from its proper use.

From applications in industry, fuzzy theory moved into disparate medical specialties. These include neurology,[53-55] anesthesiology,[49] nuclear medicine,[56,57] oncology,[58] biomedical engineering,[59,60] psychiatry,[61,62] clinical pharmacology,[63] surgery,[64-66] infectious disease epidemiology,[67] veterinary medicine,[68,69] and nutrition,[70] among others.[71]

Even if fuzzy sets analysis provides a transitional opinion about a disease and better subsequent clinical decisions, some important questions remain unanswered. If the patient is diagnosed with a disease, he is treated. If the patient is probably sick, the decision to treat will depend on treatment effectiveness, cost, and adverse effects noted in healthy, "semi-ill," and definitely sick patients. The treatment may carry multiple risks if the patient is healthy or suffers from another disease. In many situations, a practitioner will require a clear identification of who is sick and who is not, as well as who is a candidate for treatment.

If fuzzy systems act as universal approximators for the handling of complex, nonlinear, imprecise, and often conflicting relationships in multidimensional systems with a minimum of rules,[68] an ensuing **fuzzy decision-making theory** and its application must still be perfected.

We are currently working within the framework of three theories: probability and uncertainty, chaos, and fuzzy sets. These theories are complementary rather than competing. Let us not make the mistake of pitting one against another. Griffiths and Byrne[72] state, "*There are two current trends in general practice research that may appear contradictory: the promotion of evidence-based practice with a high value given to numerical outcome research; and the increasing interest in qualitative research. The theories of chaos and complexity help us understand the link between qualitative research, where the results are categories of data and interpretation of meaning, and quantitative research, where outcome is measured."* All these old and new paradigms and theories may apply both to human biology and to health care. Human heart activity as well as the functioning of emergency services or walk-in clinics may indeed be "chaotic."

Probability theory served us well and continues to do so. Only the future and more experience with these new approaches to health problems will show how chaotic and fuzzy the world is and how much is uncertain and probable. The impact of chaos on science and society, however, is widening.[73,74] For the moment, a disproportionate volume of experience lies in the area of probability theory. To correct such an imbalance, fuzzy theory and fuzzy logic must continue to prove themselves as practical tools in daily medical thinking, practice, and decisions. This is not an easy task.

3.8 CONCLUSIONS: IMPLICATIONS OF LOGIC FOR MEDICINE

Do we not need the elements of logic when making a diagnosis, searching for causes, or assessing the effect of treatment? If logic is a methodology of reasoning, discussion, and argument, do we not use it during clinical rounds, when making a differential diagnosis during consultations, or when preparing research grant applications? Definitely! Correct reasoning and arguments are vital to all decisions in prevention and care.

In medicine, fortunately, we are much less inclined to appeal to emotions, but we are still tempted to rely on the opinions of specific persons and authorities, less substantiated claims, political or economic pressures, cultural traditions, religion, parental attitudes, and so on. We continue to be tempted by ambiguity, non sequitur (a conclusion that does not follow from the premises), circular reasoning (a chain of arguments whose final conclusion is the same as the starting premise), or deficiencies in causal reasoning such as *post hoc, ergo propter hoc* (if it happens after something, it must be because of that which preceded it).

On **floor rounds**, we discuss how we made a diagnosis in a patient, what speaks for the diagnosis, and what pleads against it. We propose our treatment plan, balancing its benefits and risks. We try to establish a realistic prognosis. In our **specialty reports (consults)**, we usually go beyond one case, but in both situations, uses of evidence must be logical—as good as the evidence itself.

In the area of **cause-effect relationships** (eg, causes of disease or improvements in health and disease due to treatment and/or care), we must necessarily go beyond the classical canons of causality as outlined in philosophy by John Stuart Mill (1806–1873):[35,75,76] agreement, difference, agreement and difference, residues, concomitant variation. This is because classical philosophers and logicians were mostly observers but not experimenters skilled in trials. We are already well aware that correlated events are not necessarily related, that they may have a "third" common cause (another event), that one may be a cause of another, and that causes may be multiple and complex. Analytical methods in epidemiology and biostatistics take these realities into account.

Another instance of the use of evidence falls within the realm of **social relationships and law**.[28,77] Patients, their doctors, and ultimately lawyers present claims of compensation for injury and work-related chronic problems to various entities: employers, trade unions, compensation boards, and courts. They are all interested in decisions on whether some tort was inflicted on an individual or a community, by whom it was inflicted, and how. Cases must be logically explained on the basis of relevant evidence. Both lawyers and decision makers, as well as presenters of cases, must "be on the same wavelength." They must all know not only the solidity and weight of evidence but also ways to use it properly in argumentation and in reaching conclusions. Unfortunately, health professionals are often much better prepared for producing and evaluating evidence itself than for its logical uses. It is possible for proponents of the problem to arrive at false conclusions when using good evidence (premises), to arrive at correct conclusions despite inadequate evidence (premises), or, in the best case, to arrive at correct conclusions based on the right evidence. Needless to say, the last instance remains an ideal to strive for. (We find out more about medicine, logic, and law in Chapter 7.)

There are peculiarities of human biology and medicine, but neither human biology nor medicine escapes the fundamental rules of thought, reasoning, and decision making in general. The basic logical paradigms from Chapters 2, 3, and 4 of this book and the basics of good evidence covered in the second part of this reading must now be brought together to form an organic entity.

Diagnostic workups, choices of treatment, and making prognoses are all, in fact, a sequence of reasoning. Their premises and conclusions should be as solid as possible. Ideally, the premises should be the best evidence available, leading to an equally best-evidence-based conclusion.

For example:

Premise A: *Experience and clinical trials show that antibiotics prevent complications of streptococcal throat infections* (eg, rheumatic heart disease).

Premise B: *My patient has fiery-red nasopharynx, hypertrophied tonsils covered by white patches, and palpable submandibular lymph nodes. A throat culture confirms a streptococcal infection.* (We do not, however, always obtain sensitivity to antibiotics.)

Conclusion C: *Antibiotics will prevent complications of my patient's condition.*

According to the philosopher Bertrand Russell, there are two ways of researching in mathematics or in any other discipline[37]: one aims at expansion, the other at exploring the foundations. However, uses of logic in medicine are not metaphysical. Instead, logic helps us better understand and make decisions in practice and research.

Many elements of general logic are already present in medicine. For example, epidemiologists or other clinical researchers refer to "**class**" or "**set theory**"[37,78,79] when forming groups to compare: sick or healthy, at-risk individuals, employee categories, disease groups, and so on.

In reverse, some ideas originating in medicine have expanded into the larger framework of logic. For example, the word *semiotic* was used by John Locke in the 17th century to describe the science of signs and significations[37] related to the medical theory of symptoms. **Semiotics** is now the general science of signs and languages. Patient-doctor communication in medicine is a field of semiotics.[80,81]

In **applied logic**, one adapts elements from pure logic, such as syllogisms, and applies them to beliefs or commands such as clinical orders or public health program choices and implementations.

Pure logic is not interested in the persuasive power of arguments. The correct pathway of reasoning and the link between premises and conclusions are of main interest. Salmon[35] stresses that "*. . .since the logical correctness or incorrectness of an argument depends solely upon the relation between the premises and the conclusion and is completely independent of the truth of the premises, we can analyze arguments without knowing whether the premises are true—indeed, we can do so even when they are known to be false.*" He is right. However, in health sciences and their practice, we need more. **In medical applications of logic, we cannot afford not to pay equal attention to the quality and solidity of evidence supporting conclusions,** these being medical decisions and recommendations followed by actions. **Acceptable medical reasoning relies on the combination of our way of thinking and the evidence supporting it.**

Just as there is a *logic of understanding* is there a *logic of commands* when it comes to instructions or clinical orders? One can reason based on a set of commands: "Do not give these severely ill patients less than three drugs and do not give them more than four!" This might imply that the patients should receive three or four drugs. The logic of medical orders in practice still remains poorly understood and has not yet been adequately studied. This should be remedied since illogical orders can obviously be detrimental to patient health.

At this point, readers might like to view floor rounds as a build-up of sequences of logical arguments in order to assess the fundamental quality of clinical reasoning and decisions. They might also like to look at the kind of evidence that is used to reach correct or incorrect conclusions.

So how should we view the **connection between medical logic and EBM?**

Until now, **EBM focused mainly on the search for, evaluation of, and application of evidence. Medical logic shows the gnostic mechanisms of how to use evidence by integrating it effectively into clinical and scientific reasoning in health sciences.**

Good medicine requires success in both evidence and logic, as well as in their uses. **It is one of EBM's tasks to ensure the truthfulness of premises and conclusions.** It is EBM's additional task to use them wisely in a logically correct manner. Physicians must see that their reasoning and arguments respond to the common laws of formal logic *and* that their premises are based on the best possible evidence, be it an experimental proof, solid clinical experience, or both.

Why is this so? Physicians may harm the patient under clinical care and entire communities in public health in three ways:

- If their conclusions do not follow from the information they have.

- If their premises are based on weak and unacceptable evidence, which does not reflect the reality to which it is supposed to be applied.

- If both the reasoning and supporting evidence are bad.

For example, is our reasoning correct if we say the following?

Premise A: *All physicians wear a white coat.*

Premise B: *Mary-Ann wears a white coat.*

Conclusion C: *Mary-Ann is a physician.*

Certainly not! One may immediately argue that other health professionals, laboratory technicians, and many employees in the food and electronic industries wear white coats, too. One may also state that not all physicians wear white coats, since many do not.

Hence, reasoning and argument may be both formally or structurally incorrect and unsupported by satisfactory evidence of the full reality of the problem. With such defects, it is only an accident if the conclusion turns out to be true.

Similar discrepancies between reasoning or supporting evidence and the reality of the problem may occur anywhere in medical practice and research. We would certainly refute some clinical novice's argument that:

Premise A: *Sore throats in younger persons are often caused by β-hemolytic group A streptococci.*

Premise B: *Undesirable late complications of "strep throats" such as rheumatic heart disease may be prevented by antibiotics.*

Conclusion C: *All patients with a sore throat must receive penicillin.*

In such an argument, cases, causes, differential diagnosis, and treatment indications are poorly defined and based on poor criteria. Also, the considerations adduced are not exhaustive of the reality of sore throats, their candidates, and the whole spectrum of clinical management of this problem. For example, are all cases of sore throat a "strep throat" (ie, caused by a bacterial infection treatable with antibiotics)? If not, how many patients experience late complications when not treated with antibiotics? Is there enough evidence available on how many of these patients benefit from treatment by antibiotics? Our novice also extends what is true of younger sufferers from sore throats to all sore throat sufferers, whatever their age may be.

These examples and comments relating to them all show that skillful execution of clinical diagnostic and therapeutic maneuvers must be based on the mastery of reasoning leading to their selection and to their real and expected performance.

References

1. West HR. Logic. *Microsoft Encarta Online Encyclopedia 2004.* Seattle, Wash: Microsoft Corporation; 1997–2004. Available at: http://encarta.msn.com/encyclopedia_761554437/Logic.html.

2. Jenicek M. *Foundations of Evidence-Based Medicine.* New York, NY: The Parthenon Publishing Group; 2003.

3. Cutler P. *Problem Solving in Clinical Medicine: From Data to Diagnosis.* 2nd ed. Baltimore, Md: Williams & Wilkins; 1985.

4. Damer TE. *Attacking Faulty Reasoning.* 2nd ed. Belmont, Calif: Wadsworth Publishing Co; 1987.

5. Helicon Publishing Ltd, ed. *Instant Reference: Philosophy.* (Teach Yourself Books.) London, England and Lincolnwood, Ill: Hodder Headline PLC and NTC/Contemporary Publishing; 2000.

6. Reese WL. *Dictionary of Philosophy and Religion: Eastern and Western Thought.* Amherst, NY: Humanity Books; 1996.

7. Audi R, ed. *The Cambridge Dictionary of Philosophy.* 2nd ed. Cambridge, England: Cambridge University Press; 1999:651–654.

8. Sleigh JW. Evidence-based medicine and Kurt Gödel. *Lancet.* 1995:346:1172.

9. Sleigh JW. Logical limits of randomized controlled trials. *J Eval Clin Pract.* 1997;3:145–148.

10. Polychronis A, Miles A, Bentley P. Evidence based medicine: Reference? Dogma? Neologism? New orthodoxy? *J Eval Clin Pract.* 1996;2:1–3.

11. Upshur R. Certainty, probability and abduction: why we should look to CS Peirce rather than Gödel for a theory of reasoning. *J Eval Clin Pract.* 1997;3:201–206.

12. Toulmin SE. *The Uses of Argument.* Cambridge, England: Cambridge University Press; 1958:95–135.

13. Toulmin S, Rieke R, Janik A. *An Introduction to Reasoning.* 2nd ed. New York, NY: Collier Macmillan Publishers; 1984.

14. Engel SM. *The Chain of Logic.* Englewood Cliffs, NJ: Prentice Hall; 1987.

15. Venn J. *Symbolic Logic.* London, England: Macmillan; 1881.

16. Seech Z. *Logic in Everyday Life: Practical Reasoning Skills.* Belmont, Calif: Wadsworth Publishing Co; 1987.

17. Harrison FR III. *Logic and Rational Thought.* St Paul, Minn: West Publishing Co; 1992.

18. Rosenberg AM. Advanced drug therapy for juvenile rheumatoid arthritis. *J Pediatr.* 1989;114:171–178.

19. Leckman JF, Weissman MM, Prusoff BA, et al. Subtypes of depression: family study perspective. *Arch Gen Psychiatry.* 1984;41:833–838.

20. Avery D, Winokur G. Suicide, attempted suicide and relapse rates in depression. *Arch Gen Psychiatry*. 1978;35:749–753.

21. Ennis RH. *Ordinary Logic*. Englewood Cliffs, NJ: Prentice Hall; 1969.

22. Ennis RH. *Critical Thinking*. Upper Saddle River, NJ: Prentice Hall; 1996.

23. Bowell T, Kemp G. *Critical Thinking: A Concise Guide.* London, England: Routledge; 2002.

24. Popkin RH, Stroll A. *Philosophy Made Simple.* 2nd ed rev. New York, NY: Broadway Books; 2001.

25. Albert DA, Munson R, Resnik MD. *Reasoning in Medicine: An Introduction to Clinical Inference.* Baltimore, Md: The Johns Hopkins University Press; 1988.

26. Thomas SN. *Practical Reasoning in Natural Language.* 2nd ed. Englewood Cliffs, NJ: Prentice Hall; 1981.

27. Moore BN, Parker R. *Critical Thinking: Evaluating Claims and Arguments in Everyday Life.* Palo Alto, Calif: Mayfield Publishing Co; 1986.

28. Aldisert RJ. *Logic for Lawyers: A Guide to Clear Legal Thinking.* 3rd ed. Notre Dame, Ind: National Institute for Trial Advocacy; 1997.

29. Hitchcock D. Enthymematic arguments. *Informal Logic*. 1985;7:83–96.

30. Hitchcock D. Does the traditional treatment of enthymemes rest on mistake? *Argumentation*. 1998;12:15–37.

31. Nolt J, Rohatyn D, Varzi A. *Schaum's Outline of Theory and Problems of Logic.* 2nd ed. New York, NY: McGraw-Hill; 1998.

32. Nolt J. *Logics*. Belmont, Calif: Wadsworth Publishing Co; 1997.

33. Forbes, G. *Modern Logic: A Text in Elementary Symbolic Logic*. New York, NY: Oxford University Press; 1994.

34. Berriman M, Moor J, Nelson J. *The Logic Book With Student Solutions Manual*. 3rd ed. New York, NY: McGraw-Hill; 1998.

35. Salmon WC. *Logic.* Englewood Cliffs, NJ: Prentice Hall; 1987.

36. Osborne R, Van Loon B. *Introducing Eastern Philosophy.* Cambridge, England: Icon Books and Totem Books; 1996.

37. Hughes GE, Wang H, Roscher N. The history and kinds of logic. In: McHenry R, ed. *The New Encyclopaedia Britannica, Macropedia.* Vol 23. Chicago, Ill: Encyclopaedia Britannica, Inc; 1992:226–282.

38. Last JM, ed. *A Dictionary of Epidemiology.* 4th ed. Oxford, England: Oxford University Press; 2001.

39. Murphy EA. *The Logic of Medicine.* 2nd ed. Baltimore, Md: The Johns Hopkins University Press; 1997.

40. Bayes T. An essay towards solving a problem in the doctrine of chances. (Read 23 December 1763.) *Biometrika.* 1958;45:296–315.

41. Goodman SN. Probability at the bedside: the knowing of chances or the chances of knowing? *Ann Intern Med*. 1999;130:604–606.

42. Siegmund DO. Probability theory. In: McHenry R, ed. *The New Encyclopaedia Britannica Macropedia.* Vol 26. Chicago, Ill: Encyclopaedia Britannica Inc; 1992:135–148.

43. Steele JM. Probability theory. In: Armitage P, Colton R, eds. *Encyclopedia of Biostatistics.* Vol 5. New York, NY: John Wiley & Sons; 1998.

44. Sox HC, Blatt MA, Higgins MC, Marton KI. *Medical Decision Making.* Boston, Mass: Butterworth-Heinemann Medical; 1988:27–65.

45. Dawson NV. Physician judgments of uncertainty. In: Chapman GB, Sonnenberg FA, Arkes HR, Lopes L, Baron J, eds. *Decision Making in Health Care: Theory, Psychology, and Applications.* Cambridge, England: Cambridge University Press; 2000:211–252.

46. Denton TA, Diamond GA, Helfant RH, Khan S, Karaguezian H. Fascinating rhythm: a primer on chaos theory and its application to cardiology. *Am Heart J*. 1990;120:1419–1440.

47. *The New Encyclopaedia Britannica Micropaedia*. Vol. 7. Chicago, Ill: Encyclopaedia Britannica Inc; 1992.

48. Steinmann F. Fuzzy set theory in medicine. *Artif Intell Med*. 1997;11:1–7.

49. Asbury AJ, Tzabar Y. Fuzzy logic: new ways of thinking in anaesthesia. *Br J Anaesthesia*. 1995;75:1–2.

50. Zadeh LA. Knowledge representation in fuzzy logic. In: Yager RR, Zadeh LA, eds. *An Introduction to Fuzzy Logic Applications in Intelligent Systems.* Dordrecht, The Netherlands: Kluwer Academic Publishers; 1992:1–26.

51. Sadegh-Zadeh K. Fundamentals of clinical methodology: Differential indication. *Artif Intell Med*. 1994;6:83–102.

52. *The Columbia Encyclopedia* [online]. 6th ed. New York, NY: Columbia University Press; 2002. Available at: www.bartleby.com/65.

53. Helgason CM, Malik DS, Cheng SC, Jobe TH, Mordeson JN. Statistical versus fuzzy measures of variable interaction in patients with stroke. *Neuroepidemiology*. 2001;20:77–84.

54. Helgason CM, Jobe TH. Causal interactions, fuzzy sets and cerebrovascular 'accident': the limits of evidence-based medicine and the advent of complexity-based medicine. *Neuroepidemiology*. 1999;18:64–74.

55. Dickerson JA, Helgason CM. The characterization of stroke subtype and science of evidence-based medicine using fuzzy logic. *J Neurovasc Dis*. 1997;2:138–144.

56. Simmons M, Parker JA. Fuzzy logic, sharp results. *J Nucl Med*. 1995;36:1415–1416.

57. Shiomi S, Kuroki T, Jomura H, et al. Diagnosis of chronic liver disease from liver scintiscans by fuzzy reasoning. *J Nucl Med*. 1995;36:593–598.

58. Keller T, Bitterlich N, Hilfenhaus S, Bigl H, Loser T, Lenohardt P. Tumor markers in the diagnosis of bronchial carcinoma: new options using fuzzy logic-based tumour marker profiles. *J Cancer Res Clin Oncol*. 1998;124:565–574.

59. Rau G, Becker K, Kaufmann R, Zimmermann HJ. Fuzzy logic and control: principal approach and potential applications in medicine. *Artif Organs*. 1995;19:105–112.

60. Ament C, Hofer EP. A fuzzy logic model for fracture healing. *J Biomech*. 2000,33:961–968.

61. Ohayon MM. Improving decision-making processes with fuzzy logic approach in the epidemiology of sleep disorders. *J Psychosom Res*. 1999;47:297–311.

62. Naranjo CA, Bremner KE, Bazoon M, Turksen IB. Using fuzzy logic to predict response to citalopram in alcohol dependence. *Clin Pharmacol Ther*. 1997;62:209–224.

63. Sproule BA, Bazoon M, Shulman KI, Turksen IB, Naranjo CA. Fuzzy logic pharmacokinetic modeling: application to lithium concentration prediction. *Clin Pharmacol Ther*. 1997;62:29–40.

64. Sawyer MD. Invited commentary: fuzzy logic—an introduction. *Surgery*. 2000;127:254–256.

65. Buchman T. Invited commentary: fuzzy logic, clear reasoning. *Surgery*. 2000;127:257.

66. Amin AP, Kulkarni HR. Improvement in the information content of the Glasgow Coma Scale for the prediction of full cognitive recovery after head injury using fuzzy logic. *Surgery*. 2000;127:245–253.

67. Massad E, Burattini MN, Ortega NR. Fuzzy logic and measles vaccination: designing a control strategy. *Int J Epidemiol*. 1999;28:550–557.

68. Bellamy JE. Medical diagnosis, diagnostic spaces, and fuzzy systems. *J Am Vet Med Assoc*. 1997;210:390–396.

69. Bellamy JE. Fuzzy systems approach to diagnosis in the postpartum cow. *J Am Vet Med Assoc*. 1997;210:397–401.

70. Wirsam B, Uthus EO. The use of fuzzy logic in nutrition. *J Nutr*. 1996;126: 2337S–2341S.

71. Sadegh-Zadeh K. Advances in fuzzy theory. *Artif Intell Med*. 1999;15:309–323.

72. Griffiths F, Byrne D. General practice and the new science emerging from theories of 'chaos' and complexity. *Br J Gen Pract*. 1998;48:1697–1699.

73. Grebogi C, Yorke JA, eds. *The Impact of Chaos and Science and Society*. New York, NY: United Nations University Press; 1997.

74. Pruessner HT, Hensel WA, Rasco TL. The scientific basis of generalist medicine. *Acad Med*. 1992;67:232–235.

75. Hughes W. *Critical Thinking: An Introduction to the Basic Skills*. 3rd ed. Peterborough, Ontario: Broadview Press; 2000.

76. Mill JS. *System of Logic*. Vols. 7–8. In: Robson JM, ed. *Collected Works of John Stuart Mill*. Toronto, Ontario: University of Toronto Press; 1963.

77. Waller BN. *Critical Thinking: Consider the Verdict*. Englewood Cliffs, NJ: Prentice-Hall; 1998.

78. Lipschutz S. *Schaum's Outline of Theory and Problems of Set Theory and Related Topics*. 2nd ed. New York, NY: McGraw-Hill; 1998.

79. Haight M. *The Snake and the Fox: An Introduction to Logic*. London, England: Routledge; 1999:193–218.

80. Burnum JF. Medical diagnosis through semiotics. Giving meaning to the sign. *Ann Intern Med*. 1993;119:939–943.

81. Nessa J. About signs and symptoms: can semiotics expand the view of clinical medicine? *Theor Med*. 1996;17:363–377.

CHAPTER 4

Critical Thinking in a Nutshell

What Is "Critical" and What Is Not?

IN THIS CHAPTER

*Believers, if an evil-doer brings you a piece of news,
inquire first into its truth, lest you should wrong others
unwittingly and then regret your action.*
QUR'AN (THE CHAMBERS—AL HUJARAT), 610–632 AD

*Critical thinking is an academic competency
akin to reading and writing.*
GEORGE HANFORD, 1992

*Even highly trained experts can be misled when they rely
on personal experience and informal reasoning . . .
the realization that shortcomings of perception, reasoning,
and memory incline us toward comforting, rather than true,
conclusions . . . led the pioneers of modern science
to substitute controlled observations and formal logic
for the anecdotes and surmises that can so easily lead us astray. . . .
Those who advocate therapies of any kind have an obligation
to prove that their products are both safe and effective.*
BARRY L. BEYERSTEIN, 2001

*Uncertainty is not a sin. Ignoring it
and doing nothing about it is.*

Do we need to think critically? If so, what is needed to become a critical thinker in health sciences? What must we learn and master? This chapter delves into the various factors on which we should focus. It shows us how to apply what we have learned to the challenge posed by so-called complementary and alternative medicine (CAM).

Many health professionals benefit from not only medical education but also advanced research training leading to the Doctor of Philosophy (PhD) degree. In following such a program of study, they receive superior instruction in various research methodologies. Most often, however, their training in philosophy itself (especially logic and critical thinking) occurs on the job and is interspersed across biostatistics, epidemiology, health research methodology (whatever this means from one place to another), on-hand data collection and analysis, and offerings in other clinical and community medicine specialties. Yet critical thinking in health sciences is becoming a new additional and relatively independent methodological domain, perhaps on an equal footing with already existing and well-established disciplines.

In recent years, critical thinking, through the efforts of several philosophers, has undergone a great methodological development. This has led it to become not some abstract rules, but rather an eminently practical and relevant tool for everyday life everywhere: politics, print and electronic media, academic experience, and elsewhere. As proof of this, we need only to notice the sheer number of monographs bearing the title of *Critical Thinking* that have appeared over the past two decades.[1-7]

As cited by Fisher,[7] for George Hanford,

"critical thinking is an academic competency akin to reading and writing."

In the practice of medicine, for us, it is **a professional competency involving knowledge, attitudes, and skills.**

Given this, what is critical thinking, and does it differ from logical reasoning, as outlined in Chapter 2? Let us define it now as well as we can, then describe it and understand it through some practical examples and applications.

4.1 DEFINITION OF CRITICAL THINKING

In 1910, the American philosopher, John Dewey,[8] presented the concept of critical thinking, under the label "reflective thinking," as an

"active, persistent, and careful consideration of any belief or supposed form of knowledge in the light of the grounds that support it, and the further conclusions to which it tends."

For Dewey, such thinking arose in response to a suggested resolution of some specifically occasioned perplexity.

*"If the suggestion that occurs is at once accepted, we have uncritical thinking, the minimum of reflection. To turn the thing over in mind, to reflect, means to hunt for additional evidence, for new data, that will develop the suggestion, and will either, as we say, bear it out or make obvious its absurdity and irrelevance. . . . Reflective thinking, in short, means **judgment suspended during further inquiry**. . . ."*[8]

In essence, Dewey's reflective thinking is the systematic testing of hypotheses, what is sometimes called the **scientific method**. This involves definition of a problem, proposal of a hypothesis or hypotheses, observation, measurement, quantitative and qualitative analysis, experimentation (if necessary), interpretation, and testing tentative conclusions by further experiments. Its primary focus is the consideration of hypotheses suggested as possible solutions to the perplexities that people face. What many people now identify as critical thinking—the scrutiny of arguments and assertions produced by others—is at best a minor part of reflective thinking thus conceived, an activity hardly mentioned in Dewey's book.

Inspired by Dewey, the Progressive Education Association in the United States promoted over the next 40 years what they called critical thinking, a criterion used in the association's landmark Eight-Year Study in the 1930s. Another outgrowth of the progressive education emphasis on critical thinking was the pioneering development in 1939 by Edward Glaser[9] of the *Watson-Glaser Critical Thinking Appraisal*, a shortened version of which lives on today.

Glaser[10] characterized critical thinking as including:

*"**An attitude of being disposed to consider in a thoughtful way the problems and subjects that come within the range of one's experience; knowledge of the methods of logical inquiry and reasoning; and some skill in applying these methods. Critical thinking calls for a persistent effort to examine any belief or supposed form of knowledge in the light of the evidence that supports it and the further conclusions to which it tends.**"*

The last-quoted sentence uses almost the same words as Dewey's definition of reflective thinking. Glaser specified this basic conception with a list of abilities, including those involved in systematic problem solving. A guide to teaching critical thinking in the social studies published in 1942 likewise identified the components of critical thinking in terms of the elements of problem solving.[11]

The first introductory textbook known to contain the word *critical thinking* in its title appeared in 1946[12]; its subtitle was "*An Introduction to Logic and Scientific Method.*" About a decade later, the concept of critical thinking received an appraisal-only sense somewhat more limited than Glaser's conception:

*"Now if we set about **to find out what** . . . [a] statement means and to deter-mine whether to accept or reject it, we would be engaged in thinking which, for lack of a better term, we shall call critical thinking."*[13]

Influenced by this conception, Robert Ennis[14] defined critical thinking in a landmark 1962 article as:

*"the **correct assessing of statements**."*

Ennis identified 12 aspects of this activity and gave criteria for their correct performance. In keeping with the linguistic focus of much of the Anglo-American philosophy of the immediate post-war period Smith and Ennis reformulated as statements the "belief or supposed form of knowledge" that Dewey and Glaser took to be the starting point of reflective or critical thinking.

The 1980s brought an explosion of educational interest in critical thinking, including a mushrooming of college and university courses in informal logic or reasoning, which were conceived as alternatives to introductory symbolic logic courses. With this explosion of interest came new conceptualizations of critical thinking:

- The appropriate use of **reflective skepticism** within the problem area under consideration[15]

- Using the **standards of reason** in deciding what to believe and what to do[1]

- **Reflective and reasonable thinking** that is focused on deciding what to believe or do[4,16]

- **Skillful, responsible thinking** that facilitates good judgment because it relies on criteria, is self-correcting, and is sensitive to context[17]

- **Thinking (and acting)**, which is appropriately moved by reasons[18]

- **Disciplined, self-directed thinking** that exemplifies the perfection of thinking appropriate to a particular mode or domain of thinking[19,20]

None of these conceptions is an appraisal-only sense of critical thinking. In particular, Ennis has abandoned his earlier restriction to appraisal, partly to reflect the way the term is used, partly because the skills involved in correctly assessing statements overlap extensively with those involved in deciding reasonably and reflectively what to believe or do. Another change in the 1980s was increased attention to the attitudes and dispositions of a critical thinker; previous conceptions had focused almost exclusively on skills.

In 1990 Facione[21] presented to the Committee on Pre-College Philosophy of the American Philosophical Association a statement of expert consensus on critical thinking for the purposes of educational assessment and instruction. This report, which represented the consensus of 48 experts (including psychologists and educational researchers as well as philosophers), characterized critical thinking as:

> *"purposeful, self-regulatory judgment which results in interpretation, analysis, evaluation and inference, as well as explanation of the evidential, conceptual, methodological, criteriological, or contextual considerations upon which that judgment is based. . ."[21]*

The report specified the core skills and subskills constitutive of the kind of judgment described in this general characterization. It added a list of mental habits of the "ideal critical thinker" (eg, being inquisitive, open-minded, orderly, focused, and persistent) that has much in common with Ennis' list[16,22] of the dispositions of the ideal critical thinker. Like the definitions from the 1980s quoted earlier, the experts' consensus eschews an appraisal-only sense of critical thinking. Indeed, it includes among critical thinking skills categorizing situations, decoding graphs and paraphrasing statements, as well as the more familiar skills of devising testing strategies, formulating alternative solutions or hypotheses, judging the acceptability of premises and inferences, and drawing conclusions.

More recently, Fisher and Scriven[23] have devoted an entire monograph to the definition and assessment of critical thinking. They define critical thinking as the:

> *"skilled and active interpretation and evaluation of observations, communications, information and argumentation."*[23]

In the field of nursing, Snyder[24] has proposed the following conception of critical thinking:

> *"The ability to solve problems by making sense of information using creative, intuitive, logical and analytical mental processes."*

What are we to make of this confusing sequence of apparently competing definitions? First, we should not be surprised by the apparent absence of consensus. New domains—such as medical technology assessment, evidence-based medicine (EBM), and critical thinking itself—are normally the subjects of numerous definitions before a broad consensus is reached. Although in a state of flux, the views in these domains are comparable to our already well-established views in other basic or applied sciences, such as epidemiology, biostatistics, and various specialties in clinical and community medicine.

Second, amid the variety of definitions we can detect considerable commonality:

- Critical thinking is a type of thinking.

- Critical thinking applies to all subject matters.

- Critical thinking involves reflection, looking back, and suspending judgment.

- Good critical thinking is reasonable.

- Critical thinking involves a careful consideration of evidence.

- Critical thinking is oriented toward making a definite judgment.

- The ideal "critical thinker" thinks critically whenever appropriate.

- Being a critical thinker involves knowledge, skills, attitudes, and dispositions (behavioral tendencies).

In fact, **EBM can be considered an application of critical thinking in medicine.**

We can also detect certain key differences among the conceptions of critical thinking:

- Some conceptions[1,8,10,13,14,23] treat critical thinking as concerned only with the appraisal of already existing intellectual products (eg, hypotheses, statements, arguments). Others[16,19,20,22,25] treat it more generally as applying also to the creation of intellectual products (eg, solutions to problems, explanations of perplexing phenomena, answers to difficult questions).

- Some conceptions[1,10,14] focus on skills, others[20,26] emphasize attitudes, and still others[4,16,18,22,25] emphasize both.

- Some conceptions[4,10,14,20,25] treat at least some aspects of critical thinking as highly general, whereas others[15] treat critical thinking as necessarily subject-specific.

Third, as with EBM, the important thing is not the general definition, but the specification of standards. Hence, it is more useful to look beyond the definitions to descriptions of critical thinking skills and the attitudes and behavioral tendencies of a "critical thinker."

Table 4-1 lists the component skills of critical thinking identified by Glaser,[10] Ennis,[25] Facione,[21] and Fisher.[7] Along with Fisher and Scriven,[23] these writers have the most developed published conceptions of the skills components. In particular, Ennis[14,25] and Facione[21] have provided elaborate descriptions of subskills.

Looking at Table 4-1, we can identify the following commonalities in the various proposals for the **component skills of critical thinking**:

- Clarify meaning

- Analyze arguments

- Evaluate evidence

- Judge whether a conclusion follows

- Draw warranted conclusions

TABLE 4-1

Component skills of critical thinking

Glaser[10]	Ennis[25]	Facione[21]	Fisher[7]
Recognize problems	Focus on a question	Categorize	Identify the elements in a reasoned case
Find means for solving problems	Analyze arguments	Decode significance	Identify and evaluate assumptions
Gather information	Ask and answer questions of clarification and challenge	Clarify meaning	
Recognize assumptions		Examine ideas	Clarify and interpret expressions and ideas
Use language clearly and accurately	Judge source credibility	Detect arguments	
		Analyze arguments	Judge the acceptability and credibility of claims
Interpret data	Observe and judge observation reports	Assess claims inductions	
Appraise evidence		Assess arguments	Evaluate arguments
Evaluate arguments	Deduce and judge deductions	Query evidence	Analyze, evaluate, make explanations and decisions
Recognize relation-ships between propositions	Induce and judge	Conjecture alternatives	Draw inferences
	Make value judgments	Draw conclusions	Produce arguments
Draw warranted conclusions		State results	
Test one's conclusions	Define terms and judge definitions	Justify procedures	Clarify meaning
			Analyze arguments
Reconstruct one's beliefs	Identify assumptions	Present arguments	Synthesize considerations
	Decide on an action		

A critical thinker not only possesses critical thinking skills but also exercises them when (and only when) it is appropriate to do so. Such tendencies are called *dispositions*, and they are reflected in a person's mental attitudes. Table 4-2 lists the component dispositions and attitudes of a critical thinker identified by Glaser,[10] Ennis,[4] and Facione.[21] These writers have the most developed published conceptions of the dispositional and attitudinal components.

Looking at Table 4-2, we can identify the following commonalities in the various proposals for the **component dispositional and attitudinal characteristics of a critical thinker**:

- Open-minded
- Fair-minded
- Searches for evidence
- Tries to be well informed
- Attentive to others' views and their reasons
- Proportions belief to the evidence
- Willing to consider alternatives and revise beliefs

A list of component skills and attitudes is not yet a set of standards. There must be criteria for the possession of each skill or attitude and standards for meeting

TABLE 4-2

Attitudinal and dispositional components of a critical thinker

Glaser[10]	Ennis[4]	Facione (partial list)[21]
Wants evidence for beliefs	Seeks, and is open to, alternatives	Cares to be generally well informed
Reasonable	Endorses a position to the extent justified by the information available	Trusts processes of inquiry
Thoughtfully considers problems and subjects in the range of one's own experiences	Tries to be well informed	Confident in one's own ability to reason
	Seriously considers points of view other than one's own	Open-minded on world views
	Is clear about the intended meaning of what is communicated, seeking the precision the situation requires	Flexible in considering alternatives
		Fair-minded in appraising reasoning
	Determines, and maintains focus on, the conclusion or question	Honest in facing one's biases
	Seeks and offers reasons	Prudent in suspending, making, or altering judgments
	Takes into account the total situation	Willing to reconsider views
	Is reflectively aware of one's own basic beliefs	Clear in stating a question or concern
	Discovers and listens to others' views and reasons	Diligent in seeking information
		Persistent in the face of difficulty
		Precise to the degree possible

each criterion in a satisfactory way. Of the authors whose views are summarized in Table 4-1, only Ennis[14] has produced criteria, let alone standards. However, Glaser,[10] Ennis and coworkers,[27,28] and Facione[29,30] have produced standardized tests of critical thinking skills that implicitly provide criteria. Additionally, Fisher has developed for the University of Cambridge Local Examinations Syndicate an examination in critical thinking, which thousands of 17-year-olds take in the United Kingdom each year.[31] Fisher's[7] monograph serves as a textbook for the course leading to this examination. Each of the standardized tests has norms derived from previous administrations of the test, which can be used as the basis for at least comparative standards. Table 4-3 lists the types of items in each of these four standardized tests of critical thinking skills. (The Advanced Subsidiary General Certificate of Education in Critical Thinking has a written component as well as the multiple-choice component

TABLE 4-3

Types of items in standardized tests of critical thinking skills

Watson-Glaser Critical Thinking Appraisal[9]	Cornell Critical Thinking Test Level Z[27]
Inference: Given some data, is a statement definitely true, probably true, indeterminate, probably false, or definitely false?	**Deduction:** Does it follow necessarily, contradict, or neither?
Assumption recognition: Does a statement presuppose another statement?	**Fallacies:** Why is given thinking faulty?
Deduction: Does a given statement follow necessarily from other given statements?	**Credibility:** Which is more believable?
Interpretation: Does a statement follow beyond a reasonable doubt from other given statements?	**Relevance:** Do data support a conclusion, go against it, or neither?
Inference evaluation: Assuming the premise true, is a given argument strong or weak?	**Experimental design:** Which statement is the best prediction for planning an experiment?
	Definition: Which definition best states how a speaker uses a term?
	Assumptions: Which statement does the argument assume?

California Critical Thinking Skills Test[29]	General Certificate of Education in Critical Thinking[31]
Evaluation: Given some premises, is the conclusion definitely true, probably true, probably false, or definitely false?	**Identification:** Identify reasons and conclusion.
Interpretation: Which statement means the same as a given statement?	**Evaluation of claims:** What is relevant to evaluating a given claim?
Analysis: What role does a statement play in a given passage?	**Credibility:** Is the source of this information credible? Why (not)?
Inference: Which statement must be true if given information is true?	**Analysis:** What is the pattern of reasoning?
Explanation: Which is the best evaluation of the speaker's reasoning?	**Evaluation of inferences:** How well do the reasons if true support the conclusion?
Note: Some subsections have one or two items of other types.	**Assumptions:** Identify and evaluate them.
	Clarification: Clarify and interpret expressions and ideas.

whose item types are listed. The written component focuses on evaluating reasoning of different kinds and on presenting arguments.)

Comparing the four lists, we can identify the following skills tested (the number in parentheses indicates the number of tests with such items):

- Evaluation of inferences from given statements to a given conclusion (4)

- Identification of an assumption implicit in a given statement or argument (4)

- Clarification of meaning (3)

- Evaluation of the credibility of a statement (2)

- Analysis of the structure of argumentation in a passage (2)

- Evaluation of what follows from given information (1)

- Judgment of how to evaluate a given claim (1)

- Identification of fallacies (1)

Of the four tests, the Cornell Critical Thinking Test Level Z is the most comprehensive.

The skills listed in Table 4-3 do not just summarize the experience of those researchers who structured critical thinking and made its methodology operational. The listed skills are also relevant and important in clinical practice and medical research. For example, as we see in Chapter 6, these skills must be found and recognized in argumentation at clinical rounds if we wish to know whether our colleagues' recommendations are sound products of critical reasoning. In research, as we see in Chapter 5, the reading and critical evaluation of medical articles should apply such skills. Another domain is the writing and evaluation of research projects and applications for grants (research financing). Applications for research grants are defensible if they reflect and respect the skills listed in Table 4-3. Clear research questions and the required impeccable statistical methods (sampling, univariate or multivariate analysis, etc) must be anchored in an overall critical thinking, which produces an explanation and justification of the research project.

Is critical thinking synonymous with logical analysis of arguments or is it something more than that? Logical analysis of arguments certainly covers many core critical thinking skills. But these skills go beyond logical analysis to include such things as the evaluation of evidence and searching for additional information. In this respect, critical thinking is broader than the logical analysis of arguments. On the other hand, critical thinking comes into play only with "judgment suspended during further inquiry," to quote Dewey's[8] original formulation. Much reasoning and argument is routine; an example is the decision to prescribe antibiotics for a streptococcal infection. Critical thinking in a clinical context occurs only occasionally, for example, when we make a differential diagnosis or work out a plan of treatment when there is a great deal of uncertainty about prognosis or the patient's wishes conflict with our initial recommendation. Also, critical thinking typically involves consideration of many arguments, whereas the techniques described in

Chapters 2 and 3 apply to single arguments. Hence, if we were to make a "Venn diagram" of logical reasoning and argument on the one hand, and critical thinking on the other, the two circles would overlap. Some, but not all, logical analysis of argument is critical thinking. And some critical thinking, but not all, is logical analysis of argument.

We may already feel, and rightly so, that critical thinking is a bit different from logical reasoning and argument alone. In fact, it is really more than that, and this is what defines its *raison d'être*. We not only want to find out if a single piece of reasoning or argument is good or bad. We want to know more about its context and see it in a broader framework of alternative choices or ways. We want to trace the best path toward our understanding of a health problem and make the best decision about it. **In EBM and evidence-based public health, we also look at the extent to which all our judgments and decisions about health promotion and disease protection, prevention, cure, and care are supported by evidence while also examining the quality of this evidence.**

The key to developing critical thinking skills and dispositions is to become aware of how we think and to work consciously at improving our thinking with reference to some model. This conscious drive to improve involves an overall assessment of our own thinking—a "thinking about our own thinking," commonly known as *metacognition.*[7]

4.2 A CHECKLIST FOR CRITICAL THINKING

A list of skills and attitudes, even if accompanied by criteria and standards for their attainment, gives little guidance on how to deploy the skills and attitudes included in the list when one thinks critically about a particular problem, hypothesis, or argument. For this purpose, a checklist provides a helpful framework. Such checklists can be found in some writings about critical thinking. Three of them are summarized in Table 4-4, the first two taken from the cited sources, the third our own adaptation of the task of thinking critically about a health problem.

A **critical thinking process** has the following components:

- **Problem identification and analysis:** The problem (the main question or the main point) is identified and, if necessary, broken up into its components.

- **Clarification of meaning:** The meaning of terms, phrases, and sentences is clarified where necessary. This component includes clarification of the problem to see how it should be investigated, as well as operationalization of key terms in an investigation.

- **Gathering the evidence:** Evidence relevant to the problem is obtained.

- **Assessing the evidence:** The quality of the evidence is judged.

- **Inferring conclusions:** Conclusions are drawn from the best evidence, or inferences drawn by others are evaluated.

- **Other considerations:** Other relevant information is considered. Examples include possible exception-making circumstances, situational factors, implications of one's tentative conclusions, alternative positions and their justification, alternative explanations of results, and possible objections and criticisms.

- **Overall judgment:** Some sort of overall judgment on the problem is reached, taking into account all the components of the critical thinking process.

These seven components and related questions, which Fisher[7] termed a thinking map, should be regarded as a checklist rather than a sequence. A given critical thinking process can jump around from one point on the checklist to another, and back again. For example, it may be necessary to clarify meaning at more than one stage of the process. The seven components should be understood as in Sections 4.2.1 to 4.2.7 that follow.

4.2.1 Problem Identification and Analysis: *What's in Focus?*

It is important to identify the central focus of our critical thinking. It may be a problem or question, either open-ended or restricted to specified alternatives. It may be a hypothesis suggested as an explanation of some phenomenon. It may be the main conclusion of an array of connected arguments.

Sometimes, a problem is so vast that it needs to be "**atomized,**" broken into components that can be separately treated. Such an analysis of a complex problem is part of the critical thinking component of identifying the focus.

TABLE 4-4

Checklists for critical thinking

The OMSITOG approach[1] says:	The FRISCO approach[4] says:	This reading's approach says:
1. Get an **O**VERVIEW of the message.	1. Identify the **F**OCUS: the main point or main problem.	1. Identify and analyze the problem.
2. Clarify **M**EANING.		2. Clarify meaning.
3. Portray **S**TRUCTURE of argumentation, if any.	2. Identify and evaluate the relevant **R**EASONS.	3. Gather the evidence.
4. Check whether **I**NFERENCES are sound.	3. Judge the **I**NFERENCES.	4. Assess the evidence.
5. Evaluate the **T**RUTH of claims not supported by argument (assess the evidence on which conclusions are based).	4. Attend to the **S**ITUATION: aspects of the setting, which provide meaning and rules.	5. Infer conclusions, or judge inferences to conclusions.
6. Consider **O**THER relevant evidence and arguments.	5. Obtain and maintain **C**LARITY in what is said.	6. Consider other relevant information.
7. **G**RADE the message.	6. Make an **O**VERVIEW of what you have discovered, decided, considered, learned, and inferred.	7. Make an overall judgment about the problem.

Within the discussion of a complex problem, one may find terms such as *excerpt, passage, topic,* or **link** identifying a "component." What do such terms mean? In the line of thought and chain of arguments, they mean simply a fraction of a complex problem—its **atom.** An "atom" is a coherent ensemble of statements about a health question whether it is spoken at medical rounds, presented at a medical convention, or written in medical journals or books. It often "*makes a single main point about that topic.*"[1]

In health sciences, the focus may be some morphologic or functional characteristics in human biology, occurrence of disease, risk (causal) factors, treatment, prognosis, or decision making. Justification and explanation of cause-effect relationships may be perhaps the most challenging domain of critical thinking. In medical articles, such topics and their coverage are found in the Introduction section (justification of the article) and in the Discussion/Conclusions section (explanation of findings).

Identification and analysis of the problem naturally are found at the beginning of a critical thinking process. Sometimes, however, it is necessary to come back to this component in order to reformulate the problem or analyze it differently (or for the first time). And it is important throughout the critical thinking process to maintain one's focus on the central problem or thesis, so as not to wander off into irrelevancy.

4.2.2 Clarification of Meaning: *What Kind of Study for What Kind of Question? What Does This Mean?*

For further evaluation and an eventual judgment, we must grasp the meaning of the problem. Suppose we are thinking critically about an article in a medical journal. We should ask:

- Is it a description of an observation (raising questions about sampling and representativeness)? *Is Lyme disease epidemic or endemic on the East Coast of North America?*

- Is it a comparison of two or more sets of observations to explore a cause-effect relationship? *Does passive smoking increase the risk of respiratory diseases in restaurant employees?*

- Is it a comparison of two or more groups in a controlled (randomized, double-blind) experiment or clinical trial to study treatment effectiveness? *Does a corticosteroid such as fluticasone propionate inhalation reduce symptoms and exacerbations of asthma in young adults?*

- Is it a search for factors of good or bad prognosis in an experimental or observational study? *Do various levels of overcrowding of hospital emergency rooms affect outcomes of noncritical injuries in the elderly?*

- Is it a comparison of alternative treatment methods? *Should sore throat cases in family practice be treated with antibiotics without laboratory testing for streptococcal infection, simultaneously tested and treated, or treated only according to the test result?*

In all these instances, the types of warrants that are applicable, and thus the type of relevant reasoning and argument, will differ.

Clarification of meaning goes beyond classifying the problem and inferring the appropriate method of investigation. It can involve clarification of terms and concepts used in the statement of the problem (hypothesis, main conclusion, etc) or in any part of the evidence, reasoning, or argument brought to bear on it. An important component of clarifying meaning in an evidence-gathering critical thinking process is to operationalize vague terms such as *depressed* or *feeling tired*. Although clarifying meaning comes naturally at the beginning of a problem-solving type of critical thinking, it can occur at any stage of a critical thinking process.

4.2.3 Gathering Evidence: *What Basic Relevant Information Can We Obtain?*

Besides the earlier-mentioned meaning of the problem as a focus of study, the logical "architecture" of the problem and of evidence relevant to its solution must be elucidated. Once this material is reconstructed from the natural language, is it a classical Aristotelian argument, a chaining of several arguments, or some kind of nontraditional argumentation?

Reasoning, as stated previously, is thinking directed to a conclusion. It must begin from premises that are not themselves conclusions of previous reasoning. These may be assumptions, established scientific theories, and the like. In regard to a health problem, they will typically include data, that is, primary observations, and their transformation into information. Such observations are the evidence on which our thinking should be based.

If the critical thinking is critical appraisal of an array of already produced arguments (eg, an article in a medical journal), the evidence will be the data reported in the ultimate premises of these arguments. In that case, the task of gathering evidence is one of analyzing the structure of the arguments in the text being appraised, so as to identify their ultimate premises.

If the critical thinking is reflective thinking about an open problem, gathering evidence will involve conducting the sort of study indicated by the classification of the problem at the stage of clarifying its meaning.

4.2.4 Assessing Evidence: *How Good Is Our Basic Information?*

Let us consider the following syllogism in a simplified clinical situation. *Nonimmunized individuals who contract measles manifest an enanthema called Koplik spots; this nonimmunized child has Koplik spots in his mouth; therefore, this child has measles.*

The diagnostic value of Koplik spots must be known from studies showing that there is no exception to their diagnostic power. (In reality, not all patients with measles have Koplik spots; only about 30% of them do, and these spots also may be found in other diseases.) The clinician who examines the child must know what Koplik spots look like and he must not miss them (or "find" them when they are not there). The diagnosis is made after all differential diagnostic considerations (if applicable) to this case are made.

These requirements illustrate the important critical thinking component of assessing the evidence. The ultimate premises relevant to the critical thinking problem must be checked to determine whether they are true, by seeing whether they are justified. In health sciences, general claims such as the premise about all young non-immunized individuals who contract measles would typically receive their justification from well-designed analytical studies, graded according to the hierarchy that is standard in EBM. (Such general claims more usually function as implicit warrants.) In EBM, evidence of treatment effectiveness increases from anecdotal evidence, case reports, and case series studies, through observational analytical studies and controlled clinical trials up to valid systematic reviews and research synthesis from the earlier-mentioned original sources. Particular claims such as the one about the nonimmunized child typically rest on observation, whether immediately or through the interpretation of data as information.

A "pure" logician will focus mainly on the quality of the inferences involved, but for critically thinking physicians, evidence is equally important. Good evidence must complement good inferences.

As illustrated in Figure 4-1 (in a complementary way to Chapter 2), good critical thinking must have as grounds equally good evidence.

FIGURE 4-1

A good argument needs *both* good evidence *and* a good inference

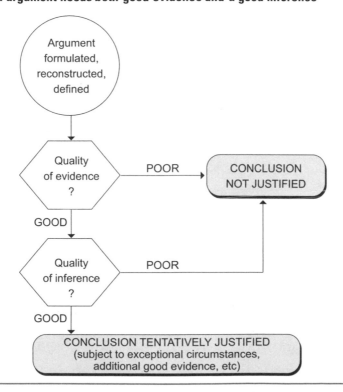

4.2.5 Inferring Conclusions: *What Follows?*

Besides assessing the evidence, we must determine what follows from it. If we are critically appraising an array of arguments, our question is whether each inference in the array is justified. Is the path from the premises to the conclusion right? Do the premises really lead to the stated conclusion? Are premises and conclusions held strictly within a predefined problem and question? As already described in detail in Chapter 2, the basic question is whether there is a justified warrant that applies to the inference from premises to conclusion in each single argument. If the warrant is not universal, but only presumptive or probabilistic, a further question is whether there are exceptions (contraindications, rebuttals) in the particular case that dictate a rejection of the conclusion.

If we engage in constructive critical thinking in which we ourselves gather evidence, we must use justified warrants in drawing conclusions from our good evidence. These warrants must be kept in mind in designing the systematic observation or experiment in which the evidence is gathered. Thus, in evidence-gathering critical thinking, the inferential component both precedes and follows the evidence-gathering and evidence-assessing components.

4.2.6 Other Considerations: *What Else Is Relevant to the Problem?*

One way in which critical thinking goes beyond the logical appraisal of a single argument or piece of reasoning is to look to other considerations, which are not mentioned in a text being critically appraised, or not explicitly part of gathering and assessing evidence and drawing inferences from it. In designing a study of some question, these other considerations will include a critical review of the relevant peer-reviewed literature. In evaluating the inferences in an array of existing arguments, they will include attention to possible exception-making circumstances (rebuttals). They also include consideration of challenges that could plausibly be raised regarding the conclusion one wants to draw—for example, other possible explanations of the data one has gathered, objections to and criticisms of one's premises or inferences, situational factors that put the evidence in a new light. The implications of the conclusion may also need to be taken into account, as Dewey[8] pointed out in his original 1910 definition of **reflective thought**. We may ask whether our conclusions are probable in the light of other well-established information (knowledge). We may also be interested in whether our conclusions confirm or improve our existing understanding of the problem. Finally, we may ask ourselves whether our conclusions provide some new insight into the problem of interest.

4.2.7 Overall Judgment: *What Is Our Stand on the Problem?*

Finally, the critical thinker must take a stand on the main question or problem. If it is a question of what to believe, some judgment (possibly qualified) should be reached on the basis of all the components of the critical thinking process. If it is a question about what to do, some decision should be made on what is the best path among all the options under consideration.

Here it is worth noting that a critical appraisal that finds serious flaws in an array of arguments for some conclusion does not necessarily show that this conclusion is false. A series of examples will exhibit the delicate relationship between truth (evidence) in premises, soundness of inference, and acceptability of conclusion. As one of us[1] points out, showing a premise to be false or an inference to be unsound does not establish the falsehood of the conclusion.

Figure 4-2 illustrates an argument in which one false and one true premise may still yield by way of deductively valid inference a true conclusion.

Figure 4-3 shows an example of a totally unsound (ie, deductively invalid) inference from one false and one true premise leading to a true conclusion.

The argument in Figure 4-4 shows correct premises and a correct conclusion linked, however, by an unsound (deductively invalid) inference.

Figure 4-5 offers an extreme, if not caricatured, example of false premises driven through an unsound (deductively invalid) inference to a true conclusion.

Finally, Figure 4-6 gives an example of a true statement (conclusion) as a product of a deductively valid inference from true premises.

These and other types of reasoning occur daily in clinical practice (see Chapter 6), often in the Discussion and Conclusion sections of medical articles (see Chapter 5), or when dealing with problems in non-medical forums (see Chapter 7).

The evaluation of a chain of arguments is even more challenging, as we see in Section 4.3.

FIGURE 4-2

One false premise, one true premise, deductively valid inference, true conclusion: a false premise does not necessarily mean a false conclusion

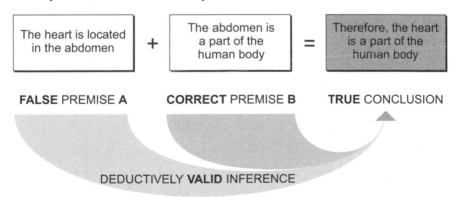

FIGURE 4-3

One false premise, one true premise, deductively invalid inference, true conclusion: a false premise combined with an invalid inference does not necessarily mean a false conclusion

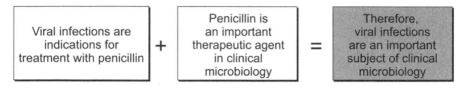

Viral infections are indications for treatment with penicillin	+	Penicillin is an important therapeutic agent in clinical microbiology	=	Therefore, viral infections are an important subject of clinical microbiology

PREMISE **A** IS **FALSE**   PREMISE **B** IS **CORRECT**   CONCLUSION IS **TRUE**

DEDUCTIVELY **INVALID** INFERENCE

FIGURE 4-4

True premises, deductively invalid inference, true conclusion: deductive invalidity with true premises does not necessarily mean a false conclusion

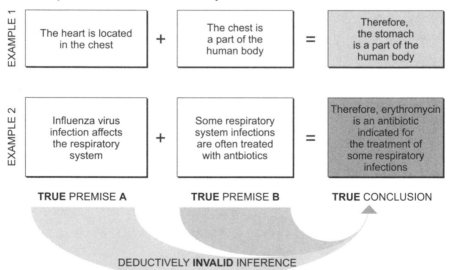

EXAMPLE 1

The heart is located in the chest	+	The chest is a part of the human body	=	Therefore, the stomach is a part of the human body

EXAMPLE 2

Influenza virus infection affects the respiratory system	+	Some respiratory system infections are often treated with antbiotics	=	Therefore, erythromycin is an antibiotic indicated for the treatment of some respiratory infections

TRUE PREMISE **A**   **TRUE** PREMISE **B**   **TRUE** CONCLUSION

DEDUCTIVELY **INVALID** INFERENCE

The moral of these examples is clear: **If in your critical thinking you determine that an argument has a bad premise or a bad inference (or both), you have not thereby shown that the conclusion is false.** You have only shown that this argument does not establish its truth.

FIGURE 4-5

False premises, deductively invalid inference, true conclusion: even an argument with everything wrong with it can have a true conclusion

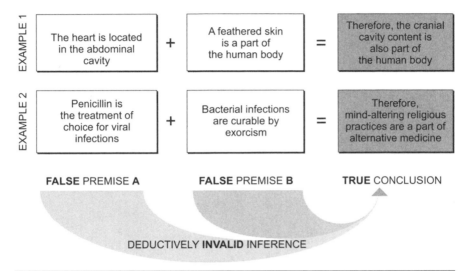

FIGURE 4-6

True premises, deductively valid inference, true conclusion: when the premises are all true and the inference deductively valid, the conclusion must be true

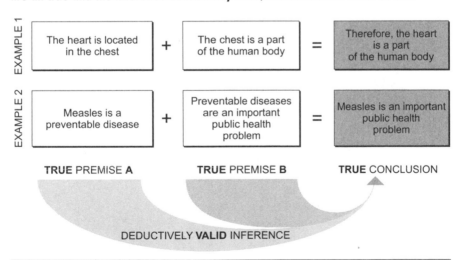

It would be desirable to complete a critical thinking process by some sort of grading of how well the process was conducted. A summary of the correctness or incorrectness of all the earlier-mentioned components of the critical thinking process must be made. Is the **overall** process good or bad? What are its strongest and weakest points?

For the moment, there is no directional categorical scale to score a particular critical thinking analysis of a given problem, which would be comparable to such scales used to evaluate evidence in EBM.

All in all, there are three major differences in medicine between logical appraisal and critical thinking:

1. Critical thinking in medicine extends well **beyond a single argument**, just as general critical thinking does.

2. There is a **creative component** represented by proposing and evaluating alternatives as well as choosing the best of them. This is also a shared characteristic with general critical thinking.

3. Critical thinking in medicine couples with an equally **critical assessment of evidence itself**, its choice and uses, as has become customary in EBM. Such a critical assessment, selection, use, and evaluation of evidence is specific to an evidence-based approach, be it in medicine, other health sciences, or elsewhere.

4.3 PRACTICAL EXAMPLE OF CRITICAL THINKING TO SOLVE A HEALTH PROBLEM: THE CHALLENGE OF COMPLEMENTARY AND ALTERNATIVE MEDICINE

Critical thinking does not apply solely to a single argument. A sequence or array of arguments may also be in focus, as a comprehensive attempt to solve a complex problem. We have already discussed single arguments in Chapters 2 and 3. Let us see here how a more complex topic might be subject to critical thinking of the type outlined in Section 4.2. Let us look at the problem of CAM and how it is handled by the collective critical thinking of the medical community with all its strengths and weaknesses. Our brief critical reflection about CAM can, of course, only scratch the surface of a vast and complex domain, giving some indication of what critical thinking looks like when applied to a complex problem. The following discussion includes all the components of a critical thinking process mentioned in Section 4.2 but jumps around them, coming back more than once to the same component (eg, clarification of meaning). In this chapter's concluding remarks, we connect our example to the components of Section 4.2.

4.3.1 Identification of the Problem

How should medicine respond to the challenge of CAM? Should CAM be treated as an annoying burden or as an asset in the domain of health and disease?

Health maintenance and effective treatment of ailments are goals for both patients and health professionals. Modern medicine (variously described in the medical literature as "scientific," "conventional," "mainstream," "Western," or "allopathic" medicine) grew from traditional medicines of various types, which are still practiced either alone or together with modern medicine. (We define "traditional medicines" as systems of prevention, diagnosis, and treatment of medical conditions that are handed down in a local cultural and historical context from generation to generation, without substantial change and without accompanying scrutiny of their evidential basis.) In many parts of the world, especially in Asia and Africa, tradition, poverty, and lack of modern medical human and material resources make traditional medicine the only kind available. Or it may work together with today's medicine. Even in the world of high-tech medicine in wealthy countries, patients who have incurable medical problems seek solace in so-called alternative medicine and perhaps a "miraculous" cure or improvement. Others are making "natural" prevention and treatment part of what they consider "a healthier lifestyle." Their numbers are important. It is estimated that 25% to 50% of adults in industrialized countries seek CAM and their providers[32] in various ways. In some groups (eg, pediatric oncology),[33,34] up to 84% of patients receive some form of CAM. Sometimes, patients who would benefit from modern treatment are driven away from it by seeking refuge in a mystical world of belief and faith.

Complementary and alternative medicine is even more widespread in the health care of animals. Some veterinarians exclusively practice acupuncture, homeopathy, and/or chiropractic veterinary medicine (especially in horse breeding, care, and racing). Others combine it with mainstream veterinary medicine.

Another part of CAM is an ever-growing industry of "natural," "healthy," "additive-free," "gentle," and other adjective-labeled dietary supplements and herbal remedies. The products of this industry are of unequal quality; in fact, quality control itself is questionable in this domain, which is much less rigorously controlled than the modern pharmaceutical industry that produces prescription drugs and scientifically validated over-the-counter drugs.

This situation stimulated a more critical and much needed look at CAM by physicians and other health professionals.[35] If we look at CAM through the eyes of critical thinkers, what is it worth?

During the last decade, the need for more critical assessment produced several articles reviewing the CAM reality in each of at least six leading medical journals (presented here in order of their citation in the reference list): *Annals of Internal Medicine*,[35-41] *Academic Medicine*,[42-50] *Seminars in Oncology*,[51-53] *JAMA*,[54-63] *American Family Physician*,[64-66] and the *Medical Journal of Australia*.[67-73] Complementary and alternative medicine has even entered the world of EBM.[74-76] Original research and its systematic reviews of CAM are published in ever-increasing numbers.

Modern medicine has at least four options:

1. Sweepingly label CAM as garbage, quackery, unethical, and unscientific poisoning of lay minds, and an unscrupulous drain on the limited means of people in search of higher values in life.

2. Ignore CAM altogether.

3. Embrace all or some forms of CAM as legitimate complements and alternatives to modern scientific medicine, which medical practitioners and their patients

can choose along with or instead of interventions accepted in scientifically based medicine, as they see fit.

4. Submit CAM to the same degree of critical appraisal as we would expect in the case of a new medical technology.

We argue that medical research would be wise to choose the last of these options, even if some awakenings might be rude.

4.3.2 Analysis of the Problem

How can we understand the problem? It has many dimensions:

- What exactly does "complementary and alternative medicine" mean? What is "in" the scope of this phrase and what is "out"?

- How important is CAM? That is, how often do people use it, and how serious are the conditions for which they turn to it as a remedy?

- What are the possible causes, motives, and reasons for its popularity?

- How does CAM work in practice within the community?

- What are the outcomes of interest in CAM?

- How do the consumers of CAM reason about it?

- How can CAM providers reason about it?

- Would studying the philosophy, practice, and uses of CAM explain what is wrong with so-called mainstream medicine?

- What should health professionals do about it? Forbid it? Encourage and expand it? Improve it? Follow it up and evaluate it? Integrate it somehow with mainstream medicine?

Critical thinking about an all-encompassing problem such as CAM as a whole is difficult, if not impossible. Breaking it into more manageable and better-defined parts, as listed above, makes possible more successful and concrete thinking about it. Understanding the problem relies on available evidence supporting the answers to the above-mentioned questions. Each question requires a specific ad hoc research protocol, assessment, evaluation, and interpretation of findings.

In what follows, we begin by clarifying the meaning of "complementary medicine" and "alternative medicine." Then, we analyze and evaluate in a schematic way the kinds of arguments given by proponents of various CAM interventions. The weakness of these arguments naturally raises the question of why CAM interventions are so popular; we consider some possible explanations. Having found the arguments for CAM interventions generally wanting and having explained away the widespread belief in their safety and effectiveness, is our task of critical thinking finished? No! Even bad arguments may have correct conclusions. So we look at how to scientifically and rationally investigate claims made by proponents of CAM. How should studies of CAM interventions be designed? How should evidence gathered in such studies be assessed? What kind of cause-effect reasoning is appropriately applied to such evidence? How should systematic reviews and meta-analyses of CAM studies be conducted? Our answers to these questions adhere to the models generally accepted in EBM. Since some proponents of CAM challenge these models, we consider their objections and describe possible alternative methods of testing CAM claims. Finally, we sum up the results of the preceding reflections. Because our thoughts focus on medical research, we leave as exercises for the reader the issues of how medical education and medical practice should respond to the claims of CAM proponents.

4.3.3 Clarification of Meaning: What Is CAM?

Complementary medicine and *alternative medicine* are general terms like *oak tree* and *postmodern architecture.* Such terms have two dimensions to their meaning:[77]

- The **connotation** of the term, the single set of characteristics that a person who understands the meaning of the term grasps. Similar terms to *connotation* are *intension, comprehension,* and *sense.* Many general terms have a loose connotation, perhaps best explained by a set of criteria, none of which is necessary for the application of the term; in medicine, *schizophrenia* is an example of such a term.

- The **denotation** of the term, the individual objects to which the term applies. Similar terms to *denotation* are *extension* and *reference.* The denotation of *oak tree* is the set of oak trees, which might be indicated by enumerating its main kinds: live oaks, white oaks, blue oaks, black oaks, scarlet oaks, pin oaks, and so on.

It is also important to pay attention to the emotional associations of such general terms, especially when they are used in disputes. "Terminating a pregnancy" and "killing an unborn child" may have the same connotation and the same denotation, but the emotional associations of the two terms are quite different.

In trying to understand and explain the meaning of the terms *complementary medicine* and *alternative medicine,* we focus first on the denotation or extension: what kinds of interventions are covered by these terms? Then, we turn to their emotional associations, as indicated by the literal meaning of their components. Finally, we address their connotation, and the connotation of the related terms *integrative medicine* and *unconventional medicine.*

Complementary and alternative medicine may be seen as a heterogeneous ensemble of health trends in several open-ended categories:[37]

1. **Professionalized medical systems** are organized movements with distinctive theories, practices, and institutions: ***chiropractic, osteopathy, homeopathy, naturopathy, massage therapy, Ayurveda,*** and ***traditional Chinese medicine,***

including acupuncture and acupressure. To this category also belong **dual-training health practices** such as classically trained physicians practicing acupuncture.

2. **Popular health reform and "healthy" lifestyle practices** espouse various vegetarian and nonvegetarian **diets**, only cooked foods, only raw foods, with or without dietary supplements, and so on. *Aromatherapy* also belongs in this category.

3. **New Age healing** as another rather heterogeneous group is based on a philosophy of unrestricted self-expression and unlimited abundance. It overlaps with various religious and healing movements. *Therapeutic touch, laying on of hands,* and *spiritual healing by clairvoyant health protagonists* all fall into this category.

4. **Psychological interventions of "mind-cure" and mind-body medicine** include both **mind-cure movements** (eg, Deepak Chopra or Bernie Siegel—harnessing mind forces will solve your health problem) and *cognitive-behavioral therapies such as biofeedback, hypnosis, guided imagery,* or *relaxation techniques.*

5. **Nonnormative scientific enterprises** emerge in the face of frequently incurable diseases, such as cancer. Sophisticated pharmacologic agents such as antineoplastons, biological substances such as pleomorphic bacteria cancer vaccine and chelation therapy, or such diagnostic methods as hair analysis and iridology are advanced as counterparts of mainstream methods, techniques, and agents.

6. **Herbal medicines**[45] include biological agents whose active agent is known (eg, digitalis in foxglove, vitamins in fruits or vegetables, or "natural health byproducts" such as bark), as well as natural vehicles of yet unknown mystical substances ("well-being boosters"). The former agents are much more justified than the latter. Colchicine to treat gout, digitalis for congestive heart failure, opium and its derivatives as analgesics, antimalarial quinine, vinblastine and vincristine from the Madagascar periwinkle, antibiotics from molds and bacteria (actinomycins and others), and some agents from animal sources (interferons, interleukins, or steroids)[44] have proved their effectiveness in formal clinical trials comparing them and their alternatives according to the methods of scientific proof.

Besides CAM, another more historical place is occupied by **parochial unconventional therapies** such as *ethnomedicines* (voodoo), *religious charismatic healing* in various churches ("stand up and walk" healing), and *folk-medicine practices* (magnetic bracelets for musculoskeletal and other disorders, chicken soup for influenza, a wide array of amulets, fashion-friendly or not, and many others).

What is the connotation of the terms *alternative medicine* and *complementary medicine* when used as labels for this heterogeneous set of health practices? It is worth noting, first of all, that these are the labels assigned by proponents of these practices. By using the word *medicine,* they implicitly confer the respectability of the art and science of medicine on their favorite nostrums. In the debate over what medicine should do about these practices, the use of the labels "alternative medicine" and "complementary medicine" in the scientific medical literature already prejudices the debate in favor of their acceptance as alternatives or complements. If these practices are medicine, then clearly they should be subjects of medical research, part of the medical school curriculum, and components of medical practice. As already mentioned, the connotation and denotation may be the same for the phrases "killing an unborn child" and "terminating a pregnancy," but the emotional associations are different. The same holds when referring to the just-mentioned heterogeneous collection of practices as "complementary and alternative medicine." In fact, there is something questionable about dignifying the above collection with the name "medicine." A sign that this name is misplaced comes when we ask: Alternative to what? Complement to what? We cannot just say "medicine," because then the alternatives and complements could not be dignified with the same label. So various qualifiers are invented for the term *medicine*. From the point of view of practitioners of traditional Chinese medicine and Ayurveda, medicine is "Western medicine." From the point of view of homeopaths, medicine is "allopathic medicine." From the point of view of proponents of herbal and other "natural" remedies, medicine is "biochemical medicine." None of these qualifiers accurately describes the institution of medicine in rich, technologically advanced countries. There is nothing parochially Western about the scientific basis of contemporary medicine in human anatomy and physiology on the one hand, and in biochemistry and pharmacology on the other. Most scientifically proven treatments in contemporary medicine are neither homeopathic nor allopathic. Nor is contemporary medicine exclusively oriented to synthetically produced drugs as a means to health. Diet, exercise, stress reduction, not smoking, and moderation in the use of alcohol and other mind-affecting drugs have all been studied as methods of maintaining health and preventing or curing ailments, and are part of the armamentarium of physicians in daily practice. Medical students do not go to schools of "Western medicine," "allopathic medicine," or "biochemical medicine"; nor are their degrees so qualified; they go to medical school and earn the degree doctor of medicine. If the heterogeneous practices listed earlier are to be dignified with the name "medicine" (in order for medicine to acquire some qualifying label to distinguish itself), let the label be "contemporary scientific medicine." Alternatively, reserve the term *medicine* for medicine and call the practices listed above "unproven practices used to treat health problems." The latter label can be justified by a consideration of the evidence adduced by proponents of such treatments. If it were adopted, then the list would be reduced by the deletion of proven remedies (colchicine, digitalis, opium and its derivatives, quinine, vinblastine, vincristine, antibiotics from molds and bacteria, interferons, interleukins, and steroids—for the previously listed conditions). In fact, plant-derived prescription drugs generally receive at most passing mention in books on herbal remedies produced for the general public.[78,79] On the other hand, the Canadian Pharmacists Association and Canadian Medical Association's book on herbs[80] and some other serious references[81-84] are examples of a good systematic critical and structured approach to the health effects of various herbs.

We may accept as a meaningful and working definition of alternative medicine the one proposed by Eskinazi:[60]

Alternative medicine is

"a broad set of health practices (ie, already available to the public) that are not readily integrated into the dominant health care model, because they pose challenges to diverse societal beliefs and practices (cultural, economic, scientific, medical, and educational)."

Eisenberg et al[33] define **alternative medical therapies** as

"interventions neither taught widely in medical schools nor generally available in US hospitals."

The words *alternative* and *complementary* are used for an entire system of practices or even for the whole gamut of possible systems. They are meant to suggest that one or more systems could be used as a replacement for medical treatment directed by a physician, or as an addition to it. If applied to a particular proposed remedy, they have clear implications for the design of studies on the remedy's safety and/or effectiveness.

"**Complementary**" means "*added to something.*" Hence, the study of a proposed "complementary" remedy would imply a study of its additional effect when combined with some proven remedy accepted in contemporary scientific medicine. In practice, for example, it would mean carrying out a clinical trial comparing the effectiveness of a medically accepted, proven remedy with that of the same intervention when joined by an additional CAM intervention.

"**Alternative**" means "*instead of something.*" Hence, a study of a proposed "alternative" remedy would assess how well it replaces an already proven, accepted medical intervention. In practice, for example, it would mean carrying out a clinical trial comparing a proposed "alternative" action (as a kind of experimental group) with the accepted medical intervention (as its control group).

In both cases, "alternative" and "complementary" compete with a proven, medically accepted intervention for the same expected beneficial outcome, such as disease prevention or its cure.

"**Integrative**" medicine appears as an additional alternative to CAM. For some,[85,86] integrative medicine is a comprehensive primary care system that emphasizes wellness and the healing of a person as a whole. It goes well beyond the handling of the patient's chief complaint and its solution. It is supposed to facilitate healing and to give patients some empowerment over their condition and fate.

Consequently, "integrative" medicine may be either "complementary" or "alternative." In addition, its desired objective and outcomes are different. Its focus is "the person as a whole." The person as a whole then becomes a new dependent variable in a research hypothesis under scrutiny. Integrative medicine's claim[86] to originality in its multifactorial approach to disease or health causes is questionable, since epidemiology already adopted long ago the concept of webs of causes.[87] The inclusion of "soft data" in clinimetric terms as dependent or independent variables under study is not original either; psychiatry has historically worked with many soft data.

Hence, the additional challenge in integrative medicine research is how soft data are properly defined, measured, analyzed, and interpreted.[87]

Therefore, the practical challenge in the evaluation of "integrative medicine" is the evaluation of outcomes. They may be multiple and are often poorly defined.

"Unconventional medicine" is a term amenable to more than one meaning. It includes anything not taught at schools of medicine, anything provided by an uncertified health professional within his or her professional mandate, anything not endorsed by an official professional health body such as a college of physicians or nurses, or anything not covered by health insurance. Anything goes.

Before any study of CAM is attempted, its definition within the study should be specified and clearly worded.

4.3.4 Arguments for CAM Interventions

In a comprehensive survey such as the present exercise, we can only look schematically at the types of arguments given in support of various CAM interventions. These can be classified under the following headings: theoretical rationales, anecdotal evidence, appeal to naturalness, and appeal to traditional, analytical studies.

Theoretical rationales are given for comprehensive systems of treatment such as chiropractic, homeopathy, and acupuncture and acupressure. The core idea of homeopathy, for example, is that "like is cured by like": a substance which in large doses causes symptoms of an illness will in very small doses cure that illness. The small dose is supposed to act as a stimulus to restore balance in the body's "vital force." The doses in question are obtained by successive dilutions, which may leave not a single molecule of the supposed active ingredient in the "medicine" that the patient consumes; each dilution involves putting one drop of the previous product into a mixture of alcohol and water.[78] Acupuncture and acupressure are supposed to restore balance to the body's *chi*, energy which flows through invisible channels called meridians. Correct touch or stimulation of points on the body where these channels terminate is supposed to relieve pain and speed healing.[78]

These theoretical rationales are unsupported by any direct observation and run contrary to basic well-confirmed theories of contemporary natural science. Not only is there no justification for accepting these theories, there is very strong justification for rejecting them. There is very strong reason to doubt that you can get some benefit from a supposedly curative substance by drinking a liquid that contains not a single molecule of that substance; to the best of our knowledge, no testable hypothesis about how the substance could have any effect in such circumstances has been proposed. And there is very strong reason to doubt that there are meridians carrying *chi* through the human body; to the best of our knowledge, no contemporary textbook in scientific anatomy shows such meridians, nor has any method been proposed for directly testing their presence. Unless some rationale consistent with well-confirmed highly general scientific theories can be found, researchers will justifiably refuse to accept even positive results from apparently impeccable meta-analyses of apparently impeccable randomized trials of proposed remedies grounded in scientifically false theories.[39]

Anecdotal evidence is ubiquitous in the popular literature publicizing various forms of CAM. "My daughter has a communication disorder. She used to feel very intimidated in the classroom, afraid to raise her hand even though she knew what the answer was. Since she started taking this organic food concentrate, she has become more focused and motivated. She sleeps much better at night. She is much happier." Such testimonials are worthless as evidential support. If they come from the seller of the CAM product, as they usually do, they may be pure inventions. If they are genuine, they are, of course, selected. We have no idea how frequently the reported change occurred after customers started taking the CAM product. Most importantly, we do not know that any ingredients in the CAM product caused the change. To infer that some of them did is to commit a post hoc fallacy: "the change happened after I started taking the product, so something in the product caused the change." There are other possibilities. Maybe the change was going to happen anyway, and it was a coincidence that it happened when you began to take the product. Maybe the belief that you were taking something effective caused the change; the placebo effect is very powerful, and belief in the effectiveness of advertised alternative "natural" remedies is a recurrent theme in testimonials about them. Maybe you did something else when you began taking the CAM product, and it was the something else that caused the change. To rule out these alternatives, well-designed analytical studies (ideally, randomized clinical trials) are needed.

Appeal to naturalness is a common theme in literature promoting CAM, as the very titles of such books indicate.[78] So is the **appeal to tradition**. "People are turning to natural healing—simple, traditional, low-tech methods of preventing illness and solving everyday problems." This single sentence manages to combine four appeals at once: to popularity, to naturalness, to tradition, and against high technology.

Although persuasive, such appeals are irrelevant to whether a given recommendation is safe and effective for the intended purpose. Popularity is irrelevant; individual practices for warding off illness come and go as fads quite independently of any rational basis for them. Naturalness is irrelevant; in fact, most synthetic prescription drugs have a much better evidential basis for their safety and efficacy than most "natural" remedies, largely because natural products have received little of the careful testing required for licensing a new prescription drug. Also, many "natural" products are chemically complex and vary in chemical composition from one sample to another. Tradition is irrelevant; many traditional practices, such as bloodletting and treatment with heavy metals such as mercury, persisted for many generations before being proved ineffective or dangerous. In addition, the sophistication of the technology involved is irrelevant; there is no reason to think that being low-tech makes an intervention safer or more effective than a high-tech intervention.

Analytical studies potentially provide the best evidential support for a proposed complementary or alternative prophylaxis or remedy. As recent articles in medical journals indicate,[40,52,62,64-66,69,73] such analytical studies are increasing in frequency and sophistication. Unfortunately, many of them are poorly designed, as these articles point out. When they are well designed, they tend to show no statistically or clinically significant difference between the CAM intervention and the control one.

As far as we can tell from our survey of the medical literature, most CAM interventions have little or no evidence supporting them, and certainly not

enough to justify a belief that they are safe and effective for their intended purpose.

The reasoning glorifying CAM is often based on something other than logical argumentation, such as:[42]

- **The will to believe.** Our comfort and self-esteem are at stake.

- **Logical errors and shortcomings of judgment.** Fallacy of equating sequence or correlation with cause is frequent.

- **Wishful thinking.** Patients receiving CAM and therapists performing CAM remember things as they wish they had happened, rather than the way in which they really occurred.

Most of the evidence cited by proponents of CAM interventions can be explained by reasons other than their effectiveness:[42,88]

- Interventions occur at a **favorable moment.** The disease may have run its natural course, other much more effective and proven treatments preceded the CAM maneuver, the intervention occurred at the downturn of cyclic diseases, such as arthritis, allergic disorders, or migraines.

- The **placebo effect** of many CAM interventions is a reality. The combination of suggestion, expectancy, and cognitive reinterpretation is a culprit. However, if the placebo works, keep it (after a proper evaluation).

- **Spontaneous remissions** may occur. Without acceptable explanation, they even become miracles in more than one faith.

- Justified or unjustified **worrying about one's own wellness** may be relieved by a gentle CAM maneuver. People **somatize:** "*My doctor told me that nothing is wrong with me, but there must be this or that . . .*"

- Protagonists of CAM may try to improve their credibility by referring to themselves as **complementary and/or integrative practitioners** instead of **alternative.**

- **Misdiagnosis** may make the CAM treatment effective. It might be otherwise, if the diagnosis were correct at the onset. For example, a patient may be treated for a problem with a better prognosis.

- **Derivative benefits** according to Beyerstein[42] refer to a patient's perception of well-being subsequent to exposure to charismatic CAM providers. The charismatic providers' messianic attitudes and power of conviction may even improve the patient's health-related habits more than a family physician's advice in a busy practice.

- Let us add to this the **poor or nonexistent operational definitions of variables under study and the rest of clinimetrics.**

- Diseases that are treated using CAM are most often self-limiting, not yet preventable or curable, or subject to frequent spontaneous remissions.[88] Even a unique, amazing, unexpected, and/or unexplained successful outcome, with or without serious side effects, is enthusiastically welcomed and accepted independently of its frequency and lack of analysis.

If all these additional factors are important, nobody has yet studied them as independent variables (causes) related to improvement of the patient's health, and even less in competition with mainstream scientifically proven treatments.

Protagonists of CAM are well aware of several limitations in the evidence-based approach to their interventions:[85]

- Therapies are often multimodal, as in traditional Chinese medicine or Indian Ayurveda. Randomized, double-blind, controlled clinical trials are best suited to evaluate single interventions.

- It may be difficult to recruit participants for certain randomized, double-blind, controlled trials. Some remedies, for example, mistletoe in Germany, are so widely used that patients refuse randomization.[88]

- Remedies are not standardized enough.

- Finding placebo medications or sham interventions, especially "active" placebos (imitating a procedure and some effect, adverse or other, of the experimental intervention), may be difficult or impossible.

- Remedies are already currently available over the counter everywhere, and their uncontrolled use by participants in trials may "contaminate" trial results in both groups under comparison.

- The adverse effects of CAM interventions are still poorly known. Complementary and alternative medicine interventions are not innocuous. Chiropractic, acupuncture, and herbal medicine[89] all have potential adverse side effects.

Obtaining informed consent is a requirement for not only physicians[53,57,74] **but all health care providers,**[86] including healers of all kinds, without exception. Obtaining informed consent for a CAM intervention is exigent. The patient's decision must be based on information that includes evidence about the effectiveness of a proposed treatment, realistic expectations from it, adverse reactions, and other risks. Also, alternatives must be offered, including those from mainstream medicine, and the justification of the health provider's preference must be explicit. How many healers obtain a patient's consent in this way?

4.3.5 Explanations of the Popularity of CAM

According to Beyerstein[42] the state of the CAM domain, including its popularity, is due to several factors: poor scientific literacy, anti-intellectualism and antiscientific attitudes, vigorous marketing and extravagant and unsubstantiated claims, social malaise and antidoctor backlash, dislike of the delivery of scientific biomedicine, a romantic perception of CAM safety, and idealistic conviction of the absence of CAM side effects (even CAM has them).

4.3.6 Methods of Investigating Claims Made by CAM Proponents

Should medicine then ignore the claims made by CAM proponents, dismissing them all as quackery? Not necessarily. *Absence of evidence is not evidence of absence. Bad reasoning and bad argument may by chance have a true conclusion.* A CAM intervention for which there is only poor anecdotal evidence may turn out, on careful investigation, to be safe and effective for the intended purpose; in fact, this has happened, as in the case of St John's wort, a herb used as a treatment of depression, as commented recently by Hoffer.[75] Importantly, once such unequivocal evidence emerges, the intervention leaves the world of alternative medicine and becomes part of mainstream medicine.

Let us make the vague concept of complementary and alternative medicine more precise. If we, as already suggested, define a complementary intervention as one proposed in addition to the accepted treatment and an alternative intervention as one proposed instead of the accepted treatment, then research evaluating CAM interventions involves two distinct methods.

First, **to test an "alternative" intervention**, we need a clinical trial in which an experimental group receiving the alternative medicine is compared with a control group of subjects treated with a substance or technique of mainstream medicine whose effectiveness is known. Comparing an experimental group receiving an unconventional treatment with a control group receiving a placebo tests only the effectiveness of the unconventional treatment per se, unless similar trial results comparing mainstream interventions with a placebo are available for an indirect comparison.

Second, in the evaluation of the **effectiveness of a complementary medicine**, we would need a trial involving an experimental group (a complementary medicine added to either a mainstream intervention or another complementary medicine or both) and a control group receiving the same combination without the complementary medicine being tested.

Similar reasoning applies to all alternatives to randomized, double-blind, controlled trials, such as single-patient trials (n-of-1 trials) and sequential trials.

Manageable questions

Once the fundamental direction is traced for the problem, it must be given a manageable meaning and paths to reach the desired answers. As already mentioned, usable answers require manageable questions. The CAM challenge cannot be advanced by an overencompassing approach.

A CAM problem requires two paths of structuring:

1. Structuring the **topic requiring evidence**: diagnosis, treatment, prognosis, correct decision making. Evidence-based medicine addresses these problems in more detail.[87] Is the CAM problem well defined? Do we wish to assess the internal or external validity of diagnoses, the effectiveness of treatment, or something else?

2. Structuring the **path, means, and ends of logical reasoning and argument.** The whole process of inference is also at stake.

Such topical and logical structuring still remains rudimentary or even nonexistent in the CAM world.

4.3.7 Assessment of Evidence in CAM Studies

The primary problem of missing or poor quality evidence in CAM begins with various degrees of ignorance of **clinimetrics**[87,90] (path from clinical observation to diagnosis).

It concerns *initial states.* What does it mean to have low energy? Or to feel as if one does not have control of oneself?

It concerns *maneuvers.*[38] How can we define by acceptable inclusion or exclusion criteria an "electromagnetic power, life force, universal innate intelligence, psychic, parapsychological agent, psi, astral, spiritual vital force, energy flow" or even "giving more time to the patient"?

It concerns *subsequent states* and *outcomes* such as " well-being," "better control of myself and my fate." Such ill-defined outcomes are sometimes used "to show these docs that their work is worthless." Moreover, a cure is often not the desired outcome. It may be empowerment and/or instant gratification of any kind.

Clinimetrics means a process from clinical observation to clinical explanation (diagnosis).[87] Its success relies on good definition and measurement not only of *hard data,* such as body temperature or blood cell counts, but also, and most importantly, of *soft data*: their operational definition, challenge of their measurement, quantification, and classification.[90] Wherever it is relevant, the "hardening of soft data"[87,90] is mandatory and should be attempted.

If a psychiatrist is able to give a clinimetric dimension to such phenomena as "mood" or "aggressive behavior," protagonists of integrative medicine are equally responsible for giving meaningful clinimetric dimension to notions such as "the person as a whole" or "empowerment." Without it, the best intention remains in the realm of faith and belief. It is impossible to give it some scientific basis and credibility because of cloudy meanings and impossible measurement.

Without a clear clinimetric view of the problem, there is no clear problem for which the scientific method could be used. A hypothesis of what? The measurement of what? An evaluation of what? Or is there some other mystical scientific method other than the one already well defined by philosophy and science? (See Section 4.1.)

It is possible to judiciously handle soft data. For example, pain is nowadays much more clinimetrically assessed than other states of body and mind.

Without clinimetrics, there are no other usable components and tools of science. One may argue that chiropractic and homeopathy are scientific because they use radiography or magnetic resonance imaging as diagnostic methods (chiropractic), because they use knowledge of chemical substances (homeopathy), or because they use manual skills, technological procedures, or laboratory analyses and tests. But such proficiencies are only the trappings of science, not its core.

Some CAM protagonists are not trained or experienced in clinical epidemiology and clinimetrics. Some may find it easier not to try to improve clinical epidemiologic and clinimetric challenges of CAM by shrouding CAM in the aura of uniqueness, mysticism, and sacrosanct wholeness of the CAM domain. Some, on the other hand, may accept the challenge of critical thinking and EBM and support well-designed analytical studies of their favored interventions.

4.3.8 Cause-Effect Reasoning in CAM Studies

Another source of lack of clarity is poor **cause-effect reasoning** in CAM studies. Many variables under consideration and study may be independent (causes) and dependent (consequences) at the same time. A "higher energy flow" may be a consequence of "spiritual healing," but "higher energy flow" may produce better mental and spiritual health. It is often unclear in CAM studies if a given phenomenon is an independent or dependent variable.

The demonstration of a cause-effect relationship requires more evidence than biological plausibility. Some advocates defend the value of a CAM intervention solely on the basis of its biological plausibility (if it has any). Others draw their conclusions based on different criteria without discussing biological plausibility and without proposing other types of explanation in a clear and operational manner (alternative reasoning itself). Even if such an explanation were obtained in the best-ever trials, the grounds would remain obscure.

Evidence-based medicine proposes a hierarchy of cause-effect proof, with single clinical trials and their research integration as the most probative, followed by observational analytical studies, descriptive occurrence studies, case series, single case reports, narratives, and expert opinions, in that order. The volume of evidence for various CAM interventions appears for the moment to be inversely correlated with that order. In other words, the stronger the type of evidence for a CAM cause-effect relationship, the less there is of it.

At this time, we know practically nothing about the effectiveness of various CAM interventions in the case of multiple health problems (comorbidities) and multiple treatments for these problems (cotreatments for comorbidities). Sometimes, CAM protagonists tout the "**holistic effect of CAM.**" Let us remember the varying connotations of "holistic": treatment for known or unknown comorbidity, webs of consequences[87] of exposure to some undesirable or suspicious factor, psychiatric support, treatment of neuroendocrine body regulations, solving the patient's social problems as well as those of his or her family, and treating anything else beyond the patient's chief complaint and the physician's main diagnosis. For now, we do not have an operational and measurable definition of a "patient as a whole" that we would be able to study and use as a dependent variable in cause-effect studies.

Complementary and alternative diagnostic methods (CAD) such as evaluating a patient's health and disease from coffee sediment or hair analysis remain an even less known entity than CAM.

The problem of evaluating CAM effectiveness is further compounded by an increasing number of narrative overviews, systematic reviews, and meta-analyses.[37,38,87] Such research integration is not always based on well-designed original studies to review and integrate. Poor clinimetrics at the start result in poor overall understanding, conclusions, and ensuing recommendations (garbage in, garbage out). Today, CAM strongly needs a systematic assessment of the complexity, heterogeneity, and missing information and findings of available original studies.

Even historically well-rooted and widely used herbal medicines, such as complementary mistletoe therapy for cancer in German-speaking countries, may prove non-beneficial in survival, quality of life, or cellular immune changes in some cancers.[89]

Can CAM be evidence-based? Tonelli and Callahan[48] believe that it cannot. These authors go so far as to claim that clinical trials in CAM do not represent a scientific necessity but rather a philosophical demand. Is this because they cannot be performed in some cases or situations? What are the alternatives? A randomized, double-blind, controlled clinical trial is not the only source of evidence, and it is not synonymous with EBM itself. This type of clinical trial can be a gold standard of experimental proof of causality, but there are alternatives to it, if for some reason it cannot be done. Circumstantial observations, narratives, case studies, and case reports or case series, as well as observational descriptive and analytical studies, all have their place in the hierarchy of evidence. Only their meaning, relevance, limitations, and impact in a given context and need of specific decision making are different, and they carry a varying degree of convincing force from one medical question to another.

In his much more realistic view of evidence-based CAM, Bloom[49] quotes not only the increasing number of clinical trials in CAM but also their overall quality, which in many cases still does not reach that of trials in mainstream medicine. These trials, however, will likely multiply and improve with time.[62,91-97]

4.3.9 Systematic Reviews and Meta-Analyses of CAM Research

Systematic reviews and meta-analyses of evidence in CAM are encouraged.[54] They are possible, as shown by Wilt et al[91] in their meta-analysis of the effectiveness of saw palmetto extracts in the treatment of benign prostatic hyperplasia and by Neil et al[98] in their assessment of garlic powder in the treatment of moderate hyperlipidemia. Another example is Ernst's[99] review of a proven treatment (chelation therapy) in heavy metal poisoning if applied with a variety of adjuvant therapies to another diagnostic entity (peripheral arterial occlusive disease).

Consequently, CAM has three choices to make: (1) improve itself as a science, (2) explain clearly and demonstrate that it is a "special science," or (3) remain as a subject of faith and belief, escaping the rules and scrutiny of logic and critical thinking.

If some forms of CAM are solely faith or belief, there is nothing bad about this. Moreover, the beneficial impact of faith and belief on humanity is monumental. However, if this is the case, CAM cannot be termed logical or scientific. If they are termed as such, the validity of this claim must be proved. To quote a fast-food advertisement, we can still ask ourselves with regard to CAM: *Where's the beef?*

4.3.10 Alternative Methods of Evaluating CAM Claims

A simple acceptance or denial of CAM phenomena is not enough. If CAM escapes consideration by mainstream logic and assessment of evidence, are there other ways to evaluate evidence in the CAM domain[48]? Is it subject to some special kind of production and assessment of evidence, or to some special kind of logic, inference, and critical thinking? We doubt it.

If special methods of reasoning and assessing evidence are appropriate for CAM interventions, they should be not only explained but also justified. Sheer intellectual cogitation, however refined it might be, is not enough.

As an example of alternative ways of thinking, let us examine the problem of clinical trials in CAM.

Are there alternatives to the experimental evaluation of CAM? One, as reviewed by Nahin,[100] uses **best case series** to obtain disease course and desirable outcomes and to compare them with some historical controls such as hospital follow-up examinations of patients who received mainstream interventions. However, to compare natural histories and clinical courses in both groups may prove very difficult given the different quality and complexity of relevant observations and findings.

4.3.11 Summary Remarks About CAM

An evidence-based approach and critical thinking are both possible and necessary when reflecting on CAM. It is easy for a commercially motivated or mentally lazy person to claim that CAM is so special that it escapes common logic, critical thinking, and evidence assessment.

Fontanarosa and Lundberg[59] rightly conclude:

"There is no alternative medicine. There is only scientifically proven, evidence-based medicine supported by solid data or unproven medicine, for which scientific evidence is lacking. Whether therapeutic practice is 'Eastern' or 'Western,' is unconventional or mainstream, or involves mind-body techniques or molecular genetics is largely irrelevant except for historical purposes and cultural interest."

Mainstream medicine may benefit enormously from the CAM experience.[48] What are we doing wrong that even the best care and cures available are not enough for human beings? If our care and cures are not the very best, how can we improve them and drive them toward their best direction? What is missing in our care in view of patients' expectations? Are we providing enough good-quality information to our patients about how they can maintain their own health through healthy diet, regular exercise, regular sleep patterns, stress reduction, and other proven healthful practices? Patient health remains fourfold: physical, mental, social, and spiritual. In many cases, the contribution of CAM to these four aspects of health still remains to be seen. There is an unquestionable demand for CAM, whether its foundation is cultural, social, or economical. The sheer volume of CAM providers, services, and consumers as well as their spending and revenues show it.[33,34,37,38]

If the scientific method cannot measure hope, divine intervention, or the power of belief,[50] let us handle faith and belief separately from science if we do not succeed in giving them an acceptable clinimetric dimension. We should do this equally well within the framework of faith and belief as we already try to do in the domain of evidence itself. Like science, faith, marvelous in itself, is one of the most important qualities of human beings and of being human. One does what the other does not.

If the reader is interested in further discussion of CAM, there are books that sum-marize and review CAM, which have been reviewed.[55] Ad hoc periodicals are avail-able (*Alternative Therapies in Health and Medicine, Complementary Medical Research, Complementary Therapies in Medicine* [online], *Integrative Medicine*). Institutions are devoted to the task of evaluating CAM activities and driving them in the best direc-tion (US Office of Alternative Medicine at the National Institutes of Health becoming the National Center for Complementary and Alternative Medicine, among oth-ers).[58,60] The Cochrane Collaboration is also interested in CAM.[55]

The debate about alternative, complementary, and integrative medicine contin-ues.[76,101-103] The Quackwatch Web site is well worth the reader's attention.[104] It was not the purpose of this schematic critical appraisal of CAM to solve all the problems and challenges of CAM. Our remarks illustrate only the practical application of critical thinking to a specific health and disease phenomenon with its multiple unresolved problems and unanswered questions.

4.3.12 Complementary and Alternative Medicine in Medical Education and Practice

The preceding discussion has focused on the evidential basis for CAM interven-tions and the way in which research on their safety and effectiveness should be con-ducted. It has had little to say, except by implication, about how medical education and medical practice should respond to the challenge of CAM. Critical thinking about those two questions is left as an exercise for the reader. We offer some refer-ences and a few hints on how to conduct that critical thinking process.

As to medical education, the educational establishment in mainstream medicine has recently decided that CAM should be offered as part of a physician's formal training.[39,41,43,44,46,47] The main argument supporting this decision is that physicians need to know about "medical" interventions that their patients are using on their own. However, there are debates about how exposure to CAM practices should be incorporated into the medical curriculum. Should learning about CAM be a stand-alone option or integrated within a required curriculum? Should it be taught from a CAM perspective or from the perspective of critical appraisal and EBM? Before any knowledge, attitude, or skill pertaining to one of the CAM approaches, however justified this might be, is offered to health professionals, they should first under-stand and master critical thinking about it, since they are already in increasing con-tact with CAM in mainstream medicine.

Teachers and their students must realize that CAM is "too big to chew off in one bite" and that "it has too many flavors." It must be atomized in manageable pieces of teaching, learning, and understanding. It must be understood first.

As to medical practice, there is a growing peer-reviewed literature with advice for the practicing physician.[40,57,61,101] Surveys show that most US residents who use some CAM intervention do not inform their physician of that fact, partly because they fear that their physician will not approve.[33,37] Such data indicate a need for physicians in their discussions with patients to adopt a nonjudgmental attitude toward patients' independent attempts at health maintenance and self-healing. The challenge is to combine an atmosphere of open communication with good information provided to the patient about the evidential basis of particular CAM practices. All this must be done within the constraints of medical ethics[61] (especially its first maxim, "do no harm") and the law.[56] A further question is how to decide which CAM interventions one's patients should be discouraged from using under specified circumstances, which ones should be accepted, and which ones should be recommended.[40]

If you decide to take CAM into account in your practice of medicine, you should remember the following:

- Practice evidence-based CAM (provided that meaningful evidence is available).

- If meaningful evidence is not available, do not harm patients by an unsubstantiated faith in CAM.

- Do not comply with patient-pleasing practices as a money-making provision of questionable health services.

- All canons of medical ethics apply to the field of CAM.

4.4 CONCLUSIONS

A justified conclusion requires good evidence and a warranted inference. Is good-quality evidence coupled with its equally good logical uses?

It is much easier to grade the evidence that enters the critical thinking process than the result of the critical process itself.

As already mentioned, the quality of evidence for a cause-effect relationship ranges in EBM from anecdotal observations or case reports to rigorous clinical trials and systematic reviews of evidence. As reviewed elsewhere,[87,105,106] quality checklists, scoring systems, and criteria were proposed for practically all major types of observational and experimental studies, including clinical trials and meta-analyses with all their strengths and weaknesses.

In the assessment of evidence, a single "fatal blow" may be discovered that invalidates the whole study despite a better overall result on a scoring system. An extremely large attrition of the number of eligible and enrolled participants may invalidate the conclusions of even the best-conceived randomized, double-blind, controlled trial. A similar "fatal blow" may occur at any moment in the critical thinking process.

Any grading of a hypothesis subjected to a critical thinking process, whether by a simple dichotomy such as "acceptable/unacceptable" or "valid/invalid," or by some degree of strength or weakness, must also identify weak and even missing components of critical thinking. Ultimately, ways to improve weak components and to complete the missing ones must be proposed.

Critical thinking is much more than appraisal of a single argument. It may be simpler if one tackles a pinpoint and precise question such as the effectiveness of some preventive measure, or of some therapeutic drug or surgical procedure, in a clinical trial. It may be more difficult when trying to answer more complex problems such as the meaning and value of CAM.

Proponents of EBM[87,105,106] have already produced a wide array of checklists to evaluate well-defined problems: the validity of diagnostic methods, effectiveness of treatment, causation in the domain of risk, realistic prognosis, and many others. Behind these attempts lies a common thread of a more general thought, which we presented in the general critical thinking checklist in Section 4.2. To illustrate how the common thread is present in a specific context, we relate our schematic critical thinking about CAM in Section 4.3 to the critical thinking checklist of Section 4.2:

- **Identify and analyze the problem.** We identified the problem in Section 4.3.1 and indicated in Section 4.3.2 how it could be broken down into more specific and more manageable questions.

- **Clarify meaning.** We devoted Section 4.3.3 to clarifying what was meant by complementary medicine and by alternative medicine. We came back to the component of clarifying meaning in Section 4.3.6 when we considered how one would investigate a claim that a particular intervention was an alternative or a complement to a conventionally accepted intervention.

- **Gather the evidence.** In considering in Section 4.3.4 the arguments found in popular advocacy of CAM interventions, we attended to the evidence cited by CAM proponents. In Section 4.3.6, we considered how one would gather evidence about some specific alternative or complementary intervention.

- **Assess the evidence.** In Section 4.3.4 we evaluated the types of evidence found in popular advocacy of CAM interventions. We devoted Section 4.3.6 to clinimetric issues in assessing evidence for CAM claims.

- **Infer conclusions or judge inferences to conclusions.** In Section 4.3.4, we evaluated inferences in popular advocacy of CAM. In Section 4.3.8, we discussed the quality of cause-effect reasoning in CAM studies.

- **Consider other relevant information.** In Section 4.3.5, we considered how one could explain widespread belief in the efficacy of CAM interventions when the popular arguments for their effectiveness were in general so weak. In Section 4.3.9, we considered how one could put together the results of good-quality peer-reviewed studies of a CAM intervention in a systematic review or meta-analysis. In Section 4.3.10, we addressed the challenge of some CAM proponents to the methodological assumptions of EBM.

- **Make an overall judgment about the problem.** In Section 4.3.11, we concluded that claims by CAM proponents either should be appraised by the standards of EBM or should be relegated to the realm of faith and belief. A CAM proponent cannot consistently claim scientific validity for some intervention and refuse to have it appraised by scientific standards.

A critical thinking checklist may be useful both in investigation, when one decides how to think critically about a health problem, and in appraisal, when one looks at the already available results of good or questionable critical thinking. Any medical article is a product of critical thinking. So is any decision or order relating to prevention or treatment in a clinical or community context.

As in any other domain of the arts and sciences, critical thinking in health sciences shows not only the strengths and weaknesses in the handling of a particular health problem but also the directions to take in the future.

We physicians and other health professionals as well need to master critical thinking as well as the basic and clinical sciences, biostatistics, epidemiology, or public health. The present state of the art and science of medicine and our own performance in research and practice already give us good reason to do so.

References

1. Hitchcock D. *Critical Thinking: A Guide to Evaluating Information.* Toronto, Ontario: Methuen Publishing; 1983.

2. Moore BN, Parker R. *Critical Thinking: Evaluating Claims and Arguments in Everyday Life.* Palo Alto, Calif: Mayfield Publishing Co; 1986.

3. Little JF, Groarke LA, Tindale CW. *Good Reasoning Matters! A Constructive Approach to Critical Thinking.* Toronto, Ontario: McClelland & Stewart, Inc (M&S); 1989.

4. Ennis RH. *Critical Thinking.* Upper Saddle River, NJ: Prentice Hall; 1996.

5. Waller BN. *Critical Thinking: Consider the Verdict.* Englewood Cliffs, NJ: Prentice Hall; 1998.

6. Hughes W. *Critical Thinking: An Introduction to Basic Skills.* 3rd ed. Peterborough, Ontario: Broadview Press; 2000.

7. Fisher A. *Critical Thinking: An Introduction.* Cambridge, England: Cambridge University Press; 2001.

8. Dewey J. *How We Think.* Boston, Mass: D. C. Heath; 1910.

9. Watson G, Glaser EM. *Watson-Glaser Critical Thinking Appraisal, Forms A and B.* San Antonio, Texas: The Psychological Corp; 1980.

10. Glaser EM. *An Experiment in the Development of Critical Thinking.* New York, NY: Advanced School of Education at Teachers College, Columbia University; 1941.

11. Anderson HR, ed. *Teaching Critical Thinking in the Social Studies.* 13th Yearbook of the National Council for Social Studies. Washington, DC: National Council for Social Studies; 1942.

12. Black M. *Critical Thinking: An Introduction to Logic and Scientific Method.* New York, NY: Prentice-Hall; 1946.

13. Smith BO. The improvement of critical thinking. *Progressive Education.* 1953;30:129–134.

14. Ennis RH. A concept of critical thinking: a proposed basis for research in the teaching and evaluation of critical thinking ability. *Harvard Educ Rev.* 1962;32:81–111.

15. McPeck J. *Critical Thinking and Education.* New York, NY: St Martin's Press; 1981.

16. Ennis RH. A logical basis for measuring critical thinking skills. *Educ Leadership.* 1985;43,2:44–48.

17. Lipman M. Critical thinking: what can it be? *Analytic Teaching.* 1988;8:5–12.

18. Siegel H. *Educating Reason: Rationality, Critical Thinking and Education.* London, England: Routledge; 1988.

19. Paul RW. Critical thinking in North America: a new theory of knowledge, learning and literacy. *Argumentation.* 1989;3:197–235.

20. Paul R. *Critical Thinking: What Every Person Needs to Survive in a Rapidly Changing World.* 3rd ed rev. Santa Rosa, Calif: Foundation for Critical Thinking; 1993.

21. Facione PA. *Critical Thinking: A Statement of Expert Consensus for Purposes of Educational Assessment and Instruction.* Research findings and recommendations prepared for the Committee on Pre-College Philosophy of the American Philosophical Association. Newark, Del: American Philosophical Association. ERIC Document #ED 315-423;1990.

22. Ennis RH. Critical thinking: a streamlined conception. *Teaching Philosophy.* 1991;14:5–24.

23. Fisher A, Scriven M. *Critical Thinking: Its Definition and Assessment.* Point Reyes, Calif: Edgepress and Norwich, UK: Centre for Research in Critical Thinking, University of East Anglia; 1997.

24. Snyder M. Critical thinking: a foundation for consumer-focused care. *J Contin Educ Nurs .* 1993;24:206–210.

25. Ennis RH. A taxonomy of critical thinking dispositions and abilities. In: Baron JB, Steinberg RJ, eds. *Teaching Thinking Skills: Theory and Practice.* New York, NY: WH Freeman; 1987:9–26.

26. Paul R. Teaching critical thinking in the "strong" sense: a focus on self-deception, world-views, and a dialectical mode of analysis. *Informal Logic Newslett.* 1982;4,2:2–7.

27. Ennis RH, Millman J, Tomko TN. *Cornell Critical Thinking Tests Level X & Level Z.* 3rd ed. Pacific Grove, Calif: Midwest Publications; 1985.

28. Ennis RH, Weir E. *The Ennis-Weir Critical Thinking Essay Test.* Pacific Grove, Calif: Midwest Publications; 1985.

29. Facione PA. *California Critical Thinking Skills Test, Forms A and B.* Millbrae, Calif: California Academic Press; 1998.

30. Facione PA. *California Critical Thinking Skills Test—2000.* Millbrae, Calif: California Academic Press; 2000.

31. Oxford, Cambridge, and RSA Examinations. *OCR Advanced Subsidiary GCE in Critical Thinking (3821)*. Cambridge, England: OCR; 2000. Available at www.ocr.org.uk/OCR/WebSite/Data/Publication/Specifications%2c %20Syllabuses%20%26%20Tutors%20Handbooks/cquartetOCRTempFile PQX1nq3frB.pdf.

32. Davidoff F. Weighing the alternatives: lessons from the paradoxes of alternative medicine. *Ann Intern Med*. 1998;129:1068–1070.

33. Eisenberg DM, Davis RB, Ettner S, et al. Trends in alternative medicine use in the United States, 1990-1997. Results of a follow-up national survey. *JAMA*. 1998;280:1569–1575.

34. Kelly KM, Jacobson JS, Kennedy DO, Brandt SM, Mallick M, Weiner MA. Use of non-conventional therapies by children with cancer at an urban medical center. *J Pediatr Hematol Oncol*. 2000;22:412–426.

35. Bagley CM Jr, Shaugnessy AF, Ganguly A, Ernst E, Kaptchuk TJ, Eisenberg DM. Alternative views on alternative medicine [letter]. *Ann Intern Med*. 1999;131:229–230.

36. Eisenberg DM, Kaptchuk TJ, Laine C, Davidoff F. Complementary and alternative medicine—an Annals series. *Ann Intern Med*. 2001;135:208.

37. Kaptchuk TJ, Eisenberg DM. Varieties of healing. 1: medical pluralism in the United States. *Ann Intern Med*. 2001;135:189–195.

38. Kaptchuk TJ, Eisenberg DM. Varieties of healing. 2: taxonomy of unconventional healing practices. *Ann Intern Med*. 2001;135:196–204.

39. Vandenbroucke JP, de Craen AJ. Alternative medicine: a 'mirror image' for scientific reasoning in conventional medicine. *Ann Intern Med*. 2001;135:507–513.

40. Weiger W, Smith M, Boon H, Richardson MA, Kaptchuk TJ, Eisenberg DM. Advising patients who seek complementary and alternative medical therapies for cancer. *Ann Intern Med*. 2002;137:889–903.

41. Wetzel MS, Kaptchuk TJ, Haramati A, Eisenberg DM. Complementary and alternative medical therapies: implications for medical education. *Ann Intern Med*. 2003;138:191–196.

42. Beyerstein BL. Alternative medicine and common errors of reasoning. *Acad Med*. 2001;76:230–237.

43. Grollman AP. Alternative medicine: the importance of evidence in medicine and medical education. Is there wheat among the chaff? *Acad Med*. 2001;76:221–223.

44. Marcus DM. How should alternative medicine be taught to medical students and physicians? *Acad Med*. 2001;76:224–229.

45. Talalay P, Talalay P. The importance of using scientific principles in the development of medical agents from plants. *Acad Med*. 2001;76:238–247.

46. Sampson W. The need for educational reform in teaching about alternative therapies. *Acad Med*. 2001;76:248–250.

47. Frenkel M, Ben Arye E. The growing need to teach about complementary and alternative medicine: questions and challenges. *Acad Med*. 2001;76:251–254.

48. Tonelli MR, Callahan TC. Why alternative medicine cannot be evidence-based. *Acad Med*. 2001;76:1213–1220.

49. Bloom BS. What is this nonsense that complementary and alternative medicine is not amenable to controlled investigation of population effects? *Acad Med*. 2001;76:1221–1223.

50. Puchalski CM. Reconnecting the science and art of medicine. *Ann Intern Med*. 2001;76:1224–1225.

51. Curt GA. Complementary and alternative medicine cancer treatment. *Semin Oncol*. 2002;29:529–530.

52. White JD. Complementary and alternative medicine research: a National Cancer Institute perspective. *Semin Oncol*. 2002;29:546–551.

53. Powers Monaco G, Smith G. Informed consent in complementary and alternative medicine: current status and future needs. *Semin Oncol*. 2002;29:601–608.

54. Ezzo J, Berman BM, Vickers AJ, Linde K. Complementary medicine and the Cochrane Collaboration. *JAMA*. 1998;280:1628–1630.

55. Books, journals, new media: (Physio-medicalism, alternative medicine). Reviews (various reviewers). *JAMA*. 1998;280:1634–1636.

56. Studdert DM, Eisenberg DM, Miller FH, Curto DA, Kaptchuk TJ, Brennan TA. Medical malpractice implications of alternative medicine. *JAMA*. 1998;280:1610–1615.

57. Udani J. Integrating alternative medicine into practice. *JAMA*. 1998;280:1620.

58. Jonas WB. Alternative medicine—learning from the past, examining the present, advancing to the future. *JAMA*. 1998;280:1616–1618.

59. Fontanarosa PB, Lundberg GD. Alternative medicine meets science. *JAMA*. 1998;280:1618–1619.

60. Eskinazi DP. Factors that shape alternative medicine. *JAMA*. 1998;280:1621–1623.

61. Sugarman J, Burk L. Physician's ethical obligations regarding alternative medicine. *JAMA*. 1998;280:1623–1625.

62. Margolin A, Avants SK, Kleber RD. Investigating alternative medicine therapies in randomized controlled trials. *JAMA*. 1998;280:1626–1628.

63. National Institutes of Health, Office of Alternative Medicine (OAM), OAM Clearinghouse. Alternative choices: what it means to use nonconventional therapy. *JAMA*. 1998;280:1640.

64. Morelli V, Zoorob RJ. Alternative therapies: Part I. Depression, diabetes, obesity. *Am Fam Physician*. 2000;62:1051–1060.

65. Morelli V, Zoorob RJ. Alternative therapies: Part II. Congestive heart failure and hypercholesterolemia. *Am Fam Physician*. 2000;62:1325–1330.

66. Morelli V, Naquin C. Alternative therapies for traditional disease states: menopause. *Am Fam Physician*. 2002;66:129–134.

67. Hensley MJ, Gibson PG. Promoting evidence-based alternative medicine. *Med J Aust*. 1998;169:573–574.

68. Bowler SD, Green A, Mitchell CA. Buteyko breathing techniques in asthma: a blind randomized controlled trial. *Med J Aust*. 1998;169:575–578.

69. Liu C, Douglas RM. Chinese herbal medicines in the treatment of acute respiratory infections: a review of randomised and controlled clinical trials. *Med J Aust*. 1998;169:575–582.

70. Rey JM, Walter G. Hyperbaricum perforatum (St.John's wort) in depression: pest or blessing? *Med J Aust*. 1998;169:583–586.

71. Bensoussan A. Complementary medicine—where lies its appeal? *Med J Aust*. 1999;170:247–248.

72. Del Mar CB, Glasziou PP, Spinks AB, Sanders SL. Does drinking carrot juice affect cancer of the prostate? *Med J Aust*. 2001;174:197.

73. Davis SR, Briganti EM, Chen RQ, Dalais FS, Bailey M, Burger HG. The effects of Chinese medicinal herbs on postmenopausal vasomotor symptoms of Australian women. a randomized controlled trial. *Med J Aust*. 2001;174:69–71.

74. Reynolds T. Keeping up with alternative medicine: researchers offer evaluation criteria. *J Natl Cancer Inst*. 2003;95:96–98.

75. Hoffer J. Complementary or alternative medicine: the need for plausibility. *Can Med Assoc J*. 2003:168:180–182.

76. Wickers A. Evidence-based medicine and complementary medicine. *Evidence-based Ment Health*. 1999;2:102–103.

77. Mill, JS. *A System of Logic Ratiocinative and Inductive: Being a Connected View of the Principles of Evidence and the Methods of Scientific Investigation*. 10th ed. London, England: Longmans Green; 1879.

78. Gottlieb B, Berg SG, Fisher P. *New Choices in Natural Healing: Over 1,800 of the Best Self-Help Remedies from the World of Alternative Medicine*. Emmaus, Pa: Rodale Press; 1995.

79. Duke, JA. *The Green Pharmacy*. Emmaus, Pa: Rodale Press; 1997.

80. Chandler F, ed. *Herbs: Everyday Reference for Health Professionals.* Ottawa, Ontario: Canadian Pharmacists Association and Canadian Medical Association; 2000.

81. Ernst E, ed. *The Desktop Guide to Complementary and Alternative Medicine: An Evidence-based Approach.* St Louis, Mo: Mosby; 2001.

82. Lewith G, Jonas WB, Wallach H, eds. *Clinical Research in Complementary Therapies: Principles, Problems and Solutions.* London, England: Churchill Livingstone; 2002.

83. Barnes J, Anderson LA, Phillipson JD. *Herbal Medicines: A Guide for Health Care Professionals.* 2nd ed. London, England: Pharmaceutical Press; 2002.

84. Fetrow CW, Avila JR. *Professional's Handbook of Complementary & Alternative Medicines.* 3rd ed. Philadelphia, Pa: Lippincott Williams & Wilkins; 2004.

85. Snyderman R, Weil AT. Integrative medicine: bringing medicine back to its roots. *Arch Intern Med.* 2002;162:395–397.

86. Bell IR, Caspi O, Schwartz GER, et al. Integrative medicine and systemic outcomes research: issues in the emergence of a new model for primary care. *Arch Intern Med.* 2002;162:133–140.

87. Jenicek M. *Foundations of Evidence-Based Medicine.* New York, NY: The Parthenon Publishing Group; 2003.

88. Brewin TB. Complementary medicine—is there a reasonable basis for dialogue? *J R Coll Physicians Lond.* 1996;30:406–409.

89. Richardson MA, Straus SE. Complementary and alternative medicine: opportunities and challenges for cancer management and research. *Semin Oncol.* 2002;29:531–545.

90. Feinstein AR. *Clinimetrics.* New Haven, Conn: Yale University Press; 1987.

91. Wilt TJ, Ishani A, Stark G, MacDonald R, Lau J, Mulrow C. Saw palmetto extracts for treatment of benign prostatic hyperplasia: a systematic review. *JAMA.* 1998;280:1604–1609.

92. Bove G, Nilsson N. Spinal manipulation in the treatment of episodic tension-type headache: a randomized controlled trial. *JAMA.* 1988;280:1576–1579.

93. Cardini F, Weixin H. Moxibustion for correction of breach presentation: a randomized controlled trial. *JAMA.* 1998;280:1580–1584.

94. Bensoussan A, Talley NJ, Hing M, Menzies R, Guo A, Ngu M. Treatment of irritable bowel syndrome with Chinese herbal medicine. *JAMA.* 1998; 280:1585–1589.

95. Shlay JC, Chaloner K, Max MB, et al. Acupuncture and amitriptyline for pain due to HIV-related peripheral neuropathy: a randomized controlled trial. Terry Beirn Community Programs for Clinical Research on AIDS. *JAMA.* 1998;280:1590–1595.

96. Heymsfield SB, Allison DB, Vasselli JR, et al. Garcinia cambogia (Hydroxycitric acid) as a potential antiobesity agent: a randomized controlled trial. *JAMA.* 1998:280:1590–1595.

97. Garfinkel MS, Snghal A, Katz WA, Allen DA, Reshetar R, Schumacher RH. Yoga-based intervention for carpal tunnel syndrome: a randomized trial. *JAMA.* 1998;280:1601–1603.

98. Neil HAW, Silagy CA, Lancaster T, et al. Garlic powder in the treatment of moderate hyperlipidaemia: a controlled trial and meta-analysis. *J R Coll Physicians Lond*. 1996;30:329–334.

99. Ernst E. Chelation therapy for peripheral arterial occlusive disease: a systematic review. *Circulation*. 1997;96:1031–1033.

100. Nahin RL. Use of best case series to evaluate complementary and alternative therapies for cancer: a systematic review. *Semin Oncol.* 2002;29:552–562.

101. Gaudet TW, Snyderman R. Integrative medicine and the search for the best practice of medicine. *Acad Med*. 2002;77:861–863.

102. Astin JA. Complementary and alternative medicine and the need for evidence-based criticism. *Acad Med*. 2002;77:864–868.

103. Beyerstein BL, Frenkel M, Ben-Arye E, Grollman AP, Marcus DM, Sampson W. Five special theme commentaries. *Acad Med*. 2002;77:869–875.

104. Quackwatch: Your Guide to Health Fraud, Quackery, and Intelligent Decisions [Web site]. Available at: www.quackwatch.org.

105. Sackett DL, Straus SE, Scott Richardson W, Rosenberg W, Haynes RB. *Evidence-Based Medicine: How to Practice and Teach EBM.* 2nd ed. London, England: Churchill Livingstone; 2000.

106. Guyatt G, Rennie D, eds. *Users' Guides to the Medical Literature: Essentials of Evidence-Based Clinical Practice.* Chicago, Ill: AMA Press; 2002.

Part 2

Practical Applications

CHAPTER 5

Logic in Research: Critical Writing and Reading of Medical Articles

What Do These Results Really Prove?
How to Write and Read Discussion and
Conclusions Sections

IN THIS CHAPTER

*When a "scientist of the surgical unit" at a teaching
hospital was asked what the job entailed, he used
to say: "The professor removes a piece of
tissue, gives it to me, and expects me to go off
and do something scientific with it."*
MICHAEL O'DONNELL, 1985

*. . . most importantly of all,
. . .[scientific papers] stake their author's claim to the new
knowledge they contain.*
MICHAEL SHORTLAND AND JANE GREGORY, 1991

*What gets cancer—the genes, the cell,
the organism, or perhaps even the population?*
JOHN D. POTTER, 1992

*A wise man . . . proportions his belief to the evidence. . . .
[Where conclusions are not founded on an infallible experience]
he weighs the opposite experiments: he considers
which side is supported by the greater number
of experiments: to that side he inclines, with doubt
and hesitation: and when at last he fixes his judgment,
the evidence exceeds not what we properly call probability.*
DAVID HUME, 1758

*(Isn't this what we are doing today in our systematic review
of evidence and meta-analysis?)*

**In essence, any medical article is, and must be,
an exercise in logic and critical thinking
applied to obtaining, evaluating, and using
the best evidence possible.**

So you want to write or understand the Discussion of Findings and the Conclusions sections in medical articles? You want to know which ones are done well and which ones are eminently forgettable?

From a philosophical standpoint, most medical articles (especially original studies) are logical discourses. A piece of medical research produces premises for arguments, proposes a new solution to an old problem, or represents a complete argument. Arguments in a medical article must be cogent. If not, even good research findings risk being misinterpreted and misused, and good intentions left unfulfilled.

How solid is the proof that passive smoking is bad for your health? How can we justify our claim that angioplasty is better in some clinical cases than coronary bypass? Any novice in the field of research quickly finds that he or she received much better training in the production of the best possible evidence than in ways of explaining it properly. The reader (novice or otherwise) of any research article should fully understand its message.

A medical research article usually has the following sections:[1] Introduction (statement of the problem and critical review of the literature and research question), Material and Methods, Results, Discussion, and Conclusions. Most often, we are more thoroughly trained on how to produce new evidence than how to discuss and interpret it critically. "My observations and computations are fine; my mission is accomplished!" Or is it?

The research question leads to a logical argument whose conclusion must fit the stated problem (question). Other possibilities and alternatives are explored, and the weight of one view of the problem is pitted against another. The Discussion and Conclusions sections of medical articles provide the space for such a logical discourse. Writing it is as much a learned skill as performing a biopsy to gather research material or performing a statistical analysis of findings. This chapter outlines the essentials of "Discussion" and "Conclusion" reasoning for which authors and readers should be on the same wavelength. The same applies to presenters of research and their audience at scientific meetings. Verbal and written messages must follow the same rules in the critical thinking game.

The prevailing content and form of articles in the medical literature, as diversified as they may appear, are based on both science and philosophy, particularly logic.

Careful scientific observation and experimentation provide data. However, data require interpretation: What does this mean? **Data** represent the first line of gathered evidence. For example, a blood pressure reading of 180/110 mm Hg is a piece of data on blood pressure. This datum becomes meaningful **information** when it is interpreted and labeled as hypertension.

Philosophy examines the interpretation of scientific data and the logical processes by which new information is obtained from them. Such information is a product of a thinking mind encountering external evidence (data). **Information** contains both the external evidence and the mental framework by means of which the information is apprehended, and through which it is articulated. Scientists and their readers arrive at their interpretations through **logic and critical thinking**.

5.1 CLASSIFICATION AND STRUCTURE OF MEDICAL ARTICLES

Different types of medical articles bring answers to five different questions:

1. **Describing what was seen:** anatomical or functional findings, occurrence of disease in the community: *How does it look, and how much of it is there?*

2. **Describing medical technology (tools):** *What is it, how does it work, where should it be used, and what is its benefit?*

3. **Attempting to explain the cause or causes of a given problem:** *What causes disease and death in the case of a noxious factor? What controls disease and improves health and to what extent, in the case of a beneficial factor such as treatment?*

4. **Making a systematic review and synthesis of all available relevant evidence:** in one of the three above-mentioned cases: *All in all, what do we know about it?*

5. **Managing the health problem (patients, community, health professionals, society, economics, culture, faith):** *How does it work and how should it work?*

To cover any one of these five major questions, scientific articles based on original research now have a fairly uniform structure:

- **Introduction:** The problem is explained, objectives of inquiry are given, and the hypothesis or hypotheses on which the objective or objectives are based are formulated.

- **Material and methods:** Research subjects and all variables (factors, possible causes, characteristics, time, place, timetable, means) are defined and described in operational and reproducible terms as well as how such information was gathered.

- **Results:** Observations and crude findings (data) are presented.

- **Discussion:** The meaning of the findings is interpreted.

- **Conclusions:** What can be done with the findings is summarized, as are the research implications and uses of findings in practical decision making.

These sections, in varying degrees, use what we call an **object language** and a **meta-language**.[2] In fact, both medical research and clinical practice use object language and meta-language. Here are some examples, with the object-language statement in italics:

Object language:	*Drinking and driving kills.*
Meta-language:	What does it mean to say that drinking and driving kills (causes death)?
Object language:	*It is right to treat single-vessel coronary disease by percutaneous transluminal coronary angioplasty.*
Meta-language:	What does it mean to say that this treatment decision in the case of this health problem is right?
Object language:	*It is mandatory to surgically débride a dirty wound.*
Meta-language:	What does it mean to say that it is mandatory?
Object language:	*This drug will make you feel better.*
Meta-language:	What does it mean to say that it "will make me feel better"?

An object language is a language used to talk about objects in the world. A meta-language is a language used to talk about a language; it is found partly in the Introduction, but mainly in the Discussion and Conclusions sections. Medical articles primarily use an object language when they speak directly about observations. However, they use meta-language when stating a research problem, question, or hypothesis (introduction) and when examining what is said and whether or not the conveyed information accurately reflects the reality that it purports to describe. In this sense, the **Discussion and Conclusions section of medical articles is the logical and linguistic discussion of whatever precedes them in the first part of the article.**

So, you want to understand or write Discussion and Conclusions sections stemming from a research article? To do so, you need both science and logic. And logic is part of philosophy.

Do we really need to equally master both the scientific and the philosophical aspects of our work in health sciences? This double mastery is required because philosophy helps us answer two fundamental questions:

1. What is the nature of the problem? What lies beneath the sort of evidence that medicine examines? This is a metaphysical question.

2. What can we know and what do we know for sure? If we are not sure, why is this the case? What constitutes sound evidence? This is an epistemological question, focusing on knowledge.

Just as cooking a good meal depends on the use of fresh ingredients and how the cook uses them, good research and good evidence usable in practice will depend on the quality of ingredients (data) and how they are handled in terms of logical argumentation and the final explanation of their meaning. Good evidence with a minimum of uncertainty and absence of chance is more than desirable, if not necessary for good practice and further research.

Evidence is defined in evidence-based medicine (EBM) as "*any data or information, whether solid or weak, obtained through experience, observational research or experimental work (trials) used either for the understanding of the health problem or for decision making about it.*" (See Chapter 1. For definitions beyond medicine, see Feldman.[3]) Most often, evidence is subject to uncertainty.

Uncertainty is the **possibility that future observation or reflection will provide good reason to change any opinion one now has**. Decision making under uncertainty[4] is decision making in a situation in which the probabilities of different possible outcomes are not known. Chance is mainly responsible for our uncertainty in a given situation.

Chance is "*an uncalculated, and possibly incalculable, element of existence; the contingent as opposed to the necessary aspects of existence.*"[5]

Clinical data as "fresh ingredients" depend on their **measurement**—how all observations are defined according to the best operational inclusion and exclusion criteria; how they are diagnosed, quantified, interpreted, and recorded for further research. Gathering the right information from the patient will also depend on the type of **questions** asked. These may be entirely **open-ended** (*"How do you feel today?"*) or **close-ended** (*"Did you have a pain in your back preventing you from stretching your body after you finished chopping wood yesterday?"*). They may be **directive or focused** (*"How did your low back pain evolve throughout the day?"*) or **nondirective** (*"Tell me about your back pain."*). They may be **single** (*"Have you had episodes of back pain recently?"*), **double** (*"Have you recently had episodes of back pain or discomfort when twisting your body?"*), or **multiple-choice** (*"Do you get back pain at work, at rest, or in bed?"*). They can be **leading questions**, pointing to a specific answer (*"You had that back pain yesterday, didn't you?"*) or **nonleading** (*"Did you have back pain yesterday?"*). All these and other aspects of **clinimetrics**[6] will greatly determine the occurrence of problems that will be established in describing disease, comparing cases and noncases in relation to some exposure, interpreting clinical trials, or prognostic studies. The quality and completeness of data is a prerequisite for the satisfactory production, analysis, and interpretation of evidence.

Perhaps the two most important topics relating to medical articles and logic are the search for cause-effect relationships and uses of logical argumentation in the interpretation of findings. Let us look at them now.

5.2 CAUSES AND THEIR EFFECTS

In the simplest terms, a **cause** is *an event* (eg, infection by the human immuno-deficiency virus [HIV]) *without which some subsequent event* (eg, acquired immunodeficiency syndrome [AIDS]) *would not have occurred or because of* *which the subsequent event occured.* A cause is thus either a necessary condition for the effect to occur or a condition that is sufficient in the circumstances. Things become a bit more complicated, however, if we consider, as we do in epidemiology, that there is a web of causes at the origin of disease or its cure and a possible web of consequences emerging from a single cause.[6]

Causation has been defined as *"the relation between two events that holds when, proven that one occurs, it produces or brings forth, or determines, or necessitates a second. Once the first happens, the second must happen."*[7] This definition is in our view too narrow because it restricts causation to sufficient causes. In fact, two types of causes of causes are involved in causation: necessary and sufficient. An example illustrates this twofold conception before we discuss it in more detail in Section 5.2.2: Suppose that excessive alcohol consumption causes a particular traffic accident and injury. In such a case, the driver's drinking is a **necessary cause** of injury. However, some additional factors were needed to produce this effect, such as the driver getting behind the wheel while inebriated, poor visibility and road conditions, the inattentive pedestrian crossing who received the injury, or a person who did not prevent the drunken driver from operating the motor vehicle. A combination of the necessary causes and some of those additional factors as a background situation form an ensemble of a **sufficient cause** leading to a traffic accident and injury.

So how is causation viewed historically and today? The following historical milestones in causal reasoning will clarify this still open question.

5.2.1 Historical Milestones

Aristotle (384–322 BC) was the first philosopher to articulate what is generally meant by a cause. For him, there were four types of cause,[8-10] meaning a factor that is an answer to the question "why?" We illustrate his four causes with medical examples:

- The **efficient cause**: the *"primary source of the change,"*[10] the agent that begins the process leading to the effect (microbial agent, cause in modern epidemiologic terms)

- The **material cause**: *"that out of which a thing comes to be and which persists,"*[10] the affected recipient of the effect or the raw material of which something is made (the affected tissue or organ)

- The **formal cause**: *"the form or the archetype, ie, the definition of the essence and its genera,"*[10] what is produced (the disease condition in the tissue or organ)

- The **final cause**: *"end or that for the sake of which a thing is done,"*[10] the function of the thing produced or the goal for the sake of which someone has produced it (the function of some part of an organ, eg, valves in blood vessels)

Later, John Stuart **Mill** (1806–1873) was interested in methods for determining the cause of a given phenomenon (in the sense of an agent that is a sufficient condition for the phenomenon). He proposed **five "canons of induction"**[7,11] as principles regulating scientific inquiry:

1. The **method of agreement**. If two or more cases of a phenomenon share only one feature, that feature is the cause (or effect) of the phenomenon.

2. The **method of difference**. If a case in which a phenomenon occurs and one in which it does not occur differ by only one feature, the feature occurring with the phenomenon is the cause, or a necessary part of the cause, of the phenomenon, or it is its effect.

3. The **joint method of agreement and difference**. This principle combines the previous two.

4. The **method of residues**. If we subtract from a phenomenon what is already known to be the effect of some antecedent circumstances, then the remainder is the result of the remaining antecedents.

5. The **method of concomitant variation**. If an antecedent circumstance is observed to change proportionally with the occurrence of a phenomenon, it is probably the cause of that phenomenon.

However, some warning is worthy of consideration.[7,11] Although the methods may make sense, they do depend on a preceding analysis of the relevant factors, and they are not immediately applicable to cases in which causation proceeds more holistically, or in virtue of a field of interlocking factors.

5.2.2 Contributions of Present Generations

In the philosophical thinking of the 20th century, more advances in thinking regarding causation were made.[12-14] Paths in the chaining of causes were studied,[15] and experimental and other analytical methods were also developed as a gold standard for proof of a cause-effect relationship.

All these trends were studied in depth by epidemiologists, biostatisticians, and social scientists and their impressive and often-essential contribution is spread across the medical literature.[16-31] The discussion of causal criteria in health sciences remains open and the subject of further refinements.

In summary, Table 5-1 lists in its first section some basic **assumptions** (prerequisites) of causal criteria, followed in the second section by the criteria themselves. For a detailed discussion, see the companion to this book.[6(pp 186-193)]

The ensemble of general criteria[17-19,23] in Table 5-1 may require some additional criteria depending on the specific context, content, and characteristics of the problem under study. Table 5-2 summarizes such additional criteria, brought forward by Evans[23,29] for causal search in the domains of certain types of infectious and noninfectious diseases. They are, however, grouped together with the general criteria of causation as outlined in Table 5-1.

Causal criteria listed in these tables are based on both measurement and judgment. **Quantification** is needed in some cases, such as in evaluating the strength and specificity of associations. Judgment is needed elsewhere, such as in assessing the consistency or biological plausibility of findings. Quantification gives us the size

TABLE 5-1

Fundamental prerequisites and assessment criteria of cause-effect relationship in medicine*

Assumptions (prerequisites, before any causal criteria apply)

- Exclusion of the play of **chance**
- Consistency of results with **prediction**
- Even observational studies respect as much as possible the same logic and similar precautions as used in **experimental research**
- Studies are based on **clinimetrically valid data**
- Data are subject to **unbiased observations, comparisons, and analysis**
- **Uncontrollable and uninterpretable factors** are ideally absent from the study

Criteria of causation

Major

- **Temporality** ("cart behind the horse")
- **Strength** (relative risk, odds ratio, hazard ratio)
- **Specificity** (exclusivity or predominance of an observation)
  - ○ **Manifestational** ("unique" pattern of clinical spectrum and gradient as presumed consequence of exposure)
  - ○ **Causal** (attributable risk, etiological fraction, attributable risk percent, attributable hazard, proportional hazard)
- **Biological gradient** (more exposure = stronger association)
- **Consistency** (assessment of homogeneity of findings across studies, settings, time, place, and people)
- **Biological plausibility** (explanation of the nature of association)

Conditional

- **Coherence with prevalent knowledge**
- **Analogy**

Reference

- **Experimental proof** (preventability, curability)
- Clinical trial, other kind of controlled experiment or "cessation study"

Confirmation

- **Systematic review** and **meta-analysis** of evidence

* Compiled and modified from references 6, 17, 19, 23, and 24.

of an event. **Judgment** means evaluating the nature and the soundness of some information and giving it a value for subsequent decision making.

Pushing the concept of causation further, both philosophers and epidemiologists see multiple causes at the origin of a health problem (or of its improvement), also called **webs of causes.** It should be noted as well that a cause may lead to "**webs of consequences,**" to multiple outcomes. Alcohol abuse is not the sole cause of liver

TABLE 5-2

Specific causal criteria proposed for some types of disease*,†

Henle-Koch postulates for infectious disease of bacterial origin (abridged) (Koch, 1976, 1882)

Parasite occurs in every case of the disease in question

It occurs in no other disease as a fortuitous and nonpathogenic parasite

Once isolated from the body and repeatedly grown in pure culture, it can induce the disease anew

Criteria for a subclinical (inapparent) infection (Evans, 1991)

A well-defined clinical syndrome

Known and identifiable causes of syndrome demonstrable by laboratory tests (antibodies, antigen isolation or identification)

Ability to differentiate between the laboratory markers of acute and of past infection

Occurrence of subclinical cases concurrently with clinical cases, especially during an epidemic or in close contact with subclinical cases

Huebner's considerations for diseases of viral origin (abridged) (Huebner, 1957)

Virus must be a real entity (passages in animal and tissue cultures)

Virus is not a simple contaminant

Antibody response must result from active infection

Specific tissue and cell changes related to the virus are identified

The virus must be constantly present (associated) with a specific illness

Controlled trials in volunteers show inoculation followed by a specific syndrome

Distinct epidemiologic pattern of disease spread in the community exists

Disease is preventable by a specific vaccine (if available)

Material resources available for all the above criteria assessments

Causal criteria for noninfectious and occupational diseases, injuries, intoxications, and mental problems

Criteria from Table 5-1 apply

Causation in disease epidemic (Evans 1993)

Agent isolated from most cases

Agent isolated more commonly in sick than healthy individuals

Incubation period of the agent corresponds to that of the disease

A fourfold or greater increase of antibody titer during the illness

Measures to control agent, vehicles, and people prove effective

Disease and mode of spread reproducible in susceptible experimental animals

No other agent shows the same causal association

Causal criteria for a chronic disease (Yerushalmy and Palmer, 1959)

Suspected characteristic is more frequent in persons with the disease than in those without the disease

Persons with the characteristic develop the disease more frequently than do persons without the characteristic

Strength and specificity of an association with the characteristic of interest must be better than in association with other characteristics

---

*All other general criteria of causality apply.

† Compiled and modified from Evans.[23,29]

cirrhosis or fatal accidents. The latter can also be caused by the condition of the vehicle and the road, weather conditions, other interacting drivers, and so on. Alcohol abuse can nevertheless lead to a web of consequences, which may include not only liver disease but also injury, psychiatric problems, or poor social functioning.

Within a given web of causes, a distinction is made between necessary causes and sufficient causes.[22,32,33] A **necessary cause** is "*a causal factor whose presence is required for the occurrence of the effect.*"[33] A **sufficient cause** is "*a minimum set of conditions, factors or events needed to produce a given outcome. . . . A complete causal mechanism that does not require the presence of any other determinant in order for the outcome, such as disease, to occur.*"[33] For example, let us consider the problem of natural foci of disease, such as the endemic occurrence of malaria in several regions of the world. Its parasitic agent, *Plasmodium malariae,* may be considered as a necessary cause of the endemic malaria spread. In addition to it, a warm and humid climate; specific vegetation; Anopheles mosquitoes; and people entering, living, and working in such areas are all parts of a sufficient cause of malaria endemicity. As another example, possession of a firearm is a necessary condition to shoot somebody, but it is not a sufficient condition for homicide. When there is a web of causes, the distinction between necessary and sufficient causes is important from the point of view of trying to prevent or bring about the effect. If we want to prevent the effect, then we should try to find a necessary cause that we can eliminate; once it is eliminated, the effect will not occur. On the other hand, if we want to produce the effect, then we need to find a sufficient cause. We want a scaphoid fracture to heal; if surgery and/or immobilization does not produce the desired effect, some may try electrical stimulation. Since electrical stimulation alone does not always succeed in uniting the fracture, it is obviously not a sufficient cause, even given optimal circumstances (undisplaced stable fracture with early immobilization). Knowing what combination of additional circumstances is sufficient to make electrical stimulation effective would clearly help treatment decisions. Another example: We want our patients to maintain cardiovascular fitness. Many different patterns of exercise will have the desired effect. Research should try to discover patterns that are sufficient to produce and maintain a specified degree of cardiovascular fitness in people with specified characteristics.

5.2.3 How a Cause-Effect Relationship Is Demonstrated or Refuted

Studies of causes and their effects, also frequently termed *analytical studies,* are essentially based on comparisons. For example, smokers and nonsmokers are compared for the risk of respiratory problems (observational analytical studies), or patients treated or not treated by a drug of interest are compared in order to see which of them will fare better (experimental studies, controlled trials). The same criteria for causality as summarized in Table 5-1 apply equally to both observational analytical and experimental studies (trials).

Analytical studies are considered

Analytical studies in epidemiology are studies in which comparisons of two or more groups are made to demonstrate contrasts between events (consequences) occurring in groups of individuals exposed or unexposed to some putative factor. For example, one may study the effect of alcohol abuse on the occurrence of traffic- or work-related injuries. Drinkers and nondrinkers are compared. The risk of skin cancer may be analyzed by studying its occurrence in sunbathers and sunshine avoiders. In the case of a noxious factor, analytical studies are based on observation rather than experiment. Ethical reasons exclude experimental proof. Nonnoxious and possibly beneficial factors may be studied in an experimental design in which individuals are assigned by the will of the experimenter to either the experimental or control group. Statistical precautions are taken to exclude major biases (systematic errors). Randomized double-blind controlled clinical trials represent the current gold standard of causal proof that a beneficial factor (treatment) works. This methodology is described in detail in most current epidemiology and pharmacology textbooks.

Hypotheses are formulated

Hypotheses are propositions to be confirmed or refuted by an analytical study. Hypothesis testing proceeds either by induction or by deduction.

Induction in this context means generalization from observations.[4] Data are gathered first, then analyzed, and finally conclusions are drawn in terms of a hypothesis formulated on the basis of observations made. Hypotheses may be tested further by experiment and, if necessary, modified in the light of the experiment. We may argue for a theory on the basis of the preceding steps and then derive predictions by which the theory can later be confirmed or disproved.[8]

Deduction proceeds somewhat in reverse. Hypotheses are formulated first either intuitively or from experience. Then, they are tested by an analytical study designed for their refutation or confirmation. In deduction, we can apply Popper's strategy[21] for scientific progress (including causal discoveries): Science makes progress if a scientific hypothesis (one capable of being falsified) is subjected to severe tests that can show that it is false. Progress is not made by continually piling up examples of where a theory works, like indefinitely confirming studies of the same problem, such as smoking and lung cancer. Instead, progress is made by trying to find examples of where a theory fails. Any such failure leads to the formulation of new hypotheses and theories. It is clear that we need multiple studies to confirm the consistency of findings as one of the important criteria of causation.

Deductive hypothesis testing is considered more powerful in cause-effect demonstration but is still widely debated in epidemiologic circles. We should, in fact, see all cause-effect studies as an iterative process in which induction and deduction both play an important role. However, we must understand whether causal proofs are made deductively or inductively to be able to better understand and judge their value.

Multiple hypotheses may be evaluated by studying several putative factors (possible causes) at once. Today, powerful computers and software allow **multivariate analysis** of several possible causal factors at once. For example, the risk of (probability of getting) coronary heart disease may be studied in relation to dietary habits, smoking, blood cholesterol, physical activity, stressful life events, heredity, and other endogenous factors at once. This kind of analysis does not, however, make obsolete two major virtues of causation problem solving.

One consists in **atomizing the problem**: breaking it into smaller, simpler, and more manageable problems, questions, and consequent study designs. "Small is beautiful" shines even in the logic of science. "Atomized" problems may be advantageously brought together later. Potter's earlier-mentioned saying, "*What gets cancer—the genes, the cell, the organ, the organism, or perhaps even the population?*"[34] makes the problem manageable and brings together complementary competencies and experiences from various specialties. The solution to the problem as a whole may be attempted later by integrating the whole spectrum of findings.

Another virtue in causation studies is **Ockham's razor** or **principle of parsimony**: keeping things as simple as possible. William of Ockham (1287–1347), a count and Franciscan friar, is credited for the saying that *entia non sunt multiplicanda praeter necessitatem*: entities are not to be multiplied beyond necessity. For Reese,[5] the sense of this razor is to cut away useless and gratuitous ideas in explanation, and to accept the simplest hypothesis that can explain the data. This principle is, however, only a rule of thumb; sometimes a more complex hypothesis is correct and a simpler one is false. Furthermore, it is not always possible to decide which of two competing hypotheses (both explaining all known data) is simpler.

The almost ubiquitous availability of powerful computing should not be an equally powerful detractor from atomization and "Ockham's shave."

Both strategies—atomizing the problem and Ockham's razor—also speak in favor of deductive research in the context of which they can be better controlled.

In any case, **we must understand from the statement of the problem, the title of the article, and from hypotheses proposed what conclusions are at stake and what premises (evidence) would be sufficient to establish those conclusions.**

Findings from studies that have been carried on are subject to criteria assessment for causation

Some of the assumptions and criteria of causation, as summarized in Table 5-1, merit additional comments. The reader can also read much more about them in epidemiology and EBM textbooks.[6]

Researchers look for **associations** between exposure to a factor of interest and the frequency of disease by comparing events in series (groups) of exposed and unexposed subjects. Association, one of the most used and abused terms in medical literature, means any kind of co-occurrence or co-variation between two or more events, characteristics, or other variables representing possible causes and consequences. **Association does not automatically mean causation.** Causation must be elucidated beyond a single statistical analysis, however sophisticated this analysis might be.

In principle, a basic model for analysis of an association of a single suspected cause and its single suspected consequence is a fourfold (2×2) table, in which the subjects under study fall into one of four categories according to their exposure and health:

	Diseased	Nondiseased
Exposed to the cause	A	B
Unexposed to the cause	C	D

Even diagnostic test results may be seen as a product of cause-effect relationship: "Having the disease or not having it (cause) leads to (produces) positive/abnormal or negative/normal results of a test" (consequence):

	Test result (consequence) is positive (or abnormal)	Test result (consequence) is negative (or normal)
Diseased	a	b
Nondiseased	c	d

Most often, such a table is not treated as a causal relationship (it might be as well), but rather as weighing the balance between "good" (true-positive and true-negative) results, that is, a and d in the table, and "bad" (false-positive or false-negative) results, that is, b and c in the table. Sensitivity, specificity, and predictive values of test results are studied across the medical experience rather than by comparing risks, as in other etiological studies. This information is important for clinical decision making. All depends on the question asked. Is it "Does the disease cause abnormal test results?" or "How many test results correspond or not to the patient's state of health?" The former is an etiological problem; the latter is one of clinical management according to diagnosis.

In **cohort studies**, the occurrence of new cases of disease in time is compared in exposed and unexposed groups, such as the development of new cases of lung disease in smokers and nonsmokers. A group of diseased and nondiseased can also be assembled, and the frequency of exposure in both groups compared in what is called a **case-control design**. Both models are used to draw some conclusions about the strength and specificity of a possible causal association.

Before any evaluation of causation is attempted, the first step relies on statistical analysis of the play of chance in the findings. **Statistically significant findings**, the difference between compared groups in terms of P values, indicate the probability of obtaining such extreme or more extreme results as observed if the dissimilarity is entirely due to the variation in measurement or in subject response, that is, if it is the result of chance alone.[35] Nothing more, nothing less. It does not tell us at all if there is a causal relationship or not. It only tells us whether the play of chance is small enough to examine by other means if an association of interest is causal or not.

Temporality is logical if the cause precedes the effect, "if the cart is really behind the horse."

Strength of an association means the distance between two or more series of observations. A **relative risk** is used for these purposes. In cohort studies, it is a ratio of risk in the exposed and unexposed subjects, $[A/A + B] / [C/C + D]$ in the above mentioned 2×2 table. The higher the value of the relative risk, the stronger the association. Its logical equivalent from case-control studies is an **odds ratio** as an expression of the strength of association between some putative factor (exposure) and its supposed consequence (disease).

Specificity of an association tells us how a particular cause of interest prevails among other possible causes in the web of causes, which may exist at the origin of a health problem. Epidemiologists contribute to this problem in an important way by determining several expressions of **risk**, that is, the probability of a health problem developing. In cohort studies, two important estimations of specificity are **attributable risk** (also called **risk difference**), the difference between two rates $(A/A + B) - (C/C + D)$; and **attributable risk percent** (also called **etiological fraction, attributable fraction**), the proportion of such a difference among all observations in favor of the cause, that is, $[(A/A + B) - (C/C + D)] / (A/A + B)$. The greater the difference between compared rates (attributable risk, risk difference), or the more the attributable fraction approaches 100%, the greater the preponderance (importance, predominance, exclusivity) of the factor of interest among other possible causes of the health problem. Some estimation of specificity from case-control studies can be also attempted.

In the domain of **prognosis**, biostatisticians and epidemiologists handle similar probabilities, that is, what happens once the individual contracts the disease, under the term *hazard*. Cox's **hazard ratio** or **proportional hazard ratio** stands, in the area of prognosis, for their equivalents (relative risk, attributable risk, attributable risk percent) in risk research.

The remaining criteria of causation rely much more, and often exclusively, on judgment rather than on computations. Both **experimental proof**, however, and **systematic reviews** of evidence (meta-analyses) rely on judgment and quantitative analysis, both statistical and epidemiologic. More details about causation must be sought in the epidemiologic literature.

There is no way to somehow score the pros and cons of a causal relationship. One must examine all criteria of causation one by one and judge whether the whole speaks for or against a cause-effect link in the case of interest.

The history of causal proof in medicine (causes of diseases, causes of cure) is as old as medicine itself. Trials of all kinds of remedies as causes of disease cure go as far back as the Book of Daniel in the Bible,[6,36,37] James Lind's control of scurvy (1753),[38] William Watson's study of smallpox (1767),[39] and Hill's evaluation of streptomycin in the treatment of tuberculosis in the 1930s. They culminate in the current standards of randomized controlled trials as we know them today.[40] More recently, an overreliance on the brilliance of biostatistical and epidemiologic analytical methods led to criticism of the limitations of these disciplines,[41] a search for alternatives to a more rigorous causal proof[42] when this is impossible in real life, and EBM itself.[43-45] Underlying these expressions of discomfort are philosophical questions about causation.[46,47]

In all cases, reasoning and conclusions about causation must be cogent and free of fallacies.

5.3 MEDICAL ARTICLES AS ARGUMENTS

All medical articles are statements about health problems, supported by findings (evidence) from original studies or from research or opinion synthesis (meta-analyses, systematic reviews, consensus). In original studies, the way to go is fairly straightforward: The problem is formulated, currently available information about the subject is reviewed, a new hypothesis about the problem is proposed, a new study is built to confirm or disprove the new hypothesis (research question), and data stemming from this new research are analyzed and presented. The biostatistical analysis and presentation of findings can hardly be better these days. But does all this make sense?

The Discussion and Conclusion sections of medical articles (both sections are often brought together under a single heading) release authors from the constraint of data and findings. They provide an opportunity (and obligation) to argue about findings, give them meaning, outline strengths and weaknesses of the study, compare them with other findings, and stress their relevance for further research or decisions in clinical practice. Such an endeavor is no longer a question of numerical operations, but mostly a challenge of critical thinking. The latter must be as remarkable as the quantitative and other methodology that preceded it.

If we are already well experienced in our specialties and have advanced training and experience in research methodology, should we not be equally prepared and trained in how to defend our ideas? If we are the readers of medical findings, should not we readily understand the authors' interpretations and argumentation?

The next two sections (5.3.1 and 5.3.2) offer a brief summary of the link between evidence and conclusions. These comments apply not only to investigations of cause-effect relationships such as causes of disease or effectiveness of treatment or prevention but to any other kind of inquiry: descriptive, analytical observational, technology assessment, and so on. The investigation of a causal relationship will be used here for illustration.

5.3.1 Warrants for Conclusions of a Causal Relationship

In general, Toulmin's model of reasoning[48] applies entirely to the domain of medical research. Arguments about cause-effect relationships are the most frequent ways to deal with medical research questions and answers to them.

A good portion of our knowledge is acquired through **inference**, that is, the process of drawing conclusions from premises and assumptions. Hence, acquired knowledge is an **inferential knowledge**, a kind of indirect knowledge . . . knowledge based on inference.[3]

In particular, **all knowledge of general causal relationships** (smoking causes lung cancer, *Helicobacter pylori* causes peptic ulcers) **is inferential**. Conclusions about causal relationships should be warranted by the data from which they are drawn. That is, they should follow from the data in accordance with justified warrants. This is what we should find in the Discussion and Conclusion sections of medical articles. They are based on our **inference**, that is, the process of drawing conclusions from premises and assumptions.[3]

The justified warrants that apply to arguments for causal conclusions can be derived from the criteria of causation in Table 5-1. A causally relevant factor must precede its effect. In the field in which it has an influence (eg, human beings in the case of the smallpox virus, variola), its occurrence must have a positive association with its effect, assuming that other causally relevant factors are controlled. There must be a causal nexus, a chain of processes, leading in a spatially and temporally continuous fashion from the cause to the effect. There must be true scientific theories that describe the various processes that constitute this causal nexus; these theories may, however, still be unknown. The more components of the preceding requirements that are established, the greater is the support for the conclusion of a causal relationship. However, this support is never conclusive. Even seemingly well-established causal conclusions, such as the conclusion that stress causes peptic ulcers, can be overturned by new evidence and new argument. Science is an ongoing process of inquiry, whose conclusions must always be regarded as tentative and subject to revision.

5.3.2 Arguments at the Core of Discussion and Conclusions Sections of Medical Articles

The Discussion and Conclusions sections of medical articles present a string of arguments and a sort of a **meta-argument** that unites them to answer more complex and encompassing questions.

In medical articles, the message that follows the presentation of results is placed either in separate Discussion and Conclusions sections or in a single combined Discussion and Conclusions section. The discussion of the results of the study is obviously written in natural language and not as an ensemble of Toulmin's six components of good arguments. (See Section 2.4.2.) To judge if a "Discussion" is a good and complete argument, we need to read and reconstruct this section, identify the architecture of the whole argument in terms of the interrelationship between its components, and evaluate it in terms of the criteria for good arguments in Section 2.5.3.

The Discussion section in medical articles may be seen then as one huge argument. To help us understand it, we might expect that such an argument would contain all six of Toulmin's building blocks. Often, medical articles offer this kind of information. Sometimes, however, they do not. In fact, warrants, backing, and rebuttals are often left implicit. Both authors and readers should be able to determine which building blocks are present and how good they are.

Let us take a practical example, fictitious and simplified, to fit our view and explanation:

Health authorities of a rapidly developing industrial and agricultural country, in which the overwhelming majority of the adult population still smokes, analyzed last year's causes of death and found an alarmingly high mortality rate due to lung cancer. This mortality rate was determined to be significantly higher (RR = 1.5) in an industrial area with high air pollution than in the countryside. However, the authors did not at that time have information about these data (mortality, incidence, case fatality rates, air pollution, smoking practices) evolving in time (trends) or about their geographic disparities in the country. In their publication of these preliminary findings, they discussed possible cause-effect relationships such as the local role of cigarette smoking and other environmental carcinogens in a heavily polluted living and working environment in the etiology and outcomes of this disease as well as what the chances would be to control this problem if its confirmed etiological factors were brought under control by appropriate effective health measures. They also discussed directions of future research to better understand this problem.

TABLE 5-3

Discussion section of fictitious medical article in natural language and interpretation in terms of argument building blocks*

Text in natural language (simplified and abridged)	Building blocks of argument
Our data suggest that <u>air pollution</u> **may** be <u>an important causal factor contributing to death from lung cancer.</u>	Claim 1 (What do we conclude from our findings?)
	Qualifier (Indicator of the warrant strength supporting the inference from grounds to claim.)
We have found a relative risk of 1.5, meaning a *50% higher rate of death from lung cancer in industrial areas with high air pollution than in rural areas with low air pollution.*	*Grounds for claim 1*
	(What findings brought us to such a conclusion?)
The data **indicate** a <u>moderately strong causal association.</u> *The attributable risk percent of air pollution for death from lung cancer is 33%.* Hence, <u>*two thirds of lung cancer deaths may be attributed to other factors, mainly cigarette smoking.*</u>	Claim 2
	Qualifier (Indicator of warrant strength)
	Ultimate grounds for claim 2
	<u>*Intermediate conclusion linking ultimate grounds to claim 2*</u>
The possibly important role of smoking even in this study is supported overwhelmingly by **numerous studies that identify smoking as the most important cause of lung cancer.**	**Backing for warrant**
	(What evidence supports the general rule that permits us to infer our intermediate conclusion from the ultimate grounds for claim 2?)
<u>Such a possible interpretation of our findings must be confirmed in the near future by more powerful observational etiological studies in a case-control and cohort approach involving stratified and/or multi-variate analysis,</u> including measurement and quantification of **smoking and exposure to air pollution and occupational carcinogens,** together with **risk markers for lung cancer incidence and deaths.**	Claim 3
	Rebuttals
	(Circumstances undermining the force of supporting grounds, or premises, for claim 1.)
The choice of these variables for further research is justified by findings from **case-control and cohort studies in other countries,** which **confirm smoking, as well as several environmental and occupational factors, as causes of death from lung cancer.**	**Backing**
	(Body of experience and evidence that supports the warrant justifying the inference to claim 3.)

* See Section 5.3.2, and also Section 2.4.2 in Chapter 2, for details. Underscored text in first column indicates claim; boldface, qualifier, backing, or rebuttals; and italics, grounds for claim.

Table 5-3 offers a sequence of statements in natural language as it might appear in the Discussion and Conclusions section of an ensuing medical article and its translation (reconstruction) into the components of Toulmin's model, which would allow us to evaluate the completeness and quality of the whole argumentation.

In this example, we can see that all six basic elements or building blocks of an argument (claim, grounds, warrant, qualifier, rebuttals, and backing) may be identified in the text. All necessary components of an argument are here to properly answer the research question of the article.

Figures 5-1 through 5-4 display in theory (Figure 5-1) and practical applications (Figure 5-2, 5-3, and 5-4) the components of Toulmin's layout of arguments reconstructed from the fictional Discussion and Conclusions section of a medical article, as summarized in Table 5-3.

We may note that some components of Toulmin's layout may be missing from one argument to another. However, these arguments remain correct, as explained in Chapter 2.

From an EBM perspective, needless to say, the claim in Toulmin's scheme of arguments is the main conclusion based on the new evidence generated by the study. The grounds are the underlying evidence that supports this claim, that is, the results. The argument is evidence-based in the sense that the claim rests on systematically obtained observations.

To complete the evaluation of the quality of a medical article, the reader may (and should) try to make use of his or her own experience in the assessment of the

---

FIGURE 5-1

Toulmin's modern layout of arguments: application to epidemiological research (theoretical framework)*

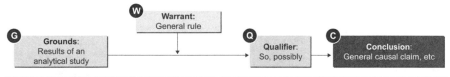

* Backing and Rebuttal(s) are missing in this example.

FIGURE 5-2

Toulmin's modern layout of arguments in epidemiological research: practical example of conclusions about a cause in a study of lung cancer and air pollution (fictitious findings)

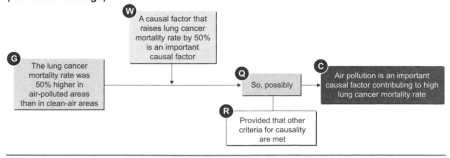

FIGURE 5-3

Toulmin's modern layout of arguments in epidemiological research: practical example of conclusions about the quantified importance attributed to a possible causal factor of interest (fictitious findings)

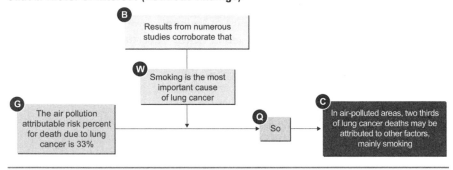

FIGURE 5-4

Toulmin's modern layout of arguments in epidemiological research: practical example of conclusions about strategies of further research (fictitious findings)

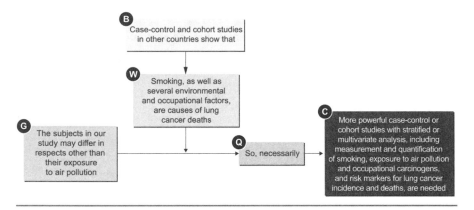

Discussion and Conclusions section of a medical article. The reader can do this by:

- Reconstructing the message into an array of arguments with a clear architecture of their relationship
- Supplying the most plausible warrant for each inference
- Evaluating the accuracy of the data (grounds)
- Evaluating whether each warrant is justified
- Considering for each argument whether good relevant obtainable information has been omitted
- Considering in each case whether there are rebuttals (exceptional conditions) that count against the conclusion drawn.

Peer reviewers and editorial boards of medical journals will increasingly evaluate not only the research question, methods, and results of research studies but also the discussion of results and ensuing recommendations by their authors.

In the Discussion and Conclusions section of medical articles, authors and their readers should pay attention to the earlier-mentioned constitutive elements of scientific argument[48] in order to answer several questions of interest. They are:

1. Can some accepted general theory be extended and applied to the problem under study?

2. Should we recognize some new phenomenon that does not fit the currently accepted theory?

3. In the case of two independent theories, is there any way to integrate them into a more comprehensive theory or system?

4. Should a comprehensive theory be split and fragmented into several different ones?

5. *"Can we find a way of restructuring our whole body of scientific theories so as to yield a tidier and better-organized overall account of the natural world?"*[48]

Focus on such arguments is as important as, if not more important than, discussing the number and characteristics of nonparticipants in a clinical trial, its sample size, or the errors and successes in the study. Where appropriate, the Discussion and Conclusions sections of medical articles should offer as clear answers as possible to these five questions.

5.4 FALLACIES IN CAUSAL REASONING AND ARGUMENT

In addition to ensuring that conclusions are inferred from good data in accordance with justified warrants, we must be on the lookout for several fallacies, especially those related to causation. Fallacies, as already defined in Chapter 2 and treated in more detail elsewhere,[49-51] are mistakes in reasoning, argument, or argumentation. Fallacies in causal reasoning, argument, and argumentation generally involve failure to observe the criteria of causation in Table 5-1. Here is a brief description of some of them.

Inferring cause from correlation

A is associated with *B,* so *A* causes *B*. A study shows a statistically significant association between the amount of alcohol consumed and the incidence of depression. Therefore, alcohol causes depression. Fallacy! The warrant "From evidence of a statistically significant association between *A* and *B,* you may infer that *A* causes *B*" is not justified. More evidence is needed to rule out other possibilities: *B* causes *A, A* and *B* cause each other, some third factor *C* causes *A* and *B,* or the association is spurious. (Even a statistically significant association can be spurious. It may disappear when other factors are controlled.) See the criteria for causation in Table 5-1.

Our fictional example in the previous section (Section 5.3.2) would have committed the fallacy of inferring cause from correlation if it had concluded that air pollution definitely causes deaths from lung cancer. The conclusion that it *may* be an important causal factor was warranted, but the fictional example was clearly correct in going on to conclude that more powerful studies would be needed to confirm the suspected causal link. We sometimes find it irritating when authors of medical articles or health journalists draw from research, for example on the causes or cure of cancer, the conclusion that *more research is needed*. The need for more research is not stressed only for obtaining more funding for the authors' research. It is often necessary for the elucidation of missing links in the chain of causal proof.

Post hoc ergo propter hoc *or "after this, therefore because of this"*

B happened after *A,* so *A* caused *B.* What follows must be due to what preceded it. This fallacy is one of the most well known to epidemiologists. "The fashion of miniskirts precedes an increase of the risk of stomach cancer. Therefore, wearing miniskirts leads to stomach cancer." A remedy to such a fallacy relies on the review of other criteria of causation, which would not support such an argument.

One may argue from case observations that spinal manipulation may cause stroke because it was observed that a stroke victim was treated by a chiropractor before the victim's stroke. The event may be biologically plausible; a presumed consequence follows a suspected cause. However, these considerations alone can never substitute for a full-fledged analytical study (case-control design or other), which would bring more answers to more causal criteria needed for the acceptance or rejection of a suspected cause-effect relationship.

Confounding necessary and sufficient cause

In the web of causes of *B,* *A* is needed. Therefore, *A* is a sufficient cause of *B.* Fallacy! A necessary cause is not also automatically a sufficient one. A ***necessary cause,*** let us remember, is one in the absence of which an event (its consequence) **cannot** occur. A ***sufficient cause*** is one whose presence guarantees that its consequence **will** occur. A microbial agent is a necessary cause, but other conditions of the host and the environment are needed to create, together with the agent, a sufficient cause for infection, disease outbreak, or endemic spread.

Argumentum ad ignorantiam *or "arguing from ignorance"*

Because we do not know that some statement is true, therefore it is false, or, because we have no proof that a certain statement is false, therefore, it is true. This form of reasoning and argument is justified only if our search for the truth has been extensive enough to uncover proof, if it exists. Advocates of "alternative medicine" sometimes use this reasoning without justification: Because it was not demonstrated that something is harmful, it is safe. (There is no evidence against it.) Chiropractic manipulations of the cervical spine do not cause cerebral hemorrhage, because nobody has proved that they do. (In other words, spinal manipulations do not lead to stroke.) Because there is no proof that they do, they don't.

This case of faulty argumentation is frequent in daily life. A dictator must not have weapons of mass destruction, because nobody has proved that he does. Or he must have them, because nobody has proved that he does not. Unidentified flying objects (UFOs) must exist, because nobody has proved that they do not. The same applies to extraterrestrials, effectiveness of miracle diets, sexual prowess and virility enhancers, antiaging cosmetic agents, infallible betting systems, and other hope inducers.

Ecological fallacy (aggregation bias)

This fallacy is also well known to epidemiologists. An association between a presumed cause and its effect on an aggregate level is not necessarily the same as one on an individual level.[33] In our earlier example of the contribution of environmental pollution, occupational factors, and smoking to the risk of cancer, an important difference may be found by comparing communities with clean air to heavily industrialized areas with polluted air. If we were to look at such regional differences by studying individual subjects living in these areas and looking at their occupation, smoking status, and exact location, our research conclusions might differ from those obtained by a simple comparison of the whole groups living in two geographic areas.

Fallacy of division (community/individual fallacy)

This fallacy is somehow an extension of the above-mentioned ecological fallacy. This fallacy occurs when it is assumed that what is true for the class (community) is also true for some specific member of that class. Geoffrey Rose[52,53] stresses rightly that what applies to a phenomenon and its explanation at the community level does not necessarily apply to a specific individual from this community. A collective risk is not necessarily a personal risk.

Fallacy of accident

A **fallacy of accident** stems from the application of a general rule to a particular case in which some special circumstance ("accident") makes the rule inapplicable.[50] This occurs when a general proposition is used as the premise for an argument without attention to the (tacit) restrictions and qualifications that govern it and invalidate its application in the matter at issue.[50] For example, in a clinical trial of a new drug, the prognostic staging of patients remains unknown for some reason. The drug proves beneficial. To conclude that this drug is beneficial for a particular prognostic subgroup would be fallacious. This fallacy is similar to the fallacy of division, except that it transfers the proposition justified for a whole group to a subgroup rather than to an individual.

Fallacy of composition

We should not automatically assume that what is true of the parts of some problem is also true for the whole problem. In the domain of prognosis, Horwitz and Feinstein[54] have shown that lidocaine prevents death by ventricular arrhythmia in patients with a prognostically poor infarction. If the problem were examined in an overall study of all cases without prognostic stratification, such an effect would not be noticed.

Also, this fallacy occurs when one incorrectly argues from a special case or situation to a general rule.[55] For example, a certain drug is proved beneficial for patients in the advanced stages of cancer. It would be fallacious to conclude that all cancer patients, regardless of the stage of their cancer, would benefit from the treatment. This fallacy can be committed if prognostic stratification and its analysis are not considered in clinical trials and interpretation of their results.

Confusion of cause and effect

This fallacy is due to the failure to recognize that there may be a reciprocal causal relation between two phenomena under study. In the study of a cause-effect relationship between depression and alcohol abuse, the problem may be seen in two ways: Either depression leads to drinking, or drinking makes an alcoholic person depressed. A working hypothesis must be clear in these cases, and the detailed review of causal criteria should help to clarify the direction of such a relationship.

Domino or slippery slope fallacy

A researcher may commit this kind of fallacy by making a cause that is responsible for a first consequence in the chain of events equally responsible for the rest of the chain. A stressful life event may lead to a panic reaction, then to drinking, then to the loss of a job, then to family disintegration, then to liver cirrhosis, and then to premature death. Every one of these claims requires a separate cause-effect assessment.

The perfectionist fallacy

In this fallacy, we reject a proposed solution, because it does not completely solve the problem.[56] Let us take this statement:

> *"The health ministry should give up plans to invest more human and material resources in an effort to control the current epidemic. It is simply impossible to bring this epidemic under control."*

In standard premise-conclusion form:

Premise: *It is impossible to eliminate this disease from the human population.*

Conclusion: *The health ministry should give up plans to invest more human and material resources in an effort to control the current epidemic.*

The conclusion follows only if we are justified in assuming some general warrant to the effect that public health officials should not invest resources to control an epidemic if it is impossible to eliminate the disease in question from the human population. But such a warrant is not justified; some improvement is better than none. A counsel of perfection is a counsel of despair.

Irrelevant conclusion (irrelevant thesis, fallacy of diversion, red herring)

The arguer tries to prove a conclusion that is not the one at issue, and thus commits a red herring fallacy. To introduce a red herring is to try to deviate the recipient of the message from the issue at hand by introducing something irrelevant. (The expression "red herring" comes from the practice, during foxhunts, of having servants drag a smoked herring across the trail of the foxes. The fish scent would divert the hunting dogs from the foxes and thus lengthen the thrill of the chase for the hunters.) For example: "*Our public health officer says that if we quarantine all contacts with an infectious disease case, we will better contain this epidemic than if we don't. He is not right, because the whole experience shows that quarantine will not eradicate the infectious disease problem.*"

Two questions underlie this problem: First, whether quarantine is the best available measure to control an epidemic and second, whether quarantine will eradicate the infectious disease. Answering the second question rather than the first means committing the fallacy of irrelevant conclusion if the question at issue is whether quarantine is the best way to control an epidemic. Even if quarantine will not eradicate the disease, this does not mean that quarantine is not effective in a given situation.

False dilemma

A false dilemma[57] is a claim that a reduced set of possibilities is the whole (complete) set. An arguer may present two options from a much wider spectrum and treat those two options as if they were the only ones in existence.

A clinical pharmacologist may carry out a trial showing better effectiveness of penicillin over another antibiotic. Is penicillin the drug of choice in this case? Not necessarily, if other equally justifiable therapeutic options are available to treat this infectious disease.

Ad populum *(appealing to the people)*

We infer a conclusion merely on the grounds that most people accept it.[56] This fallacy appears frequently in the advertising of drugs. "*Take our drug for your arthritis pain! Most family physicians prescribe it!*" Needless to say, prescribing habits do not have the same convincing power with respect to drug effectiveness as a good clinical trial. The warrant that what most people (family physicians, baseball players, etc) accept or believe deserves to be accepted or believed is justified only in special cases, where members of the group in question can be expected to have good reasons for their preference. Even in such special cases, popularity provides only weak support.

Hypostatization

The fallacy of hypostatization,[58] that is, treating something abstract as a material thing,[59] occurs if more abstract (or encompassing) words are regarded as concrete. This fallacy still occurs frequently in medicine, particularly in diagnosis. A collection of signs and/or symptoms that occurs in several people may be given a name such as insomnia, sleep apnea, or schizophrenia. We may smile at a patient who says, "I had an insomnia last night," as if some entity materialized itself somewhere inside the patient's body and caused the patient to wake up and have trouble getting back to sleep. But we ourselves use words such as *sleep apnea* and *schizophrenia* for more or less well-defined collections of symptoms, whose definition is made exact by somewhat arbitrary cutoff points or inclusion and exclusion criteria. Such collections may or may not correspond to a single disease entity such as tuberculosis, in which the common infectious agent shows that we have a real entity.

Objectionable vagueness

A word or phrase is vague if it is not clear, even in context, which individual cases fall under the phrase and which cases do not. We use vague phrases all the time without any problem. For example, if we describe a patient's complexion as ruddy, people know what we mean even though there is no exact cutoff between ruddy complexions and complexions that are not ruddy. Problems arise when it is important in context to know whether a given case falls under the phrase and the phrase does not tell us. This is objectionable vagueness. For example, researchers may claim that they "validated" a new diagnostic or screening test by reporting its good reproducibility. However, validity of a test includes not only its reproducibility (external validity for some) but also its internal validity in terms of its sensitivity, specificity, or predictive value of its positive or negative results. In another case, a clinical pharmacologist may claim (unlikely!), "*This treatment is valid.*" Does this mean that the treatment is effective, efficient, efficacious, cost-effective, affordable, accessible to the most needy, or some other quality?

Equivocation

The fallacy of equivocation occurs if the meaning of the key word in an argument changes in the course of inference. Let us take a rather caricatured, but explicit example:

Premise A: *Only man can get this infection.*

Premise B: *No woman is a man.*

Conclusion: *Therefore, women cannot get this infection.*

In premise A, *man* means human, a species. In premise B, it means a sex within a species. In the conclusion, women are referred to as a different species from man. Although this humorous example would never fool anyone, equivocation can occur in medical contexts. Consider the following reconstruction:

Premise A: *This test has good reproducibility.*

Intermediate conclusion: *This test is valid.*

Final conclusion: *This test has good specificity and sensitivity.*

Here, the vague term *valid* mentioned in the previous section is justified only in the sense of being externally valid. However, the final conclusion follows only if it is interpreted to include internal validity. The first inference requires one meaning, the second another.

5.5 CONCLUSIONS AND REMEDIES TO CONSIDER

Bilsker[60] identifies the following deficiencies in the conclusions of research articles:

- Conclusions that are based on inadequately stated hypotheses
- Conclusions that are ambiguously phrased

- Conclusions that fail to acknowledge negative findings
- Conclusions that use fallacious reasoning
- Conclusions that fail to consider alternative explanations

Such deficiencies produce conclusions that have a limited use for practical decision making. The information they contain may be misleading for patients as well as for medical decision makers.

Bilsker's critique[60] also reflects expectations from the authors of any scientific message devoted to critical thinking in health sciences, as outlined in Chapter 4.

From the critical thinking standpoint, there are currently four major points of concern in medical articles. We illustrate these weaknesses here through caricatured examples attacking poor thinkers and decision makers in medical writing and publishing today.

The first concern is an **overreliance on statistical findings at the expense of broader biological thinking.** The problem starts with noncommittal titles such as "Horse riding and low back pain" instead of "Horse riding causes low back pain" or "Horse riding does not cause horseback pain" or "Does horse riding cause low back pain?" A possible Discussion and Conclusion stating that "we have found an association between horse riding and low back pain" does not specify what the "association" means in this study and does not discuss strengths and weaknesses of causation as outlined in Table 5-1.

The second concern is **lack of specifications for use of study findings.** Are results from a clinical trial specific to a particular setting and to particular characteristics of persons, types of practice, and community? To what extent can the generalization of findings be justified? Once the internal validity (specificity, sensitivity, predictive values) or external validity (reproducibility) of a diagnostic test has been established, at what scale of clinical practice or community medicine program should we use it?

The third is **incomplete and poor arguments**. Titles of articles and introductory statements of study objectives do not present clearly enough the kinds of arguments that will follow, and the link between the starting point of the article and its conclusions can hardly be established. Subsequent arguments in the Discussion and Conclusions sections of the article are disconnected from the beginning or deviate from the main focus. Necessary premises for conclusions may be missing, or a conclusion simply does not follow.

Conclusions such as "more research is needed" may be a simple begging for research grants preceded by erroneous and/or incomplete critical thinking about the problem under study. What is the precise reason for more research?

The fourth is **narrow and uncreative critical thinking.** Alternative hypotheses are neither proposed nor assessed. Often, authors do not find it useful to outline alternative decision making in subsequent practice or research. If they do, they may omit what explanations and recommendations stem from the study itself and what conclusions are drawn from a broader framework of information (beyond the study itself) available through other information in medical literature and the authors' broader experience with the problem.

How should we look at (and write) a medical article as logicians of medicine?

- First, establish whether the message derives from simple intuition as non-inferential knowledge, which is based only on perception, memory, or introspection.
- The message should be acceptable from the clinical epidemiologic standpoint as reviewed elsewhere.[6]
- If it is, examine the title to see if it leads to what will follow as logical arguments.
- If it is not, look to see whether similar information is made explicit in the introduction of the article. If not, try to rebuild it from the available information.
- Try to understand if the discussion of results focuses on the same problem as stated in the introduction.
- If this is not clear, reconstruct all relevant statements and arguments to obtain a message whose cogency would be more suitable for understanding, assessment, and interpretation from the logical standpoint.
- Decide if the arguments are cogent, with justified premises, complete information, warranted inferences, and absence of rebuttals to the warrants.
- Conclude if the whole message makes sense from a clinical, epidemiologic, biostatistical, biological, and medical (decision-making) standpoint.
- Try for yourself to explicate better and understand what the authors did not state clearly enough.
- Accept, adopt, or reject the message of the article.

The recommendations in the previous sidebar are an application of the approach to critical thinking outlined in Chapter 4. They can also be seen as an application of the FRISCO approach due to Ennis.[61] (See Table 4-4 in Chapter 4 for a description of the components symbolized by Ennis's acronym FRISCO.)

The even wider context of development, demonstration, and acceptance of scientific ideas was applied by Thagard[62] to the shift in our views of the etiology of peptic ulcer disease and our acceptance of the *Helicobacter* infection as a necessary cofactor (cause) of this health problem, attributed historically to various noninfectious causes, such as diet or stress. His book is a worthy additional reading to this chapter.

Discussing findings and making recommendations require as much formal training and experience as the scientific handling of the problem at study itself. We are still more prepared to raise questions; carry out a study; and measure, analyze, and present **data** than to reason clearly and in a structured way while generating **information** for further understanding and uses. The ultimate goal of any research or practice information in medical communication should ideally be a better balance between the science so crucial for data production and the logic and critical thinking as pathways to valuable information.

The last blunt word in this chapter belongs to some beginners in medical research who are so impressed by today's brilliant research methodology and all new technologies supporting it. Getting a satisfactory sample size for a study, getting high-quality data, or running a multivariate analysis on them may be an absolute *conditio sine qua non*. However, **it is not enough!** What is done with all the above is equally important, if not more so.

References

1. International Committee of Medical Journals Editors. Uniform requirements for manuscripts submitted to biomedical journals. *Can Med Assoc J.* 1997;156:270–285. (See also *N Engl J Med.* 1997;336:309–315 and *Ann Intern Med.* 1997;126:36–47).

2. Gupta A. Tarski's definition of truth. In: Craig E, ed. *Routledge Encyclopedia of Philosophy* [book on CD-ROM]. London, England: Routledge; 1998.

3. Feldman, R. Evidence. In: Audi R, ed. *The Cambridge Dictionary of Philosophy.* 2nd ed. Cambridge, England: Cambridge University Press; 1999; 293–294.

4. Bullock A, Trombley S, eds. *The New Fontana Dictionary of Modern Thought.* 3rd ed. London, England: HarperCollins Publishers; 1999.

5. Reese WL. *Dictionary of Philosophy and Religion: Eastern and Western Thought.* Expanded ed. Amherst, NY: Humanity Books; 1996.

6. Jenicek M. *Foundations of Evidence-Based Medicine.* New York, NY: The Parthenon Publishing Group; 2003.

7. Blackburn S. *The Oxford Dictionary of Philosophy.* Oxford, England: Oxford University Press; 1996.

8. Helicon Publishing Ltd, ed. *Instant Reference: Philosophy.* (Teach Yourself Books.) London, England and Lincolnwood, Ill: Hodder Headline PLC and NTC/Contemporary Publishing; 2000.

9. Thompson B. *Philosophy.* (Teach Yourself Books.) London, England and Lincolnwood, Ill: Hodder Headline PLC and NTC/Contemporary Publishing; 2000.

10. Aristotle. *Physics* II.3. In: Barnes J, ed. *The Complete Works of Aristotle.* Princeton, NJ: Princeton University Press; 1984.

11. Mackie JL. Mill's methods of induction. In: Edwards P, ed. *The Encyclopedia of Philosophy.* New York, NY: Macmillan Publishing Co, Inc and The Free Press; 1967.

12. Cartwright N. Causation. In: Craig E, ed. *Routledge Encyclopedia of Philosophy* [book on CD-ROM]. London, England: Routledge; 1998.

13. Salmon WC. *Scientific Explanation and the Causal Structure of the World.* Princeton, NJ: Princeton University Press; 1984.

14. Salmon WC. *Causality and Explanation.* Oxford, England: Oxford University Press; 1998.

15. Blalock HM, ed. *Causal Models in Social Sciences.* Chicago, Ill: Aldine-Atherton; 1971.

16. Yerushalmy J, Palmer CE. On the methodology of investigations of etiological factors in chronic diseases. *J Chronic Dis.* 1959;10:27–40.

17. Surgeon General's Advisory Committee on Smoking and Health. *Smoking and Health: Report of the Advisory Committee to the Surgeon General of the Public Health Service.* Rockville, Md: US Department of Health, Education, and Welfare; 1964. Publication No. 1103.

18. Hill AB. The environment and disease: association or causation? *Proc R Soc Med.* 1965;58:295–300.

19. MacMahon B, Pugh TF. *Preventive Medicine.* Boston, Mass: Little, Brown, & Co; 1967:11–18.

20. Susser M. *Causal Thinking in the Health Sciences: Concepts and Strategies in Epidemiology.* New York, NY: Oxford University Press; 1973.

21. Buck C. Popper's philosophy for epidemiologists. *Int J Epidemiol.* 1975;4: 159–168.

22. Rothman KJ. Causes. *Am J Epidemiol.* 1976;104:587–592.

23. Evans AS. Causation and disease: a chronological journey. *Am J Epidemiol.* 1978;108:249–258.

24. Weed DL. On the logic of causal inference. *Am J Epidemiol.* 1986;123:965–979.

25. Greenland S, ed. *Evolution of Epidemiologic Ideas: Annotated Readings on Concepts and Methods.* Chestnut Hill, Mass: Epidemiology Resources Inc; 1987.

26. Rothman KJ, ed. *Causal Inference.* Chestnut Hill, Mass: Epidemiology Resources Inc; 1988.

27. Buck C, Llopis A, Najera E, Terris M, eds. *The Challenge of Epidemiology: Issues and Selected Readings.* Washington, DC: Pan American Health Organization; 1988:147–806.

28. Susser M. What is a cause and how do we know one? A grammar for pragmatic epidemiology. *Am J Epidemiol.* 1991;133:635–648.

29. Evans AS. *Causation and Disease: A Chronological Journey.* New York, NY: Plenum Medical Book Co; 1993.

30. Renton A. Epidemiology and causation: a realist view. *J Epidemiol Community Health.* 1994;48:79–85.

31. Weed DL. Epidemiologic evidence and causal inference. *Hematol Oncol Clin North Am.* 2000;14:797–807.

32. Copi I. *Informal Logic.* New York, NY: Macmillan Publishing Co; 1986.

33. Last JM, ed. *A Dictionary of Epidemiology.* 4th ed. Oxford, England: Oxford University Press; 2001.

34. Potter JD. Reconciling the epidemiology, physiology, and molecular biology of colon cancer. *JAMA.* 1992;268:1573–1577.

35. Ware JH, Mosteller F, Ingelfinger JA. P values. In: Bailar JC III, Mosteller F, eds. *Medical Uses of Statistics.* Waltham, Mass: NEJM Books; 1986.

36. Jenicek M. *Epidemiology: The Logic of Modern Medicine.* Montreal, Quebec: EPIMED International; 1995.

37. Lewis EJ. Ancient clinical trials. *N Engl J Med.* 2003;348:83–84.

38. Lind J. *A Treatise of the Scurvy: In Three Parts, Containing an Inquiry into the Nature, Causes, and Cure of that Disease: Together with a Critical and Chronological View of What Has Been Published on the Subject.* London, England: A. Millar; 1753.

39. Boylston AW. Clinical investigation of smallpox in 1767. *N Engl J Med.* 2002;346:1326–1328.

40. Meldrum ML. A brief history of the randomized controlled trial. *Hematol Oncol Clin North Am.* 2000;14:745–760.

41. Charlton BG. Statistical malpractice. *J R Coll Physicians Lond.* 1996;30:112–114.

42. Tickner JA. Developing scientific and policy methods that support precautionary action in the face of uncertainty—the Institute of Medicine Committee on Agent Orange. *Public Health Rep.* 2002;117:534–545.

43. Charlton BG. Mega-trials: methodological issues and clinical implications. *J R Coll Physicians Lond.* 1995;29:96–100.

44. Black D. The limitations of evidence. *J R Coll Physicians Lond.* 1998; 32:23–26.

45. Goodman NW. Who will challenge evidence-based medicine? *J R Coll Physicians Lond.* 1999;33:249–251.

46. Karhausen LR. Causation: the elusive grail of epidemiology. *Med Health Care Philos.* 2000,3:59–67.

47. Osterwalder JJ. The P value as the guardian of medical truth—illusion or reality? *Eur J Emerg Med.* 2002;9:283–286.

48. Toulmin S, Rieke R, Janik A. *An Introduction to Reasoning.* 2nd ed. New York, NY: Macmillan Publishing Co Inc and Collier Macmillan Publishers; 1984:313–348.

49. Damer TE. *Attacking Faulty Reasoning.* 2nd ed. Belmont, Calif: Wadsworth Publishing Co; 1987.

50. Hughes GE, Wang H, Roscher N. The history and kinds of logic. In: McHenry R, ed. *The Encyclopaedia Britannica: Macropedia/Knowledge in Depth.* Vol 23. Chicago, Ill: Encyclopaedia Britannica Inc; 1992:226–282.

51. Moore BN, Parker R. *Critical Thinking: Evaluating Claims and Arguments in Everyday Life.* Palo Alto, Calif: Mayfield Publishing Co; 1986.

52. Rose G. Sick individuals and sick populations. *Int J Epidemiol.* 1985;14:32–38.

53. Rose G. *The Strategy of Preventive Medicine.* Oxford, England: Oxford University Press; 1992.

54. Horwitz RI, Feinstein AR. Improved observational method for studying thera-peutic efficacy: suggestive evidence that lidocaine prophylaxis prevents death in acute myocardial infarction. *JAMA.* 1981;246:2455–2459.

55. Popkin RH, Stroll A. *Philosophy Made Simple.* 2nd ed, rev. New York, NY: Broadway Books; 1993.

56. Nolt J, Rohatyn D, Varzi A. *Schaum's Outline of Theory and Problems of Logic.* 2nd ed. York, NY: McGraw-Hill; 1998.

57. Bowell T, Kemp G. *Critical Thinking: A Concise Guide.* London, England: Routledge; 2002.

58. Engel SM. *With Good Reason: An Introduction to Informal Fallacies.* 3rd ed. New York, NY: St. Martin's Press; 1986.

59. Mautner T. *Penguin Dictionary of Philosophy*. London, England: Penguin Books; 1997.

60. Bilsker D. From evidence to conclusions in psychiatric research. *Can J Psychiatry.* 1996;41:227–232.

61. Ennis RH. *Critical Thinking.* Upper Saddle River, NJ: Prentice Hall; 1996.

62. Thagard P. *How Scientists Explain Disease.* Princeton, NJ: Princeton University Press; 1999.

CHAPTER 6

Logic and Critical Thinking in a Clinician's Daily Practice: Talking and Listening to Colleagues and Patients

Am I Clear Enough? You've Got It Right!

IN THIS CHAPTER

Do not follow what you know not.
Man's eyes, ears and heart—
each of his senses shall be closely questioned.
QUR'AN (THE NIGHT JOURNEY—AL ISRA), 622–632 AD

Logic is perhaps the most fundamental branch of philosophy.
All branches of philosophy employ thinking; whether
this thinking is correct or not will depend upon whether
it is in accord with the laws of logic.
R.H. POPKIN AND A. STROLL, 1993
(IT IS ALSO SO IN OUR PRACTICE OF MEDICINE.)

Correct diagnoses are based on valid reasoning,
as well as on correct information. The clinician
who disregards logic may naively assume
that he has proved a diagnosis, when
in fact he has only established
that it is possible or probable.
R.B. PRICE AND Z.R. VLAHCEVIC, 1971

In medicine, evidence and logic
together transform impressions
and beliefs into knowledge.

Never forget that "a physician proposes, the patient disposes."
It is, however, a physician's obligation to provide the patient
with the best diagnostic and other evidence available
in a meaningful argument, thus allowing him or her
to make an enlightened decision.

In essence, any clinical care, floor rounds, or medical consult is, and must be, an exercise in applying rules of logic and critical thinking to finding, appraising, and using evidence to the utmost benefit of the patient.

Let us consider the following clinical scenario in the case of a psychiatric emergency in a large teaching hospital, where a disoriented and withdrawn patient, showing waxy flexibility in posture and movement, is being evaluated by a young intern. The intern suspects chronic schizophrenia, acute drug or other intoxication, or something else.

The attending psychiatrist says the following to the intern who examined the patient: *Give him some haloperidol and admit him!* The intern replies to the attending: *I would like to understand your decision better. Can you please explain?* The intern is asking the attending for a full argument supporting these orders. If you, as an attending physician, are able to give one, you do not need to read this chapter. If you cannot, this chapter is for you.

Here is what you should realize:

We all strive to practice rational medicine,[1-4] which should be more beneficial to our patients (and health administrators as well) than medicine of an "irrational" nature. Our health sciences teachers want to make us rational in our thinking, problem solving, and decision making. But what does "rational" mean?

Webster's Dictionary defines **rational** as[5]:

1. Possessing the faculty of reasoning

2. Conformable to reason, judicious, sensible

3. Attained by reasoning

By extrapolation from the same source, a **rational physician** is capable of using his reasoning powers in patient management and community care and habitually applies them. Hence, knowledge is not enough. We need an additional learned theoretical and practical experience from the domain of logic and critical thinking. In this sense, medical education and training as a whole are intended to make an irrational freshman become a rational professional in medical care.

We encounter logic in almost all of our daily activities, such as obtaining and interpreting a patient's history, or making a diagnosis, treatment decision, or prognosis. We must see such uses of logic from two perspectives:

1. **We must know if what the patient tells us makes sense**. Is he or she logical? For example, a good part of the assessment of psychiatric patients focuses on this aspect of dealing with patients.

2. **We clinicians must be logical in our decision making** at each step of our patients' management, for the best possible clinical results, in the face of our

peers and of the patients' understanding of their problems and of our decisions concerning their health and outcomes. Patients are often smarter than we think!

Both perspectives must somehow fit together! Both of these perspectives are reflected in more than one major means of communication: with the patient; when making, keeping, and updating medical records (admission notes, progress notes, consults, discharge reports); or when sharing our experience with and seeking advice from our more experienced colleagues at the bedside, on floor rounds, or grand rounds. We communicate more or less formally over a cup of tea or coffee with our team members and other health professionals, or when teaching and coaching those who will follow in our footsteps.

Deficient reasoning and faulty logic lead to errors in not only communication but also decision making. Thus poor reasoning may harm the patient just as much as poor evidence can.

A word about common sense

Many experienced physicians will swear that common sense is a way to make clinical decisions and solve a patient's problems. "*When I work with a patient, given my experience, common sense is enough and the most important thing in my daily practice!*" Is this really the case? The answer depends on several questions and their answers:

- What does "common sense" mean, and how is it defined?

- Is it the same as a physician's experience?

- Is it really enough to solve daily problems in clinical practice?

- What are its limitations?

- Does it differ from logic and critical thinking in medicine?

Common sense is an invaluable virtue in human reasoning and decision making. It has its assets and limits as well.

In fact, the "common sense" to which we are inclined to appeal for justification of our beliefs and decisions is not well enough defined to be a touchstone. And philosophical conceptions of common sense, which are more or less clearly defined, do not give us what we need in clinical practice.

According to various philosophers, **common sense** is:

- "*The doctrine that we perceive the external world directly, that what we perceive is what there is and how things are.*"[6]

- "*The faculty responsible for coordinating the deliveries of different senses . . . the sturdy good judgment, uncontaminated by too much theory and unmoved by skepticism, that is supposed to belong to persons before they become too philosophical.*"[7]

- "... an appeal to certain innate principles of human nature that are partly con-stitutive of what it is to reason." [8]

- For the Scottish commonsense philosophy of the 18th century "... both sensa-tion and certain intuitively known general truths or principles that together yield knowledge of external objects." [9]

- "A type of reasoning studied by researchers in artificial intelligence." [10] It involves what we call "defeasible warrants," warrants that may be defeated by a rebuttal, or exceptional circumstance in which the warrant does not apply.

In everyday talk, however, common sense remains an ill-defined entity. Furthermore, common sense may even be misleading. If we were to rely on com-mon sense only, we would be convinced that the earth is flat and that the sun rotates around our planet. Common sense remains a poorly defined virtue. It does not replace valid evidence and its critical and logical uses.

In practice, an unsubstantiated certainty about evidence and its uses is often shrouded by "common sense tells us that ..." even if we are unable to specify what common sense means for its proponent. Let us see now what its alternatives and complements might be.

Moreover, Wolpert[11] reminds us that science is not founded on common sense. For Wolpert, if an idea fits with common sense, then scientifically it is almost cer-tain to be false. Probability is also often counterintuitive.

A word about intuition

Intuition means the "*quick perception of* [possible] *truth without conscious attention or reasoning ... knowledge from within; instinctive knowledge or feeling*."[5] It is an inherent part of a clinician's daily reasoning.

However, Altemeier[12] reminds us: "*Be sure you don't fool yourself. Get a full data-base before taking intuitive reasoning seriously. And trust intuitive insight only if it fits all or almost all of the data. The insight should make sense consciously, even if the information had been too complex or conflicting to put together on a purely conscious basis. Give it a try.*"

Good clinical intuition does not mean a "free-floating mind." It is grounded in clinical data and information. More about intuition follows in Section 6.2.2.

6.1 PATIENT LOGIC

Information provided by the patient is essential for our own understanding of the patient's problems and for our own ensuing clinical decision making. A patient's rea-soning may also reveal some underlying health problem such as mental retardation, schizophrenia, antisocial or criminal personality, drug abuse, or altered mental func-tioning due to acute or chronic intoxication, trauma, stroke, or congenital defect.

A conversation between a physician and a patient is typically a mixture of different kinds of dialogues: information seeking, persuasion, negotiation.[13] The physician seeks information from the patient about how the patient feels, what symptoms the patient has been experiencing, and so forth. It is important that this information be clear, accurate, and complete, so that the physician has the best possible basis (combined with data from direct observation and test results) for arriving at a diagnosis. A good physician is skilled at asking questions that elicit the required information in understandable form and at probing when more clarity or detail is needed. The patient also seeks information from the physician: what, if anything, is wrong; what the prognosis is; what treatment or treatments the physician proposes; what are the likely consequences and risks of the various options. Not all patients want to know all this; some are content to leave decision making in the hands of the physician. But it is good medicine and also respectful of the ability of human beings to make choices about their own future, to give patients the information they want about their own condition, in a form they can understand and to the degree to which they wish to be informed. It is also a good idea to check that the information has been received accurately. A patient who is actively involved in thinking and making decisions about his or her own health prospects is, at least in our culture, more likely to comply with what the physician recommends.

Persuasion dialogues (argumentation) form part of the conversation when the physician offers a justification for the diagnosis, or prognosis, or recommended treatments. As previously mentioned, what the physician proposes, the patient disposes. The patient, reasonably enough, will often expect, or even request, supporting arguments for what the physician proposes. Good argumentation, as indicated in Chapter 2 in Section 2.5.3, is addressed to the point at issue, uses premises that both the arguer and addressee are justified in accepting, and draws conclusions in accordance with justified warrants for which there are no exceptions in the particular case. The patient must be able to follow the physician's reasoning. If the patient expresses certain beliefs or preferences relevant to the treatment decision, the physician may either factor these into the argumentation or try to persuade the patient through argument that a certain belief or preference is not justified—for example, the belief of many patients that "natural" remedies have no side effects.

Negotiations differ from persuasion dialogues (argumentation) in that the goal is not to justify a conclusion to someone, but to make a deal. Such bargaining is a small part of physician-patient conversations. However, it can enter the picture if, for example, the patient strongly wants to do something, but the physician considers it inadvisable for the patient's health. The physician, aware that the patient might go ahead and do it anyway, may propose to allow the patient to do it on certain conditions, thus balancing a possibly deleterious effect on the patient's health with other factors on the plus side. (We set aside negotiations over payment by the patient for the physician's uninsured services.)

Patients increasingly seek out information about their diagnosed conditions.[14] We believe that this is a positive development, to be encouraged because it enables people to take better charge of maintaining their own health, which after all is primarily their own responsibility. The advent of the Internet has given most people immediate access to a far larger pool of information than previously. Much of this information is of dubious quality, and physicians can play a role in steering their patients to more authoritative sources on the World Wide Web. On the other hand, patients can sometimes bring to the attention of their physicians things that shed new light on diagnosis, prognosis, or treatment. Critical thinking as a general educational goal implies the development of what Mark Battersby[15] calls "*the competent layperson.*"

Competent laypeople are people who

- Have a broad understanding of the intellectual landscape

- Have strong generic intellectual abilities

- Know how to evaluate information and claims outside their area of expertise

- Can delve more deeply into an area of specialization with efficiency and appropriate confidence

- Are an informed and appreciative audience for works of human creativity

- Have an informed appreciation and understanding of nature and society

We can encourage our patients to be competent laypeople about their medical care (as well as our being competent laypeople ourselves outside our field of expertise). One well-known example of critical thinking by a competent layperson as it pertains to medical care (in this case, a diagnosis and prognosis of cancer) is an essay by the noted paleontologist Stephen Jay Gould[16] titled, "*The median isn't the message.*"

Understanding of or judgment about somebody's or one's own health, giving value to the world around, and handling one's own affairs rely on the understanding of the patient's reasoning and argumentation. Does what he or she says makes sense? A less experienced clinician might write in a patient's chart that "what he says does not make sense," but we must know why and if it's true.

Both psychology and psychiatry deal with all kinds of thinking: remembering, learning, coherence of thought and language, fitting of thought to reality. Logic focuses on reasoning as already defined in previous chapters. **The patient's perfect or imperfect reasoning provides the physician with an important part of the premises for his or her own reasoning and decision making.**

Physicians should try to better understand their patients by reconstructing their argumentation and having patients compare their reasoning with that of the clinician. This is necessary in the case of any intelligent patient. Such reconstruction and comparison improves patients' understanding of their care, their mental well-being, their compliance with care, and the overall success of treatment.

6.2 PHYSICIAN LOGIC AND REASONING

It is up to the physician to make sense of a patient's arguments in the context of a consultation for a health problem, physical examination, paraclinical data (laboratory findings), specialty consults, conservative or radical therapeutic interventions, and ensuing disease outcomes. All this may be seen as a giant logical argument about a patient's health. Let us break it down now into some manageable parts and review its characteristics and major logical points to ponder.

6.2.1 Building Up the History of the Case and Making a Clinical Examination

Listening to a patient's complaint, taking a medical history with respect to the major health problem, other past experiences with health and disease, occupational and social history and family history, and tracing the patient's trajectory through various health and social services are all invaluable sources of premises leading to both patient and doctor conclusions. These premises must be truthful, as complete as possible, and relevant to the task at hand.

On psychiatric interview and examination, we assess a patient's own reasoning and argumentation to see if it is normal or abnormal in terms of a possible affective or psychotic disorder or some other mental problem. "Does what this patient tells me make sense?" Astonishingly enough, we still do not have clear rules for such an assessment, leaving it instead to the "art" of psychiatric diagnosis.

If the patient tells us "*all my neighbors are bastards,*" what does this mean? Are the neighbors subjects of a dubious consanguinity, or do they manifest some moral flaw? Is it true? Is "*I must kill them all!*" a justified conclusion? What is our own conclusion in terms of possible psychiatric diagnosis and possible immediate restraint of the patient? Psychiatrists must find answers to such questions, often and fast.

While interviewing the patient for a somatic problem, we physicians also need truthful information, as complete and relevant as possible, within a cornucopia of premises for our own conclusions and decision making. A patient complains about shortness of breath and chest pain on exertion. Is this one of the possible premises for making a sound diagnostic conclusion? Is this a symptom as something subjectively perceived, or is it also a clinical sign as confirmed more objectively by a stress test and other components of clinical and laboratory assessment in the search for coronary heart disease?

What kind of premises are we getting? Do the patient's arguments use justified warrants? Are the patient's conclusions sound? Is my own reasoning, as the first clinical impression about the case, good (independently of the patient's arguments)?

Our discussion in Section 2.5.1 shows how to evaluate such reasoning. The premises must be justified; that is, they must be evidence-based and provide strong reasons for us to think that they are true. They must collectively include all good relevant information that is practically obtainable. Each conclusion must follow in virtue of a justified general warrant. If the warrant is not universal, the reasoner must be justified in believing that in the particular case no exceptional circumstances (rebuttals) rule out application of the warrant. For example, if the data point to a specific diagnosis but are also consistent with another diagnosis of a much less common condition, is there any reason to suspect that the patient has the less common condition? If the premises are known to match the facts, as evidence does in evidence-based medicine (EBM),[17] the premises include all good relevant information that is practically obtainable, the inferences are warranted, and no exceptional circumstances override the conclusion, then the reasoning may be considered good.

In the assessment of the goodness of one's reasoning, **modal qualifiers** such as "*usually*," "*often*," "*almost always*," or "*occasionally*" can alert us to search for exceptional circumstances (contraindications).

From the beginning of our patient care and management, logic may lead us to our better understanding of the patient and of the correctness of our own judgment about him or her.

A patient history may be taken in an unstructured way or in a structured, computer-assisted one. The resulting raw material may be the subject of formal logic later, as in clinical decision analysis (*vide infra*). The experience of Lilford and Thornton[18] shows that unstructured medical interview and information gathering work well in general practice and in specialty outpatient clinics where intuition plays a greater role and where computerized systematic interviewing may overemphasize trivial disease manifestations and symptoms. **Structured patient histories** work well in more specialized settings, such as antenatal care, infertility, or preparation for surgery.

6.2.2 Making a Diagnosis

Medical diagnosis has two meanings: A **process** leading to some finding about health or disease in a patient, like pathways leading from shortness of breath and chest pain to the suspicion of coronary heart disease. It also means a **product** of such a pathway (a case of coronary heart disease as a diagnostic conclusion).

The process of making a diagnosis may be seen as another example of a chain of reasoning. Links in the chain must be either generated or found elsewhere for subsequent reasoning.

In 1959, Ledley and Lusted[19] initiated a path leading to a better understanding of the diagnostic process by trying to understand a physician's intuitive "*information gathering—information relative importance evaluation—best fit selection from competing patterns in differential diagnosis*" as based on underlying symbolic logic, probability, and value theory.

Diagnosis is a heuristic process, that is, a way of finding things out or solving problems. *A heuristic method is a procedure for searching out an unknown goal by incremental exploration, according to some guiding principle, which reduces the amount of searching required.*[20] A diagnostic work-up of fever of unknown origin, unconsciousness, or coma or making a diagnosis by the method of the "steepest ascent"[19] (*vide infra*) may be considered a heuristic process.

Diagnosis is made by different pathways.[21-23] These pathways may be based on arguments, evidence, or nothing at all.

Ways to make a diagnosis

Seven ways of making a diagnosis will be mentioned here: intuition, pattern recognition, pattern recognition and image processing, induction, deduction, using direction-giving tools (clinical algorithms), and differentiating among several options (differential diagnosis).

DIAGNOSIS BY INTUITION

Sometimes, we reach a diagnosis by **tacit knowledge.**[24] Often, we are aware of certain objects without attention being fixed on them (Michael Polanyi, 1891–1976). Diagnosis, patient follow-up, and training in surgical skills are mastered also through tacit knowledge.

Sometimes, diagnosis is made based on intuition only. **Intuition** is a noninferential knowledge based on perception, memory, or introspection.[25] We may find intuition in diagnosis, risk assessment, or patient interview assessment. Elsewhere, parapsychology would not exist without intuition, however questionable it might be.

Intuitive decision making is more likely to occur in situations marked by uncertainty.[26]

Heuristics in diagnosis are "quick and dirty" mental shortcuts that sometimes err.[27] Intuition belongs to this kind of heuristic process. It has its advantages and disadvantages. Its disadvantages[27 (modified)] are:

- Memory construction of variable value

- Misreading of our own mind

- Misprediction of our own feelings and behavior

- Misreading of our preceding knowledge

- Inflated self-assessment

- Overconfidence in ourselves

- Illusory correlation, an intuitive perception of relationships that do not exist

It also has its good side.[27,28 (modified)] Intuition:

- Makes an everyday perception an instant parallel processing and integration of complex information streams

- Is a cognitive autopilot

- Is a learning tool in young children

- Displays knowledge that some persons cannot verbalize

- Allows us, through implicit memory, to learn something without knowing that we know

- Is a wisdom of the body in situations when instant responses are needed; the emotional and other pathways bypass the cortex, and hunches precede rational understanding

- Stimulates creativity

- Embodies heuristics, mental shortcuts or rules of thumb, which sometimes are the only ones available and at other times precede a more structured and evidence-based decision making

In the world of business, Hayashi[28] stresses that intuitive process, our "gut feeling," may be important if not essential for our decisions and that it quickly filters various options. For this author, professional judgment may be reduced to patterns and rules based on the ability to see similar patterns across disparate fields. However, one must constantly ensure that one is not seeing patterns where none exist.

Some other ways to improve intuitive decisions and actions were proposed by Shaw.[29 (modified)]

- Clarification of intention. Only action that is intended can be said to proceed from an intuition. Try to offer the reason for your intuitive action.

- Clarify and assess the consequences (outcomes) of your intuitive option.

- Would it be possible to make a trial comparing intuitive and counterintuitive options?

- In terms of Popperian falsifiablity,[30] is there any similar situation that would disprove the rightness of our intuitive action? A kind of extreme test case.

These methods detect inconsistency but do not demonstrate the rightness of an intuition.[29]

Intuitive clinical problem solving is for Greenhalgh[31] a rapid and unconscious process, which is context-sensitive; involves selective attention to small details; and addresses, integrates, and makes sense of multiple complex pieces of data. It cannot be reduced to cause-effect logic. She rightly concludes that "*... intuition is not unscientific: It is a highly creative process, fundamental to hypothesis generation in science* [and practice, we may add]. *The experienced practitioner should generate and follow clinical hunches as well as (not instead of) applying the deductive principles of evidence-based medicine....*"[31]

Even if other pathways to diagnosis prevail, the intuitive diagnostic process will always be with us. Hall[26] correctly points out that intuition and uncertainty are inescapable conditions of many instances of clinical decision making. From the point of view of theories of good reasoning and good argument, intuitive diagnoses are perfectly fine as long as the diagnostician has good reason to believe that intuition will produce the correct diagnosis in the case at hand. Evidence-based, logical medical practice does not necessarily mean reasoning and arguing logically from evidence in every particular case.

'GESTALT' OR PATTERN RECOGNITION
Pattern recognition means an instantaneous recognition that the patient's presentation conforms to a previously learned and/or experienced picture (pattern) of disease.[22]

A clinician who has seen just once a case of uncontrolled tetanus (opisthotonos, limited eyelid movement, risus sardonicus, laryngospasm, uncontrolled salivation, convulsive muscular spasms, inability to communicate with the entourage) cannot miss it the next time.

Pattern recognition is seen by some as a kind of **casuistic method**. For Shaw,[29] this technique is helpful when there is no clear intuition as to what is right in a given situation. It is analogous to the **method of case law**. The judgment made in a previous case is applied to the current problem.

Pattern recognition is also seen as an example of a **heuristic process**[32]: *"A short-cut for the generation and support of hypotheses established on the basis of adaptation of patterns from previous experience to solve similar problems. These 'rules of thumb' are based on stereotypes of disease and usually work in uncomplicated clinical situations. This method lends efficiency to the diagnostic process, but may suffer from inaccuracies when situations are wrongly interpreted as analogous, and stereotypical strategies are used by physicians for decision making."*

Ultimately, pattern recognition is not far from medieval **casuistry**, where new cases were compared with past experience. If necessary, experience was adjusted according to the new case or cases under consideration.[33] A similar process is commonly used in building up case law in a legal jurisdiction, where precedents are cited on either side of an issue to be decided and these precedents are sometimes reinterpreted by a judge in the light of a new case.[34]

PATTERN RECOGNITION THROUGH IMAGE PROCESSING

This kind of computer-assisted diagnosis may be considered wherever initial images are available (chest radiographs, EKG, EEG, etc) and information is extracted and reduced for diagnostic interpretation and classification through multivariate and multivariable analysis.[35-37]

EXHAUSTIVE PROCESS OF DIAGNOSIS MAKING: THE INDUCTIVE PATH

This kind of diagnostic process is based on induction. An impressive array of information is assembled from which various diagnostic hypotheses are drawn and an attempt to confirm is made. For example, inexperienced clinical clerks will sometimes gather all relevant and irrelevant information on clinical examination and laboratory examinations to show their elders that they have not forgotten anything (to the despair of health administrators, accountants, and economists). The staff-person will somehow figure out later what all this means. So much care and attention pleases the patient, but not health managers. Moreover, some important diagnostic hypotheses may remain unaccounted for despite all the "milking and dredging" of data.

HYPOTHETICO-DEDUCTIVE PATH

In the spirit of deduction itself, some initial and index manifestations of disease are detected. A first "impression" or "working diagnosis" (initial hypothesis) is composed to lead the clinician to an in-depth diagnostic workup. The clinician prescribes additional diagnostic tests and procedures while treating problems that cannot be delayed such as bleeding, cardiac arrest, suicidal or homicidal behavior, or premature labor. (Alternative or "competing" diagnostic possibilities for the sake of differential diagnosis may be considered at this moment.) Taking the initial hypothesis with skepticism, the clinician refines the diagnosis and consequent treatment. This "right to the point" method or "steepest ascent method"[21] is more economical and rapid than the others and often the most effective. It also makes logicians happy.

Wood[32] comments, "*It is not so much errors due to lack of knowledge or omission that lead to diagnostic failure as it is errors in judgment or interpretation applied to the hypotheses we create.*" The hypothetico-deductive path is most often used by experienced expert practitioners in novel situations and when problems occur.[31] This path also is used in situations in which the time to solve them is limited.

On the other hand, for Jonsen and Toulmin,[33] the diagnostic process means "*reasoning by analogy.*" It contains three elements:

1. A pattern of signs and symptoms includes enough elements that one diagnosis (d_1) among others $(d_2, d_3,$ etc) may be considered as presumptive.

2. These dissimilarities are considered distinctive enough to justify a particular treatment.

3. The provisional diagnosis may be reconsidered in the case of further symptoms appearing, which are possible signs of other, rarer conditions.

This application of the Toulmin model of reasoning and argument, which frames this book, combines pattern recognition with the hypothetico-deductive method.

DIRECTION-GIVING DIAGNOSTIC PATH: DIAGNOSTIC ALGORITHM

The direction-giving diagnostic path, also called by Sackett[22] the "*multiple branching*" or "*arborization*" method, is a step-by-step organization of the diagnostic steps to be followed, in which each step is defined by the result of the preceding one. The path goes unequivocally in the right direction. Figure 6-1 represents a simplified algorithm of the diagnosis of coronary heart disease and the different therapeutic indications ensuing from each diagnosis.

An elderly patient complains of rapid exhaustion on exertion, chest pain, and anxiety. His family physician prescribes an electrocardiogram and, given the anomalies found, refers him to a cardiologist. The cardiologist prescribes a stress test and other diagnostic procedures, such as an echocardiogram, a thallium or Technetium-99m sestamibi scan, and a coronary catheterization and angiogram. If the results show that the problem is a "single-vessel disease" (just one artery blocked), a percutaneous transluminal coronary angioplasty (PTCA) and stenting may be the treatment of choice. (If the patient also has diabetes, cardiologists may prefer a coronary bypass even in the case of a single-vessel disease. This is an example of an exception to Toulmin's warrant; for more information, see Chapter 2, particularly Section 2.4.2.) If "multiple disease involvement" is found, a coronary bypass may be the treatment of choice. Hence, the algorithmic diagnostic process is an **unequivocal direction-giving path to follow.**

FIGURE 6-1

Management of coronary artery disease in invasive cardiology: a simplified algorithmic approach to decision making

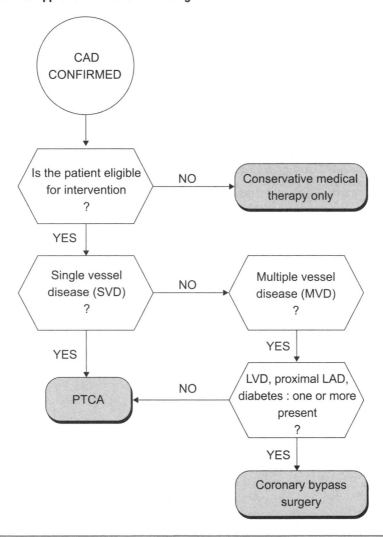

CAD indicates coronary artery disease; SVD, single-vessel disease; MVD, multiple-vessel disease; PTCA, percutaneous transluminal coronary angioplasty; LVD, left ventricular dysfunction; LAD, left atrial dysfunction.

A multiple branching method in the form of an algorithm should not be confounded with another type of multiple branching procedure developed and used in the domain of **decision analysis**. Decision analysis is not a direction-giving method. It is a **direction-finding method** about which the reader can learn more elsewhere.[17,38]

Lilford and Thornton[18] point out rightly that clinical decision analysis as an expert system means using **formal logic** to solve medical problems.

In decision analysis, as initially developed in the world of business, finance, and military arts, models of all possible decision paths are considered, as are various optional procedures to be performed, various treatments, and their outcomes. Some values (utilities) are given by the frequency and severity of outcomes weighted in clinical, financial, and other terms. Then, a best path, given by the frequency of events, their outcomes, and their value, is traced by various methods, such as *folding back* or *sensitivity assessments*. This is an evaluation method of diagnostic-therapeutic options, which leads to clinical algorithms.[17]

However, meaningful clinical algorithms should be based on a step-by-step decision analysis rather than on an "impressionistic" proposal of an algorithm based solely on its author's experience, however valuable it might be.

MAKING THE DIFFERENTIAL DIAGNOSIS

Differential diagnosis is **the process of making choices between various diagnostic options that might apply to the same patient or clinical situation**. The relevance of logic in differential diagnosis was already stressed more than 30 years ago by Price and Vlahcevic[39] in the following terms: "*To use deductive reasoning with a minimum of error we should be aware of the logical fallacies to which the diagnostician may fall prey. Correct diagnoses are based on valid reasoning, as well as correct information. The clinician who disregards logic may naively assume that he has proved a diagnosis, when in fact he has only established that it is possible or probable. Knowledge of the logical basis of proof and disproof should not only hold us to greater precision in individual diagnosis but should also provide a rational approach to devising standard diagnostic criteria.*"

These authors[39] propose to conceptualize differential diagnosis by using what they call Venn diagrams, although in fact they are Euler's diagrams. Figure 6-2 illustrates the case of manifestations that taken singly may not be specific, but in combination are unique. Epigastric pain, histamine-fast achlorhydria, and gastric ulcer may be nonspecific individually, that is, seen in more than one diagnostic entity, but in combination they are specific to cancer of the stomach.

Subcategories numbered in the common field of the three manifestations under consideration may be the subject of further analysis in the search for a more refined diagnosis within the category of stomach cancer.

The process of differential diagnosis in daily practice, which is unsupported by computing facilities, still remains poorly understood in terms of logic and critical thinking.

Fallacies in making a diagnosis

The process of diagnosis is a process of reasoning aimed at finding the **cause(s)** of a **particular** configuration of signs, symptoms, and test results in a particular patient. In other terms, we seek to establish a causal link between some unusual morphology, function, or biological, physical, chemical, or social agent and some particular manifestations of disease, illness, or sickness. As such, the process of diagnosis

FIGURE 6-2

Circle diagram of diagnostic characteristics relating epigastric pain, achlorhydria, and gastric ulcer to stomach cancer*

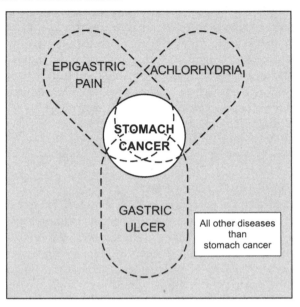

*Adapted with permission from the American College of Physicians. (Price RB, Vlahcevic ZR. Logical principles in differential diagnosis. *Ann Intern Med.* 1971;75:89–95.)

shares many features with **general** causal reasoning, which is required to establish the cause or causes of diseases and the effectiveness of treatments (see Chapter 5).

Some of the fallacies mentioned in Chapter 5 are also committed in diagnostic reasoning. We list here some common pitfalls peculiar to diagnostic reasoning.

FAULTY EVIDENCE ABOUT THE PATIENT

Some **information obtained from the patient's own reports** may be incorrect. The possibility of such errors underlines the importance of careful clinimetrics, questioning the patient, double-checking, and accurate record-keeping. The more crucial it is that the diagnosis be accurate, the more worthwhile it is to check the accuracy of the patient's reports and your interpretation of them.

Observable signs may be missed or misinterpreted. The patient's unstable gait may be taken for a possible neurologic problem, whereas he or she may be inebriated or wearing ill-fitting shoes.

Test results may be inaccurate in terms of their sensitivity, specificity, and predictive value of the positive or negative result of the test. All major reasons for such an inaccuracy are discussed elsewhere in the clinical epidemiologic literature.[16] Some reasons are technical. Either the test was done improperly (eg, with contamination of a sample from another source) or the product of the test (eg, an X-ray film) was misinterpreted or the reported result was actually the result for another patient. Reputable testing facilities have well-qualified personnel and careful proce-dures to guard against such inaccuracies, but they can occur. If a test result does not fit the pattern of other signs, symptoms, and results, it is important to make sure that the result is accurate, and a repetition of the test may be indicated.

FALSE DILEMMA

This fallacy occurs in reasoning and arguments based on exclusive and exhaustive "yes or no" considerations when other alternatives and options exist. This fallacy may occur in differential diagnosis. For example, a patient after having received a kidney transplant develops a fever. Is this due to an infection related to the surgery itself, or is it a sign of organ rejection? Are these two options the only possible ones or are there any others? May there be another concurrent new additional infec-tious disease? Drug reaction? Some other comorbidity? Infection or rejection may be the most prevalent considerations, but not the only ones. Needless to say, a dif-ferential diagnostic process should be based on all clinically important possibilities and options.

This situation is similar to a political slogan, "*whoever is not with us, is against us.*" There may be some people who are neither for nor against the ideologist in question.

ARGUMENTUM AD VERECUNDIAM

The *argumentum ad verecundiam* ("argument from bashfulness") is almost ubiqui-tous in daily hospital practice in the advancing and/or accepting of claims based solely on the prestige, status, or respect of its protagonists and proponents.

Two clinical clerks discuss the relevance of a lumbar puncture in a multiple trauma sufferer. "*Why should we do this procedure in this patient? . . . . Because the staffperson said so!*"

This is an unquestioning appeal to the prestige of someone whose dictum is unsupported by evidence, reasoning, or argument. Such appeals should be distin-guished from appeals to the legitimate authority of peer-reviewed scientific publi-cations, where data are reported and arguments are given. Of course, a clinical clerk or intern must do what the attending physician orders. But the order is not in itself a justification for doing the procedure. If one wants to know why it is the right thing to do in the circumstances, substantive reasons should be given.

The *ad verecundiam* fallacy occurs in treatment decisions and prognosis as well as in diagnosis.

OCKHAM'S RAZOR

Applied to diagnosis, Ockham's razor[40,41] can be expressed as the principle: If you can explain all the observations, reported symptoms, and test results by a condition that you know the patient has, do not bother ruling out another condition that might explain some or all of the same data. The razor is a useful rule of thumb but, as pointed out in Chapter 5, not an infallible guideline. Sometimes a patient who has suffered a fall has two broken bones, not just the one visible on the X-ray film. Sometimes a patient has two infections, not just the one identified by laboratory testing. It is a fallacy to think that knowing that a patient has a condition which explains all the data **proves conclusively** that the patient does not have some other condition as well that would explain some or all of the data. To think this way is to take something that follows inductively (probabilistically) from the data as following deductively (necessarily). Ockham's razor is a defeasible warrant, one that can be defeated by further information, not a necessary warrant.

THE "IS-OUGHT" FALLACY[42]

This fallacy is based on an assumption that if something **is** now in practice, it **ought** to be so. This assumption, or warrant, is not justified. You need some reason to think that what you are now doing has a good basis other than the fact that you are doing it. "*In our practice, the periodical examination for male patients over 50 years of age includes obtaining a chest radiograph. A chest radiograph ought to be an integral part of the periodic examination of healthy senior adults.*" (This, of course, is not the case.)

6.2.3 Treatment

Diagnoses as a process may be seen as examples of reasoning; they lead from such premises as the results of clinical examination or paraclinical tests to the conclusion that the patient has or does not have the disease under consideration. Treatment decisions can also be seen as examples of reasoning. The conclusion of the diagnostic process becomes a premise leading to the conclusion that the patient should or should not be treated, and by which therapeutic maneuver, such as drugs, surgery, support, and so on.

In essence, treatment decisions are a kind of managerial decision that can be analyzed as a categorical syllogism or, more plausibly, by Toulmin's model of reasoning (see Section 2.4.2).

Making treatment decisions

Treatment decisions are conclusions of reasoning, which may be communicated as arguments. Premises may be the findings in the patient or past experience with a treatment of interest, whereas conclusions are treatment orders in patient charts.

Premise A: *My patient has single-vessel coronary heart disease.*

Premise B: *Clinical trials and other experience show that this type of coronary heart disease is preferably treated by coronary angioplasty.*

Conclusion: *I am booking my patient for the earliest possible transluminal coronary angioplasty (PTCA).*

Typically, we reason from a diagnosis of the patient's condition, along with other information about the patient (eg, suitability for an operation), directly to a decision about treatment. Our inference is warranted if the best available evidence shows that the treatment is preferable for patients with the diagnosed condition and the particular characteristics of this patient. In the somewhat artificial example just noted, premise B states that such evidence justifies the warrant, entitling us to infer the conclusion from premise A.

The effectiveness of treatment as a cause-effect relationship is best determined by randomized, double-blind, controlled clinical trials. These trials are often based on "neat," that is, uniform, clinical cases, but in the "real" world, treatment is applied to heterogeneous patients, who differ in their demographic characteristics, stages and severity of disease, prognostic characteristics, comorbidities, treatments for comorbidity, and so on. The evaluation of clinical trials must be extended to this reality of clinical practice, which might be called phase 5 clinical trials and assessment.[17]

Where results from clinical trials or other equivalents of experimental cause-effect proof are missing, warrants for conclusions about treatment must be sought and found in other kinds of nonexperimental, analytic observational, and/or other studies.[17]

Clinical decision makers must integrate more than clinical-epidemiologic evidence in a spectrum and hierarchy adopted by EBM. Evidence from basic sciences, economic evidence, philosophical and ethical evidence (nature of clinical methods), psychological evidence (patient's values and preferences), contextual evidence (from the patient's entourage and environment), and organizational evidence (health systems in which we live)[28] make reasoning and decisions more complex if they are to be integrated.

In treatment decisions, unlike in diagnosis, intuitive thinking with or without experience is the worst (but sometimes the only available) option. Usually, enough experience from clinical trials and observational studies is available to either make an instant decision, or better, to search for the best treatment decision for a more long-term strategy through decision analysis. Clinical algorithms are also based on such analytic studies. Both decision analyses as "direction-searching tools" and algorithms as "direction-giving tools"[16] combine diagnostic, therapeutic, and prognostic steps. More about these tools may be found in our sister book.[17]

Fallacies in treatment decisions

Faulty decisions about treatment can be due to ignorance of the best available relevant evidence. Such ignorance is not a logical fallacy, but we mention it here for completeness.

IGNORING THE QUALIFICATION

A common mistake in reasoning about treatment decisions is to ignore a relevant qualification, for example, a contraindication to an otherwise preferable treatment. Penicillin is not a preferable treatment for patients who are allergic to it. To prescribe penicillin without checking whether the patient is allergic to it is to commit the fallacy of dropping the qualification, even if in the particular case the patient turns out not to be allergic. It means deciding on a certain treatment when the best available evidence indicates only that it is preferable under certain conditions, which the particular patient may not meet. For example, immunization may be a good option to prevent an infectious disease in individuals whose immunobiological state allows for the development of immunity. It may be questionable in immunocompromised patients or some people with chronic disease. The technical name for this fallacy is **secundum quid**, or more fully **a dicto secundum quid ad dictum simpliciter**, from what is said with a qualification to what is said simply. This is also known as the fallacy of **accident**.[43]

SUPPRESSING EVIDENCE

Ultimately, the treatment decision is the patient's. "*The doctor proposes, the patient disposes.*" The patient makes the treatment decision from the perspective of his or her own values and settled wishes, not from the perspective of the physician's values and wishes. The patient therefore needs to get from the physician, in a form that he or she can understand, all the information that is relevant from the perspective of his or her values and wishes. A side effect that may be so improbable or so slight from the physician's point of view as to not be worth thinking about may be a serious negative factor from the patient's point of view. If so, the physician must mention it. Courts have ruled that what should be disclosed should be considered from the point of view of what a reasonable patient would want to know in the circumstances and not from what a reasonable doctor would want to disclose.[44] To omit such information in proposing a treatment is to commit the fallacy in argument of **suppressing evidence**.[45]

POST HOC ERGO PROPTER HOC (AFTER THIS, THEREFORE BECAUSE OF THIS)

B happened after A, so A caused B. This fallacy can occur not only in writing and interpreting research reports, as discussed in Chapter 5, but also in evaluating the treatment of an individual patient. It may also mean an immediate causal explanation for an event without considering alternatives.[46] Causal claims in conclusions are not supported by their premises. For example:

- *You look great!*

- *I see that you are taking these nutrition supplements daily.*

- *They really work wonders with you!*

SLIPPERY SLOPE

A slippery slope argument is an argument against some action (or for it) based on an alleged chain reaction of steps in the wrong direction (or right steps in the good direction) leading to an undesirable (or desirable) outcome. Slippery slope arguments are cogent if the slope really is slippery, and is known to be slippery—that is, we have good evidence that each link in the chain will occur as predicted if the action (treatment) is performed. Slippery slope arguments commit a fallacy if the linkage is largely speculative:

- *If you give methotrexate or cyclosporine to this patient, you will immunosuppress him!*

- *If you immunosuppress him, he will catch a cross-infection.*

- *If he catches a cross-infection, you will not be able to control it.*

- *If you can't control it, he will die.*

One or more such premises may be false, because the outcome is presented as a certitude and not as a probability of two or more options. In these statements, one thing leads inevitably to another.

6.2.4 Prognosis and Risk Assessment

Prognosis and risk assessment are both processes of reasoning to a conclusion. The premises may include patient characteristics, past therapeutic experience or exposure to risk factors, and experience with desired and adverse effects of preventive and therapeutic interventions. The conclusion is that the patient will fare well or poorly within a defined time span.

Basic considerations: prognosis vs risk

Prognosis is one of the inherent but often unappreciated duties of the physician[47-51] and an integral and fundamental part of clinical practice. It represents a rather heterogeneous ensemble of considerations.

Intuition is even less important here than in treatment decisions and is more an attitude of faith than logic fueled by evidence.

Outcomes of disease may be studied by observational longitudinal studies to establish such and such a probability of an outcome (event) in time, such as other disease spells, occurrence of new complications, new comorbidity, cure, or death.

Elsewhere, prognostic studies are derived from a time-extended follow-up of outcomes in clinical trials or observational analytic studies. More than one group of patients are then involved and compared. Absolute and relative probabilities of outcomes are formulated as a **hazard**, absolute for a given group or relative to some other control group.

Risk as the probability of new cases of disease in the community in previously healthy subjects was already extensively discussed in the previous chapter. **Risk as assessment of disease occurrence** is essentially an evaluation of the cause-effect relationship between some **factors and disease before it occurs in individuals who do not have it and who might get it. Prognosis** means **the probability** of some events (outcomes) **in individuals who already have the disease.** For some, prognosis also includes other predictions of outcomes in individuals who still either do not have the disease or have not been treated for it or anything else. This distinction between risk and prognostic characteristics (factors and markers) is often confounded in the current literature. The reader is encouraged to read Chapter 5 of this book as well as good sources of information in epidemiologic and EBM textbooks[17] and other related literature.

Fallacies in making a prognosis

This domain of clinical considerations also has its own flaws and fallacies.

DIVISION AND COMPOSITION

Taking the truth about some whole as applying to each one of its parts or vice versa is a fallacy occurring in research, practice, and the outside world. "The prognosis of cancer is bad!" Often yes, but is it true for all of its stages, all sites, all types of medical facilities and care available? Not necessarily. Prostate cancer has a better prognosis than pancreatic cancer. Similarly, angioplasty can do marvels for single-artery coronary disease, but not necessarily in advanced atherosclerosis involving several coronary arteries.

OVERSIMPLIFICATION

This fallacy occurs if we look at prognosis too globally, without "*atomization*," a term used by logicians for breaking down a huge problem into manageable pieces. For example, a good or bad prognosis may simply mean a principal outcome of the disease of interest such as death and some of its determining clinical and other factors. Another prognosis may concern the prediction of the occurrence of additional other diseases, treatment for such comorbidity, or outcomes of the latter. To say that "a prognosis is good" or "bad" does not necessarily refer only to survival or that the patient will walk out alive from the hospital.

Fifteen basic categories of an "atomized" problem of prognosis may be found elsewhere.[18] Just saying that the prognosis in this patient is good or bad does not necessarily always mean a good or poor survival or life expectancy. For example, exposure to some prognostic beneficial factor like treatment may lead to a better prognosis in terms of a better course of the major health problem under treatment, or it may improve the course of other comorbid states (other diseases of interest). Or it may be a good prognostic factor in relation to other health problems occurring with the index health problem, such as cross-infection, new degenerative processes, or injuries—without necessarily affecting overall survival.

MISLEADING USE OF STATISTICS

Prognoses are often stated in terms of probabilities, or in terms of measures of central tendency. "*Abdominal mesothelioma is incurable, with a median mortality of only eight months after discovery*."[16] This information, extracted by the noted paleontologist Stephen Jay Gould from the technical literature soon after he received a diagnosis of abdominal mesothelioma, could easily be taken to mean that he would probably be dead within eight months. Gould's technical training in statistics enabled him to avoid drawing this dispiriting conclusion. In the first place, the expected time to death can vary according to several **prognostic markers (not modifiable) and factors (modifiable)**: in this instance, age, stage at which the disease was diagnosed, quality of medical treatment, and patient's attitude. In Gould's case, these markers and factors were all on the side of longer life expectancy. Second, cases are **not always uniformly distributed** around a median (middle-ranking) value. In this instance, the 50% of recorded patients with abdominal mesothelioma who died in eight months or less were clustered in this short period, but the 50% who lived for eight months or more were spread out over a period of several years. Third, statistical distributions **apply only to a prescribed set of**

circumstances. In this instance, the reported median applied to patients given conventional treatment, and Gould was placed on an experimental treatment protocol. In fact, he lived for 20 years after his diagnosis and died of an apparently unrelated cancer.

CONFUSION OF CONTROLLABLE WITH UNCONTROLLABLE PATIENT CHARACTERISTICS

Some patient characteristics associated with differential prognosis cannot be controlled: for example, age, sex, and past smoking and drinking history. Others can be controlled: for example, future smoking and drinking habits, treatment, future exercise regimens, and attitude. We call the uncontrollable relevant characteristics **prognostic markers** and the controllable ones **prognostic factors**. The evidence from analytic studies for the relevance of prognostic factors may not conclusively establish their causal role, but it can be good enough to establish a presumption, which can be the basis for recommendations about treatment and future patient behavior. Prognostic markers may help in communicating to a patient his or her future prospects, but by definition they cannot form the basis of recommendations directed at improving prognosis. To confuse the two types of characteristics by calling them both prognostic factors is to invite confusion on the part of the patient. Age may be a powerful prognostic marker for an elderly patient, but he or she cannot be rejuvenated to improve his or her prognosis of disease statistically related to age.

CONFUSION OF RISK FACTORS WITH PROGNOSTIC FACTORS

Further confusion may stem from a mix-up of risk factors and markers and prognostic factors and markers, as outlined in more detail elsewhere.[17] It is a fallacy to assume that a good or bad risk factor is an equally good or bad prognostic factor.

Example: A physician advises his patient, a heavy smoker in whom he has discovered advanced lung cancer, to stop smoking immediately. Heavy smoking was most probably a powerful risk factor leading to the development of the cancer, but there is no evidence that stopping smoking at this stage of disease will improve the prognosis of this patient. (Antismoking advice may, however, be given for other reasons.)

Another example: An alcoholic patient's cancer of the pancreas was alleviated by a triple bypass operation called Whipple procedure. The attending surgeons allowed the patient to continue drinking his Beaujolais wine once discharged. Even though the patient's drinking was the probable risk factor that produced his cancer, the surgeons were not faulty because continued drinking was not a prognostic factor; the patient was doomed to die soon anyway.

GAMBLER'S FALLACY

Because a chance event had a certain run in the past, the probability of its future occurrence is altered.[42] This fallacy may occur when discussing prognosis with patients. There is a 1% probability of adverse effects from a medical intervention. A patient considers having a hip replacement done at a local hospital: "*Orthopedic surgeons in this hospital operated without problem on 99 patients until now. I should not have my hip replacement done there, because I am the one who will have problems!*"

RED HERRING

This fallacy refers to attempting to hide the weakness of a position by drawing attention away from the real issue to another, not necessarily equally relevant issue. The comparison is to red cooked herring dragged across the hunting track to divert hunting dogs from their prey (or prison escapees trying to confuse police search dogs). An attending physician, for example, says to his patient: *"Mrs. Warren, don't be concerned by pain and fever after this surgery. At your age, your risk of pulmonary embolism or a cerebral-vascular accident is much greater."*

6.2.5 Making Decisions About a Particular Patient in a Particular Setting: Phronesis in Medicine?

It was Geoffrey Rose[52,53] who drew our attention to the fact that getting good evidence about some risk factor and the consequences for the whole community or a group of patients does not necessarily mean that the same risk factor will be similarly important in a specific patient and his or her specific setting. A patient may ask: *"Doctor, I know that smoking increases the risk of lung cancer eight times or more in the community. But what is the risk for me? I do smoke. But my workplace, my lifestyle, and the air I breathe all differ from what prevails in the rest of my community."* What will you say to your patient?

Good decisions in practice about a specific patient in a specific setting are the most challenging, because even if the best evidence is available, it is not sufficient to merely apply it.

For Feinstein,[54] *nothing done with nature can be all art or all science.* **Clinical judgment** is quite different from deductive logic employed in diagnosis, treatment, risk, or prognosis. Its background is clinical experience, and it depends on the knowledge of patients, the things clinicians have learned at the bedside in the care of sick people.

We may see an evidence-based approach to health problems in practice as a two-stage process. First, the question of evidence itself, which relies heavily on science (*episteme* of the ancient Greek philosopher Aristotle). Then, using it (Aristotle's *techne*) is the art of medicine. Both involve logic and critical thinking. This view stems from the latest definition of EBM: For its protagonists,[55] EBM is redefined as *"the integration of best research evidence with clinical expertise and patient values,"* where:

- **Best research evidence** means clinically relevant research

- **Clinical expertise** means the ability to use clinical skills and experience at all stages of clinical work with the patient.

- **Patient values** mean each individual's unique preferences, concerns, and expectations related to clinical decisions.[55]

Patients' personal values, their psychological state, and the familial and socioeconomic context in which they live may modify, even nullify, therapeutic decisions based on scientific certitude.[56]

Science provides "raw material"; the art of medicine arranges it in a proper manner.

Applying research evidence to a specific patient in a particular clinical setting through clinical expertise and fitting patient values has been described as **medical phronesis.**[56] The label *phronesis,* Aristotle's word for practical sense or practical wisdom, has been applied to the process in medicine of rational clinical reasoning. It is *the process of knowing and doing, experiencing and acting, undertaken by a physician on behalf of the patient.*[56] Others have defined phronesis as *"the ability to solve problems by making sense of information using creative, intuitive, logical and analytical mental process,"*[57] *"practical wisdom in dealing with particular individuals, specific problems, and the details of practical cases or actual situations."*[33] Phronesis in Aristotle's conception is a virtue that attains the truth for the sake of an action, not the truth for its own sake.

Along with others,[58] we are skeptical about this attempt to replace the traditional conception of clinical reasoning as a combination of the science and art of medicine with a conception of it as phronesis or practical wisdom. Aristotle defines phronesis as "a true state, along with reason, of acting concerning human goods."[59] The practical and wise person, in Aristotle's conception, wishes for the correct ultimate end for himself or herself, reasons well in the particular situation on how to bring about that end, and acts accordingly. In such action, which Aristotle calls **praxis,** the good of the action lies in the action itself; the ultimate end is realized in the very performance of the action. Physicians are, of course, human beings, and like any human being, they have some conception of their own ultimate goals and can develop wisdom about these goals and how to achieve them in particular situations. But the practice of medicine is not an attempt to bring about the ultimate good for the patients on whom it is practiced. It is in the service of their health, along with related goals: physical comfort, absence of suffering from illness or injury, and so on. The physician as a physician has no idea whether helping to restore a patient's health, or to preserve it, or to prolong a patient's life is, all things considered, for the ultimate good of that patient. As Plato already pointed out more than two millennia ago, health sometimes harms a person and is advantageous only if it is used wisely under the guidance of knowledge.[60] The subordinate status of health among human goods is the main reason why physicians ought to respect the autonomy of patients. It is the patient's own settled wishes that should guide treatment decisions, along with the physician's expert diagnosis, prognosis, and laying out of treatment options with likely prognosis under each.

The application of medical knowledge in particular situations is not a matter of applying "exceptionless" universal rules to particular situations in light of the unequivocal knowledge that the rule applies. Rather, it involves judgment about the particular case, judgment that is developed over time by experience. However, recognition of this fact is compatible with viewing medical practice as the exercise of a *techne* (art). Medical examination, diagnosis, prognosis, and treatment are not forms of praxis guided by practical wisdom about the patient's ultimate good. They are exercises of a *techne* or art, whose goodness lies ultimately in the product (the patient's health, comfort, etc) rather than in the performance.

In the exercise of the physician's craft, EBM meets the epistemology of clinical reasoning, the roles of knowledge, reason, and experience. Physicians in their practice deploy scientific knowledge (most often probabilistic); use statistically validated norms of human biological function; compare clinical data from the individual patient with scientifically derived concepts of the normal or abnormal, the physiological and pathological; choose the treatment; and make a "scientific" prognosis. The ultimate challenge of clinical reasoning is *the choice and pursuit of a particular course of therapeutic action in a concrete situation pervaded by uncertainty.*[56]

Figure 6-3 shows the link and complementarity between the general and the particular in clinical reasoning.[33] Figures 6-4 and 6-5 show its practical applications. Toulmin's approach to reasoning, which forms the framework of this book, accommodates both general warrants based on the best available evidence and particular facts about the individual patient (in clinical practice) or the particular community (in community medicine).

Figure 6-6 displays in a somewhat different fashion the same linkage of general and particular, including the patient's values and preferences.

The evidence part of the clinical process answers questions contained in the medieval Latin hexameter *quis, quid, ubi, quibus auxiliis, cur, quomodo, quando*—who, what, where, by what means, why, how, when. (The hexameter was developed by theologians—for example, the 13th century Danish theologian Augustine of Dacia—for use as a meditation to analyze the deviation of the soul from the path of righteousness[61] and has since been used in many contexts, including clinical practice, as a rubric for gathering all relevant information.) The practical judgment of the clinician questions "all this, in this precise case and its setting."

FIGURE 6-3

Toulmin's modern layout of arguments and its six components: theoretical model*

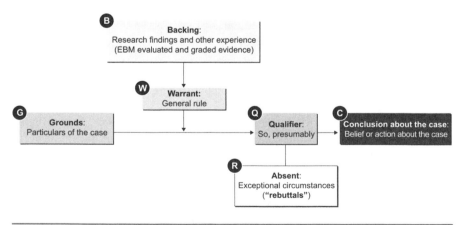

*Information adapted from Walther[61] and Bowell, et al.[62]

FIGURE 6-4

Toulmin's modern layout of arguments and its six components (clinical example: coronary artery disease management in invasive cardiology)

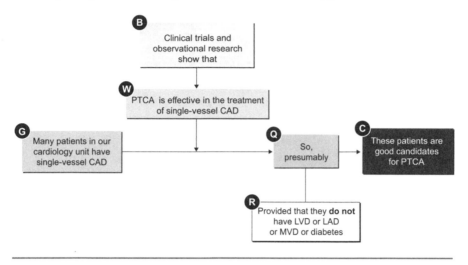

FIGURE 6-5

Toulmin's modern layout of arguments and its six components (public health and community medicine example: surveillance and control of infectious disease in the community)

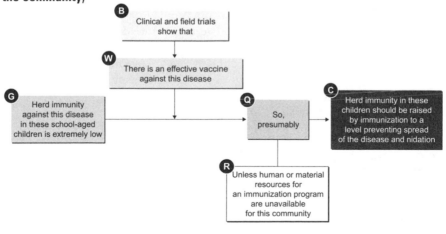

FIGURE 6-6

Integrating evidence, experience, context, medical evaluation, patient values, and preferences in decision-making in evidence-based medicine

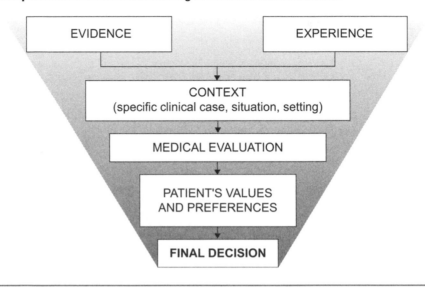

In fact, all clinical medicine is the reflective use of medical judgment in dealing with the specific conditions of individual patients—simply "applied biomedical science."[33]

Hence, any concrete clinical decision is a product of critical thinking and judgment in a concrete situation with quantified scientific evidence "looming in its background." This paradigm of clinical reasoning goes back well into the 1960s. Feinstein[54] proposes that a clinician's reasoning should be divided into two categories: **therapeutic** and **environmental**. The therapeutic decision deals with the choice of therapy in general. The environmental decision deals with the management of its particular host. The therapeutic decision answers the question about the best treatment for this ailment; the environmental decision answers the question of how this treatment should be managed and modified for a particular person in its particular clinical and extraclinical setting.

6.3 Logic in Communication with Patients

Most often, patients and their physicians reason differently. They base their reasoning and argumentation on different premises and use different warrants. As a result, ensuing conclusions may differ and may have different values for patient and doctor. Successful treatment and care needs common ground reached through back-and-forth accommodation of these differences.

6.3.1 Understanding Patients' Statements and Reasoning

Communication with a patient is a two-way discussion that may include argumentation. Patient and physician each have their own logic. Part of a physician's task is to explain to a receptive patient what is leading him or her to propose a particular diagnosis, other diagnostic procedures, treatment, or care. Before such an explanation, a physician must first "decipher" and understand the patient's statements and arguments. This is necessary not only for the apprehension of the etiology and motives of the patient's chief complaint but also for the effective prevention of similar problems and cases.

The understanding of a patient's reasoning may often require **reconstruction.**[62] In the flow of current daily communication, a rather heterogeneous ensemble of propositions (including premises and conclusions of arguments) are "hidden" in an informal language. It may be necessary for the physician to probe with further questioning to discover exactly what the patient means. Some examples:

- Patient: "*I get up often in the night to void.*" Physician: "*How many times a night in the last two or three days?*"

- Patient: "*Since I came home from the hospital after having my baby, I have had vaginal bleeding.*" Physician: "*How much blood did you lose in the last three hours?*"

- Patient: "*I've been having pain in my back.*" Physician: "*Show me where you feel the pain. Do you feel the pain all the time? How many times a day? Have you noticed what you were doing just before you felt it? How does the pain feel? Can you describe what kind of pain it is?*"

A common form of lack of clarity in patients' statements is indefiniteness about quantity (how much), frequency (how often), or nature (quality, eg, throbbing, squeezing, burning, sharp): How many? How often? How much? If quantitative and qualitative definiteness is needed, probing will be required.

Making such statements better defined, quantified, and hence more operational is termed by clinical epidemiologists "*hardening of soft data.*"[17]

Not understanding a patient's arguments may lead to an erroneous diagnosis and less effective treatment and prevention.

Fallacies in understanding patients: a complex question example

Physicians sometimes fail to "decipher" what a patient says and means, but they may also tend (wrongly) to manipulate the patient to a desired or expected answer. The following fallacy illustrates such a case.

The complex question is the fallacy generally illustrated by the trick question of the lawyer, "*Have you stopped beating your wife? Yes or no?*" Whichever answer is given assumes the truth of a proposition, which the answerer may not wish to concede ("*In the past, I beat my wife*") and which may not be true. Such loaded questions abound. In medical situations, for instance, we see: "*Have you stopped taking your blood pressure pills, yes or no?*" The question presupposes that the patient was taking blood pressure pills; perhaps the patient never started taking them, or they were not prescribed.

When taking the medical history of a patient, a clinical clerk may ask: "*Are you still a heavy drinker?*" There is no escape for the patient from such a question. He or she is without a doubt labeled as a heavy drinker in advance. An already classified individual cannot dissociate himself from the expected answer.

An additional artificial barrier is placed between the patient and the physician, thereby rendering mutual understanding more difficult.

6.3.2 Assessment and Diagnosis of Psychiatric Patients

Moreover, understanding a patient's own logic, critical thinking, and reasoning is one of the essential components of assessment and diagnosis in psychiatric patients. As a matter of fact, psychiatrists should check (ideally with some uniform and operational criteria at hand) if the patient is "uncritical." If so, is it clinically meaningful? How does it fit into the available diagnostic spectrum of interest? If it is so, how to treat the patient to become "critical" again (and check if it is worth the pain to do it)? To label any patient as "crazy" requires justification by the discovery, classification, and possible explanation of the patient's faulty thought and fallacious reasoning.

For example, a psychiatrist may notice a "flight of ideas" while looking for a psychotic disorder or an adequacy of thought content and process. What does this mean exactly and do we have acceptable criteria that would explicitly justify such an assessment?

In another example, a disorder of possible **thought content** in psychosis includes paranoid **delusions**[63-65] (mistaken beliefs that somebody wants to harm me by his thoughts and action). For example:

- Delusions of reference (special attention to the patient)

- Delusions of control or influence (control by some outside force)

- Delusions of replacement (impostors instead of real people in the patient's life)

- Delusions of jealousy

- Somatic delusions (conviction about an unconfirmed disease or poisoning)

- Grandiose delusions (having special powers and extraordinary achievements)

- Technological delusions (powers given by connection to advanced technologies)

- Religious delusions (being an omnipotent and righteous supreme being, having special powers and missions conferred by a supreme being)

- Sensory (visual, auditive, and other) hallucinations, common in affective disorders, substance abuse, or dementia

Hence, psychiatrists must assess the correctness of premises and of the patient's conclusions compared with generally accepted social, cultural, political, or religious values.

Current definitions of thought content are somehow disconnected from possible meanings in logic (see earlier statements in parentheses), and clinicians have limited guidance in the assessment of this part of a patient's mental status. What would happen *in extremis* if the patient were a master logician and the psychiatrist an *ignoramus* in logic? Who would be right and who would be the judge?

The evaluation of disorders of **thought process** remains an even greater challenge. Strictly speaking, physicians should better understand how their patients evaluate and put together their premises. How do they arrive at conclusions, be they right or wrong? How do these conclusions guide them in their value judgments and subsequent behavior?

The thought process is currently evaluated by assessing patient speech. It is left mostly to the subjective "impression" of the physician. *Disorganized speech* means looseness of associations (veering from the subject of interest) characterized by several types of association according to their severity:

1. **Circumstantiality** (making digressions): Marked by tedious and unnecessary details, but eventually reaches the point.[65] (Premises are irrelevant; inference is somehow made.)

2. **Tangentiality** (irrelevance to the subject, never reaching the point): Marked by skirting the question rather than answering it. Connections between subsequent thoughts are apparent, but a goal is never reached.[65] (The connections are open-ended: no actual well-defined inference?)

3. **Looseness of associations itself** (associative leaps): A jumping from subject to subject without apparent logical and sequential connections.[65] (Premises are fleeting. No possible inference in a clear direction?)

4. **"Word (or verbal) salad"** (changes in topic, making speech incoherent): An incoherent collection of words and phrases.[65] (No usable premises or conclusions?)

5. **Velocity clustering** (abnormality of speed or rate of thought): Ranging from complete mutism to poverty of thought (little spontaneous speech) to racing thoughts (hard to keep track of them) or a rapid flight of ideas. (Poverty or superfluity of premises, no understandable inference?)

The assessment of thought process is important not only in psychosis but especially when evaluating possible affective disorders in a patient, such as depression, mania, or a bipolar affective problem, and in substance abuse or dementia.

The assessment of a patient's thought and reasoning is important not only in the medicine of the mind but also in the medicine of the body. Our diagnosis and treatment plans depend on what the patient tells the family physician or specialist. An incorrect diagnostic workup and treatment plan may result from our misreading of the reality or truth as viewed through the patient's values and reasoning.

In the examination of any patient's mental status,[63, 65, 66] the assessment of thought process is most closely related to logic. As long as we do not develop clear operational criteria for our qualifications of thought process abnormalities, our diagnostic reasoning and ensuing diagnostic conclusions will be the result of a mostly subjective process of evaluation and will be poorly reproducible from one clinician to another. Can we have better criteria for such entities as paucity and flooding of thoughts, slowing or racing of thinking, goal directedness, circumstantiality, tangential thinking, blocking, loose associations, perseverations, neologisms, word salad, intellectual impoverishment, cultural deprivation, and others? How can we consequently support our opinion about a patient's **judgment** (capacity to make appropriate decisions and actions) and **insight** (awareness of factors influencing one's situation)? Can we really do this without assessing a patient's logic and argumentation, as outlined in Chapters 2, 3, and 4?

The only way to assess a patient's thought and reasoning less subjectively is first to look at how accurate and purposeful his statements (premises and conclusions) are and then to try to understand how they are connected together.

Such an assessment requires the reconstruction of a patient's reasoning, arguments, and argumentation.

Where are the premises and what do they mean? Where are the connectors? Are there any quantifiers, which would allow us to understand in more depth the nature of reasoning and argumentation? Where are the conclusions and what are they worth? Is it clinically meaningful?

Conversely, our perception of patients and of their health problems based on a history taking will also depend on the way we speak to them. With or without empathy? Raising open-ended questions or using closed questions that beg the answer? Inquiring in a way that makes the patient feel at ease or one that causes discomfort?

Patient-doctor communication is a two-way matter.

6.4 LOGIC IN COMMUNICATION WITH PEERS

Communication with peers is usually an exchange of views about risks, diagnosis, treatment, prognosis, and ensuing clinical decisions in specific patients or in groups of patients. Floor rounds in hospitals and consults (other specialists brought to the patient's bedside to advise about the case) are times of logical **verbal communication** between health professionals. Personal views or results from rounds or consults enter as written communication by way of hospital and office medical charts and records.

6.4.1 Verbal Communication: Rounds and Consults

Communication with peers differs from communication with the patient in that there is ideally more common ground for content and process among all parties involved. When discussing clinical cases, we are supposed to work with similar premises and arrive by similar paths at correct conclusions.

Importance of the language

The logic of communication with peers stands on common ground, but it is strongly affected by language.[67] It is language that "exteriorizes" our reasoning and thought product. In its written form (medical papers, reports, or notes), the meaning of messages is not affected by the way we speak, only by the way we write; messages are thus more straightforward.

For example, a group of gynecologists makes floor rounds and discusses the delicate decision to sterilize a younger nullipara. What does this mean if one of them suggests:

"You should not consider sterilization in this single, young, nulliparous mentally retarded woman!"

If the accent is on:	What exactly is the point that he or she wants to stress?
You	. . . but it might be done by others.
should not	. . . but I would not be surprised if you were to do it.
sterilization	. . . but other treatments might be more appropriate.
single	. . . would we consider it in a married woman?
young	. . . but sterilization in an older patient might be indicated.
nulliparous	. . . but sterilization in parous women might be considered.
mentally retarded	. . . we have an ethical problem here. How would you solve it?

This example illustrates only the complexity of spoken language in contrast with the written word. If your emphasis suggests a conclusion that is unwarranted—for example, that it would be all right to perform a hysterectomy if the patient were somewhat older—then you commit what logicians call a **fallacy of accent.**[42,67] It is difficult to control if you do not explicitly ask the proponent, "*Is that what you mean?*", such as by stating explicitly the right-hand column of the just-mentioned example.

Such rhetorical fallacies are common to other types of verbal argumentation, and they will be discussed in more detail in the next chapter. Courts of law and other social bodies that discuss health problems will also be in focus.

Analysis using Toulmin's model

Tone, accent, and emphasis of both patient and physician give direction and content to ensuing arguments. In addition, a "real meaning" of statements must be brought out from the flow of clinical communication. For example, if the patient says, "I am allergic to . . ." does it mean that he or she has a systemic reaction to some allergen, an idiosyncrasy, or a dislike for something? Both the content and the nature of communication are worthy of understanding, since this will lead to better decisions.

Communication with peers on rounds (discussing cases seen on floors or on floor rounds or doing an overview of the problem as seen across cases on grand rounds) goes well beyond the rapid, if not telegraphic, messages in medical records. Pros and cons are expected in final recommendations and consensus.

Any case of such a communication must be seen as a string of arguments and scrutinized not only for the evidence used in the premises but also for the way conclusions are drawn from them. Errors may occur in either part of the process.

Exchange of ideas, news, experience, and knowledge pertaining to patients in our care has effectively the form of an argument in Toulmin's terms, as already outlined in theory in Section 2.4.2. To evaluate our argumentation, we must draw from the clinician's natural language the components of Toulmin's model (Figure 6-3) and check for their quality and completeness as well as their uses in their proper interaction.

Table 6-1 illustrates how a dialogue in natural language on rounds led by a senior physician and a young intern (clinical clerk) may be seen as an argument in Toulmin's terms, with its basic elements and their interconnection identified.

As Table 6-1 shows, one may ask:

So what do you recommend?	Isn't it our claim?
What have you seen that led you to your recommendation?	Isn't it our **grounds**?
How does your recommendation follow from these observations?	Isn't it a **warrant**?
How strongly would you endorse your recommendation?	Isn't this question about a **qualifier**?
What special circumstances would lead you to change your recommendation?	Aren't we seeking **rebuttals**?
What evidence supports doing what you recommend in this sort of case?	This is the **backing** for our warrant.

Once having all these elements at hand, we may interconnect and structure them as illustrated by Figure 6-3 and assess whether the grounds are justified and complete, the warrant is justified, and there are no exception-making circumstances in the particular case. From the point of view of EBM, needless to say, *"no justified warrant, not a good argument!"* Good evidence (backing) is necessary to justify use of a warrant.

A generalist who requires a consult by a specialist expects not only the verdict but also the explanation of the intellectual pathway by which an experienced colleague arrived at a differential diagnosis and recommendations for treatment. Both are translated into orders in the patient's charts.

How would logicians approach the evaluation of verbal and other communication?

Logicians see all oral or written statements from a different angle, which can be summarized in three steps of reasoning. As a reminder of the logicians' methods outlined in Chapter 3, a few examples will illustrate these steps:

1. Qualifying the nature of statements and propositions

2. Reconstructing the arguments

3. Assessing the logical validity of arguments

TABLE 6-1

Clinical rounds as dialogue with identification of argument components in physicians' natural language

Question	Statement	Component of argument
Attending (to on-call physician): *"Peter, anything new on our floor?"*	Intern: *"A stroke patient was transferred to us from emergency. I have evaluated him and decided that **he is a candidate for thrombolysis**."*	*Claim:* Proposition resulting from our reasoning.
Attending: *"Can you tell me what your impression [working assessment] is about this patient?"*	Intern: *"This patient most probably had **an ischemic stroke 2 hours ago**. His **computed tomography** is **normal**. Our consulting neurologist told me to 'thrombolyse' him right away."*	*Grounds:* Basis from which we reason and argue. Facts supporting the claim.
Intern: *"Do we have some general rules to handle such cases?"*	Attending: *"As a matter of fact, as shown by our own review of evidence, **all patients newly admitted for an ischemic stroke of less than 3 hours should receive IV [intravenous] thrombolysis** to limit the ensuing neurologic deficit."*	*Warrant:* General rule that permits us to infer a claim from grounds.
Intern: *"Is this treatment mandatory, or do we have other choices? Is there anything else we should do?"*	Attending: *"This patient **must** be thrombolysed right away and further evaluated as a potential candidate for endarterectomy if carotid stenosis should prove to be an underlying problem."*	*Qualifier:* A word or phrase that indicates the strength conferred by the warrant and thus the strength of support for our conclusion.
Intern: *"Do we have some competing underlying diagnoses? What should we do to adjust treatment according to the pathology behind this patient's state?"*	Attending: *"**Further diagnostic workup based, among others, on CT scan, ultrasonography, and magnetic resonance angiography** should help us to differentiate this case from intracranial venous thrombosis, aneurysm, arteriovenous aneurysms, or subarachnoid hemorrhage."*	*Grounds:* Basis from which we reason and argue. Facts supporting the claim. Here the question is whether the grounds are correct.
Intern: *"What kind of evidence do you have available to you for your recommendations and orders?"*	Attending: *"Our **systematic review of the evidence** shows that emergency IV thrombolysis of stroke patients improves stroke outcomes like neurologic deficit. Other treatment must also be considered depending on the underlying lesion. It might be obstruction by atherosclerosis or some other type of stenosis, embolus, lacunar infarction, cerebral infarction, or intracerebral hemorrhage. Glucose and temperature control are important for all causes."*	*Backing:* Body of experience and evidence that supports the warrant.

CT indicates computed tomography; IV, intravenous; to thrombolyse a patient, to give the patient thrombolytic therapy (eg, by recombinant tissue plasminogen activator).

BY QUALIFYING THE NATURE OF STATEMENTS AND PROPOSITIONS

All simple categorical propositions (what is said by patients and their doctors) may be classified as **affirmative** or **negative**. They may be **universal** (all entities in some set are involved), **particular** (some of the entities are involved), or **singular** (a single individual or entity is in focus).

We may consider a proposition that "*all patients in the intensive care unit are critically ill.*" We may also state that "*some of these patients require a continuous monitoring of vital functions.*" Finally, we may say that "*Mrs. Fitzpatrick must be transferred to the intensive care unit.*"

According to the quantity (universal, particular, singular) and quality (affirmative, negative) of propositions, **six categories of propositions** (see Section 3.2) emerge[66]:

1. **Universal and affirmative**. Example: "All patients in our intensive care unit require a continuous follow-up of vital signs."

2. **Universal and negative**. Example: "None of the patients in our intensive care unit require transfer to another ward."

3. **Particular and affirmative**. Example: "Some patients on our ward can be transferred to other wards without a thorough assessment of their prognosis and needs."

4. **Particular and negative**. Example: "Some patients on our ward do not need a thorough assessment of their care needs and prognosis."

5. **Singular and affirmative** (treated for logical purposes as universal and affirmative propositions). Example: "Mrs. Fitzpatrick can be transferred to another ward without a thorough assessment of her prognosis and needs."

6. **Singular negative** (treated for logical purposes as universal and negative propositions). Example: "Mr. Jones does not need a thorough assessment of his prognosis and needs."

BY RECONSTRUCTING ARGUMENTS

The following steps[68] in the **reconstruction of categorical syllogisms** put our reasoning and arguments into a form in which their validity can be more easily tested:

1. Identify the subject and predicate of our own or the patient's sentences.

2. When a quantifier is missing, supply it.

3. If the predicate lacks a noun ("is vomiting," "is pale"), supply one to form the name of a class ("is a vomiting person," "is a pale person").

4. If there is no copula (no word *is* or *are*), supply it.

5. Transform sentences beginning with *only* ("*only patients with serious symptoms or negative results from other tests should be prescribed magnetic resonance imaging*") or *none but* to ones beginning with *all* and with the order of subject and predicate reversed ("*All patients for whom magnetic resonance imaging is prescribed should be patients with serious symptoms or negative results from other tests.*").

6. Replace initial negative particles such as *nothing* or *nobody* with the quantifier *no.*

7. Interpret *all . . . are not* sentences (*"all sore throats are not bacterial infections"*) as particular negative propositions (*"some sore throats are not bacterial infections"*) unless a universal negative proposition (*"no sore throats are bacterial infections"*) is clearly intended. (It is not intended in this example.)

8. Break down sentences with *except* (*"all cells except red blood cells manufacture eicosanoids*) into two categorical propositions (*"all cells that are not red blood cells manufacture eicosanoids," "no red blood cells manufacture eicosanoids"*), and use as a premise whichever one works to support the conclusion.

9. Translate sentences containing words such as *anyone, anything, whoever, the, if . . . then,* or *whatever* into universal affirmative propositions.

10. Translate sentences containing words such as *someone, something, there is,* or *there are* into particular affirmative propositions.

11. If the argument is a one-premise incomplete categorical syllogism, add as an unstated premise the weakest proposition that will produce a valid categorical syllogism.

12. Do **not** try to improve the argument by what its authors did not say. Propose instead a counterargument and compare!

BY ASSESSING THE LOGICAL VALIDITY OF ARGUMENTS
Once reconstructed, any categorical syllogism used to support a clinical decision[68] must be valid, as indicated by the Venn diagram test described in Chapter 3 (Section 3.2) or by other methods of testing categorical syllogisms for validity. If, in addition, the syllogism's premises are true, then the argument is not only valid but sound; its conclusion must be true.

Thus logicians propose three tools for evaluating everyday arguments as categorical syllogisms: qualifying the nature of statements and propositions, reconstructing arguments, and assessing the logical validity of the resulting arguments. Do physicians really use these tools of logic in daily practice? For the most part, not yet or not as often as they should, because the time constraints at work do not allow for it and physicians are not always comfortable with their use. In most cases, such painstaking analysis is not needed. However, important cases may require a more in-depth look. Moreover, if questionable cases become the subject of malpractice litigation, an analysis of the logical process of argumentation becomes mandatory and crucial for the verdict regarding correct or incorrect clinical practice.

6.4.2 Written Communication: Hospital and Office Charts and Reports

Ideally, patient records and charts in hospitals and general practice should allow any of their readers to understand how the patient thinks and what path of reasoning the patient's physician follows. However, the reality of in-house and outpatient practice beats the fiction of prefixed ideals. Health professionals are busy, pressured, and overwhelmed by an ever-changing clinical situation and priorities, shortages in human and material resources and assistance, deadlines of all kinds, and sometimes unsupportive behavior in patients and other health professionals, despite all of their good will. Written messages are short, even too short to understand their logic, and consequently their factual and decision-making value must be somehow unearthed from the daily written entries.

To put it bluntly, if we want to avoid despair at our own failure, the patient's wrath, a medical malpractice suit, or all three, let us make correct medical records. Yes, clinical practice is busy and stressful, and messages are short. Nevertheless, however short the messages may be, their author should be able to reconstruct (and share with others) the reasoning that led her or him to conclusions such as diagnosis, therapeutic orders, or further diagnostic and therapeutic workup.

There are two remedies for the tendency to be too cryptic in written messages:

1. **Try to reconstruct the reasoning from the scribbled message.** As already mentioned above, is it possible to rebuild arguments from everyday speech?

    a. What observations, reported symptoms, and test results are reported?

    b. What diagnostic "impressions" or specific diagnoses are drawn from these data?

    c. Are the inferences to these diagnostic conclusions warranted? In other words, are they evidence-based?

    d. Is the information relevant to a predetermined question about risk assessment, diagnosis, therapy, or prognosis?

    e. Do the conclusions fit the reality?

    f. Is all this relevant to answering my question?

2. **If as author of the message you cannot reconstruct the reasoning, be prepared to explain what was on your mind when you wrote what you did.**

    a. What was the question leading you to write your notes?

    b. What were your premises? (On what evidence did you base your diagnosis, treatment order, or order for a further diagnostic workup?)

    c. How did you arrive at your conclusions? (What warranted you to draw these conclusions from your data? Were these warrants evidence-based?)

    d. In what way will your conclusions contribute to the solution of the problem that you are facing?

This is something that all physicians must add to their already acquired basic knowledge, practical experience, skills of which we are rightly proud, and ability to put them into practice in a universally satisfactory way.

Fallacies in medical communication

Even routine communication in clinical practice based on good critical thinking is very challenging. The practice of medicine is fast-paced, stressful, and evolving in an ever-changing clinical environment, with an array of patients, new technologies, old and new emerging diseases, and mostly limited resources and time. Many clinicians may say by the end of the day: "*Do not bother me with philosophy, I have more important things to do.*" However, maybe we should bother with it.

There is not much space for logical argumentation when writing progress notes in patient charts. Readers of consults and discharge notes want clear conclusions, recommendations, and orders. However, the authors behind these lines must always be ready to reproduce, on request and in any situation of need, the logical reasoning and critical thinking that led them to their recommendations.

During rounds there is a bit more time, and a clear need for reflective thinking. Such thinking is part of the foundation of physician training.

The other challenge of clinical practice is communication with partners with varying degrees and scopes of knowledge, experience, attitudes, preferences, and values: patients, their relatives, peers within our specialties, other specialists, freshmen (ie, beginning medical students or physicians in training), and "old wise men and women." For the benefit of them all, our clear reasoning must be conveyed successfully and understandably using an equally clear language. Nonetheless, fallacious reasoning may still occur.

As anywhere else, some fallacies may be related to the evidence for our premises, to conclusions drawn from new evidence, and to the way evidence is handled throughout the whole process of reasoning and critical thinking.[42] From an ever growing list of fallacies,[42,45,62] some are particularly relevant to clinical practice. These include the fallacies of accent, question-begging epithets, and false analogy; the sweeping explanation; the argument *ad misericordiam;* the fallacy of equivocation; and the straw man fallacy.

Fallacy of accent

This fallacy was already illustrated in Section 6.4. The emphasis on single words may change the meaning, thus leading to more than one understanding of the message. "*Did* you *have a bowel movement this morning?*" (other patients might have one) or "*Did you have a bowel movement* this morning?" (as any other day).

Fallacy of question-begging epithets

For Engel,[45] the error lies in the use of slanted language that reaffirms what we wish to prove but have not yet proved.

"*This patient has the most serious disease known to medicine.*" From what array of diseases? What does "*the most serious*" mean?

"*The colleagues from the other hospital are referring this patient to us.*" Does this mean that "*the other hospital*" affiliated with our university is full of health professionals of dubious competency? Or is the referral a result of patient overflow in this highly credited health facility? Terms such as *name calling, loaded words, verbal suggestions,* and *mud slinging*[45] are often behind such situations and their interpretation.

Fallacy of false analogy

This fallacy occurs when the comparison distorts the facts in the case that is the subject of argumentation.[45] "*It is as necessary to hospitalize all those who suffer suicidal ideation as it is to hospitalize and watch all patients brought to us after repeated suicide attempts.*" Really?

An argument ad misericordiam, appealing to pity

This means using extenuating circumstances to justify decisions or actions. "*The intern has not yet filled out admission notes. You know, this is his first month with us.*"

Sweeping explanation

This fallacy consists in taking a common (but not universal) explanation of some condition to apply to a particular case. The particular case may, however, be an exception to the usual explanation. "*My husband John is obese. Obviously he is overeating and not exercising enough.*" Not necessarily, he may have a metabolic disorder or a thyroid condition. "*You smoked for 30 years, and now you have lung cancer. Your lung cancer is due to your smoking.*" Not necessarily, there are other causes of lung cancer, which may operate even in smokers. A frequent cause is mistakenly taken to be a necessary cause.

Fallacy of equivocation

This fallacy occurs if more than one meaning is given to the same word. "*As your family physician, I have the authority to keep you isolated at home during your disease, but I do not have the authority to keep you there.*" In the first case, the physician's authority means knowledge of the epidemiology of the patient's infectious disease. In the second statement, "*authority*" means the legal empowerment of a public health officer to keep the patient home in quarantine.

Straw man fallacy

This fallacy is based on the expectation that it may be easier to knock down a "straw man" instead of a real man. A real argument and its conclusion may be made weaker not only by simplification of the problem but also by its misinterpretation, exaggeration, or other kind of distortion. Bowell and Kemp[62] offer a good example of this kind of fallacy in the case of argumentation against the legalization of voluntary euthanasia. Suppose someone maintains that terminally ill patients should have the right to choose to die and ask their doctors to end their life. An opponent may argue in response: "*You cannot give doctors the right to end a person's life just because they decide that the person's life is no longer worth living. No one should have such power over another person's life!*" The position in favor of voluntary euthanasia is presented as more extreme than it really is. It is presented as a position in favor of compulsory euthanasia, which almost nobody supports.

These few examples of fallacies worth knowing, avoiding, and correcting illustrate that clinical training also means critical thinking in medical interpretation and decision making.

6.5 CONCLUSIONS: LOGIC IN COMMUNICATION WITH THE OUTSIDE WORLD

In any clinical setting outside the hospital, a powerful reasoning or argument must have five virtues:

1. **Premises are justified:** the best evidence available indicates that they are true.

2. **Premises are complete.** They include all good relevant information that is practically obtainable.

3. **The inference is warranted.** The conclusion follows from the premises in accordance with a justified warrant.

4. **This case is not an exception.** There are no known exceptional circumstances in this case that override or rebut the warrant.

5. **The conclusion applies** to my concrete clinical problem and my patient or my community.

If one of these requirements is not respected, the clinical decision is unsupported and based on weak reasoning. It may harm a patient in the clinical setting. Equally, health programs in preventive medicine and public health based on erratic uses of evidence may harm the entire community, or at best provide less good than expected.

Clinical knowledge, experience, and practice are vital for good medicine. In addition, good uses of logic make the best impact at all levels and domains of medical care.

The expectations from our own limited attitudes, knowledge, and skills will always exceed what we are able to deliver. However, we must understand what is expected from us beyond the realm of medicine itself and perform "to the max," as popular media and advertising tell us. These expectations are not limited to our professional environment. Outside the health sciences, we live in the world, which we share with other domains of human endeavor and with which we have a common reasoning and logic within the realm of human thinking.

In the next chapter, we explore this "outside world."

References

1. Clouser KD, Gert B. Rationality and medicine: introduction to the theme. *J Med Phil.* 1986;11:119–121.

2. Wulff HR. Rational diagnosis and treatment. *J Med Phil.* 1986;11:123–134.

3. Thomasma DC. Philosophical reflections on a rational treatment plan. *J Med Phil.* 1986;11:157–165.

4. Gatens-Robinson E. Clinical judgment and the rationality of the human sciences. *J Med Phil.* 1986;11:167–178.

5. *New Illustrated Webster's Dictionary of the English Language.* New York, NY: PAMCO Publishing Co, Inc; 1992.

6. Helicon Publishing Ltd. Ed. *Instant Reference: Philosophy.* (Teach Yourself Books.) London, England and Lincolnwood, Ill: Hodder Headline PLC and NTC/Contemporary Publishing; 2000.

7. Blackburn S. *The Oxford Dictionary of Philosophy* Oxford, England: Oxford University Press; 1996.

8. Cody CAJ. Common sense. In: Honderich T, ed. *The Oxford Companion to Philosophy.* Oxford, England: Oxford University Press; 1995:142.

9. Schneewind JB. Scottish common sense philosophy. In: Audi R, ed. *The Cambridge Dictionary of Philosophy.* 2nd ed. Cambridge, England: Cambridge University Press; 1999:822–833.

10. Horty J. Common sense reasoning, theories of. In: Craig E, ed. *Concise Routledge Encyclopedia of Philosophy.* London, England: Routledge; 1999:153.

11. Wolpert L. Science: an unnatural practice. The Samuel Gee Lecture 1995. *J R Coll Physic Lond.* 1996;30:155–160.

12. Altemeier WA III. The clinical application of intuition. *Pediatric Ann.* 2001;30(12):714–716.

13. Walton DN, Krabbe ECW. *Commitment in Dialogue: Basic Concepts of Interpersonal Reasoning.* Albany, NY: State University of New York Press; 1995.

14. Gray MJA. *The Resourceful Patient.* Oxford, England: eRosetta Press; 2002. Available at: www.resourcefulpatient.org.

15. Battersby M. The competent layperson: an educational ideal for the 21st century. Paper presented at: Learning Summit 2003, Phoenix, Ariz; March 15, 2003.

16. Gould SJ. The median isn't the message. *Discover.* June 1985;6:40–42. Available at: www.cancerguide.org/median_not_msg.html.

17. Jenicek M. *Foundations of Evidence-Based Medicine.* New York, NY: The Parthenon Publishing Group; 2003.

18. Lilford RJ, Thornton JD. Decision logic in medical practice. The Millroy lecture 1992. *J R Coll Phys Lond.* 1992;26:400–412.

19. Ledley RS, Lusted LB. Reasoning foundations of medical diagnosis: symbolic logic, probability, and value theory aid our understanding of how physicians reason. *Science.* 1959;130:9–21.

20. Beer S. Heuristic. In: Bullock A, Trombley S, eds. *The New Fontana Dictionary of Modern Thought.* 3rd ed. London, England: Harper Collins Publishers; 1999:391.

21. Murphy EA. *The Logic of Medicine.* 2nd ed. Baltimore, Md: The Johns Hopkins University Press; 1997.

22. Sackett DL. Clinical diagnosis and the clinical laboratory. *J Invest Med.* 1978;1:37–43.

23. Macartney FJ. Diagnostic logic. In: Phillips CI, ed. *Logic in Medicine.* 2nd ed. London, England: BMJ Publishing Group; 1995:59–99.

24. Porter R. Tacit knowledge. In: Bullock A, Trombley S, eds. *The New Fontana Dictionary of Modern Thought.* 3rd ed. London, England: Harper Collins Publishers; 1999:856.

25. Russell B. Intuition. In: Audi R, ed. *The Cambridge Dictionary of Philosophy.* 2nd ed. Cambridge, England: Cambridge University Press; 1999:442.

26. Hall KH. Reviewing intuitive decision-making and uncertainty: the implication for medical education. *Med Educ.* 2002;36:216–224.

27. Myers DG. *Intuition: Its Powers and Perils.* New Haven, Conn: Yale University Press; 2002.

28. Hayashi AM. When to trust your gut. *Harv Bus Rev.* 2001; 79:58–65,155.

29. Shaw AB. Intuitions, principles and consequences. *J Med Ethics.* 2001; 27:16–19.

30. Buck C. Popper's philosophy for epidemiologists. *Int J Epidemiol.* 1975;4: 159–168.

31. Greenhalgh T. Intuition and evidence—uneasy bedfellows? *Br J Gen Pract.* 2002;52:395–400.

32. Wood BP. Decision making in radiology. *Radiology.* 1999;211:601–603.

33. Jonsen AR, Toulmin S. *The Abuse of Casuistry: A History of Moral Reasoning.* Berkeley, Calif: University of California Press; 1988.

34. Levi, EH. *An Introduction to Legal Reasoning.* Chicago, Ill: University of Chicago Press; 1949.

35. Fu KS. Processing of chest X-ray images by computer. In: de Dombal FT, Grémy F, eds. *Decision Making and Medical Care.* Amsterdam, The Netherlands: Elsevier North Holland Inc; 1976:271–286.

36. Pöppl SJ. Experience in computer classification of EEGs. In: de Dombal FT, Grémy F, eds. *Decision Making and Medical Care.* Amsterdam, The Netherlands: Elsevier North Holland Inc; 1976:195–211.

37. Nadler M. Effective and cost-effective real-time picture operators for medical imagery. In: de Dombal FT, Grémy F, eds. *Decision Making and Medical Care.* Amsterdam, The Netherlands: Elsevier North Holland Inc; 1976:259–270.

38. Weinstein MC, Fineberg HV, Elstein AS, et al. *Clinical Decision Analysis.* Philadelphia, Pa: WB Saunders; 1980.

39. Price RB, Vlahcevic ZR. Logical principles in differential diagnosis. *Ann Intern Med.* 1971;75:89–95.

40. Jeffrey WH, Berger JO. Ockham's razor and Bayesian analysis. *American Scientist.* 1992;80:64–72.

41. Lo Re V, Bellini LM. William of Occam and Occam's razor. *Ann Int Med*. 2002;136:634–635.

42. Damer TE. *Attacking Faulty Reasoning*. 2nd ed. Belmont, Calif: Wadsworth Publishing Co; 1987.

43. Copi IM, Cohen C. *Introduction to Logic*. 11th ed. Upper Saddle River, NJ: Prentice Hall; 2002.

44. *Hopp v. Lepp*, 2 SCR 192 (Supreme Court of Canada 1980); *Reibl v. Hughes*, 2 SCR 880 (Supreme Court of Canada 1980).

45. Engel SM. *With Good Reason: An Introduction to Informal Fallacies*. 3rd ed. New York, NY: St Martin's Press; 1986.

46. Nolt J, Rohatyn D, Varzi A. *Schaum's Outline of Theory and Problems of Logic*. 2nd ed. New York, NY: McGraw-Hill; 1998.

47. Rich BA. Defining and delineating a duty to prognosticate. *Theor Med Bioeth*. 2001;22:177–192.

48. Wieseman C. The significance of prognosis for a theory of medical practice. *Theor Med Bioeth*. 1998;19:253–261.

49. Lucas PJF, Abu-Hanna A. Prognostic methods in medicine. *Artif Intell Med*. 1999;15:105–119.

50. Hermanek P. Prognostic factor research in oncology. *J Clin Epidemiol*. 1999;52:371–374.

51. Iwashyna TJ, Christakis NA. Physicians, patients, and prognosis. *West J Med*. 2001;174:253–254.

52. Rose G. Sick individuals and sick populations. *Int J Epidemiol*. 1985;14:32–38.

53. Rose G. *The Strategy of Preventive Medicine*. Oxford, England: Oxford University Press; 1992.

54. Feinstein AR. *Clinical Judgment*. Baltimore, Md: Williams & Wilkins Co; 1967.

55. Sackett DL, Straus SE, Richardson WS, Rosenberg W, Haynes RB. *Evidence-Based Medicine: How to Practice and Teach EBM*. 2nd ed. Edinburgh, Scotland: Churchill Livinston; 2000.

56. Davis FD. Phronesis, clinical reasoning, and Pellegrino's philosophy of medicine. *Theor Med Bioeth*. 1997;18:173–195.

57. Tyreman S. Promoting critical thinking in health care: phronesis and criticality. *Med Health Care Philosophy*. 2000;3:117–124.

58. Waring D. Why the practice of medicine is not a phronetic activity. *Theor Med Bioeth*. 2000;21:139–151.

59. Aristotle. *Ethica Nicomachea*. Oxford, England: Oxford University Press; 1894. VI. 5.1140b20-21. (Translation by the second author.)

60. Plato. *Plato Complete Works*. Cooper JM, ed. Indianapolis, Ind: Hackett Publishing Co; 1997.

61. Walther, H. *Proverbia sententiaeque Latinitatis Medii Aevi: Lateinische Sprichwörter und Sentenzen des Mittelalters in alphabetischer Anordnung.* Part 4. Göttingen, Germany: Vandenhoeck & Ruprecht; 1963. Entry 25432, variants at 25428-25432.

62. Bowell T, Kemp G. *Critical Thinking: A Concise Guide.* London, England: Routledge; 2002:155–205.

63. Carlat D. *The Psychiatric Interview: A Practical Guide.* Philadelphia, Pa: Lippincott Williams & Wilkins; 1999.

64. Task Force on DSM-IV. *Diagnostic and Statistical Manual of Mental Disorders: DSM-IV-TR.* 4th ed. Washington, DC: American Psychiatric Association; 2000.

65. Stoudemire A. *Clinical Psychiatry for Medical Students.* 3rd ed. Philadelphia, Pa: Lippincott Williams & Wilkins; 1998.

66. Hales RE, Yudofsky SC, eds. *Essentials of Clinical Psychiatry: Based on the American Psychiatric Press Textbook of Psychiatry.* 3rd ed. Washington, DC: American Psychiatric Press; 1999.

67. Hughes W. *Critical Thinking: An Introduction to Basic Skills.* 3rd ed. Peterborough, Ontario: Broadview Press Ltd; 2000.

68. Popkin RH, Stroll A. *Philosophy Made Simple.* 2nd ed rev. New York, NY: Broadway Books; 1993:237–273.

CHAPTER 7

Communicating with the Outside World

Are We on the Same Wavelength?

It's not logical, Captain!
MR SPOCK TO CAPTAIN KIRK,
ON THE SPACESHIP ENTERPRISE, THIS MILLENNIUM.
(*STAR TREK* TV SERIES)
(IF YOU DO NOT ALWAYS UNDERSTAND MR SPOCK,
YOU ARE NOT ALONE!)

Doctor, what you are saying to me
sounds important, but it doesn't make any sense.
(MAKE SENSE!)

Evidence refuted in part is evidence refuted altogether.
TALMUD, FIFTH CENTURY BC TO SIXTH CENTURY AD

If you are unencumbered with the evidence,
you can say anything you want.
E. R. MCFADDEN (PARAPHRASED), 1988

> **In essence, any dealing with civic or legal bodies
> as pertains to the handling of individual
> and community health problems is, and must be,
> an exercise subject to the rules of logic and critical thinking
> in the search for and appraisal of available evidence.**

Businesspeople, industry experts, salespersons, pharmaceutical company representatives, politicians, lawyers, economists, social workers, educators, media specialists, administrators, planners, accountants, assessors and evaluation specialists, public servants, and government decision makers all want to understand our reasoning and the decisions we make in health care.

This is not because these people are better logicians than we are. It is because we are not alone and do not live in ivory towers reserved only for health professionals. We need to make ourselves understood by non–health professionals and we must understand them. Argumentation in the world beyond health sciences is a two-way process.

Is our way of thinking the same as theirs, as it should be? Not in all matters and instances. In this chapter, we will examine some important considerations and methods of reasoning when dealing with health problems in the community. Mutual understanding among all parties involved is essential to provide good health programs and policies in the community and to make them as beneficial as possible for individuals and the general population as well.

7.1 OUR POINTS OF CONTACT IN THE COMMUNITY

Health matters concern everyone. Whatever we do in our hospitals or medical offices has an impact on the outside world, the community. An incapacitated patient after discharge from the hospital is taken care of by social services. Disgruntled patients may consult their lawyer to find out whether they should sue their physician for malpractice.

Other health matters, programs, or policies are carried out directly in the non-medical environment: screening for disease, prevention programs in occupational medicine and health, measures to control disease spread in the community, and developing legislation affecting community health.

Health professionals and their activities are critiqued for their good deeds or wrongdoings, or they participate themselves as experts helping others choose, implement, and evaluate health programs and policies. Success in any of these endeavors depends on good evidence and mutually understandable argumentation through which evidence is handled.

We can become involved in argumentative discourse about health problems with numerous partners:

- Health litigations in **courts of law** bring together physicians and lawyers and require argumentation from both sides. Most often what is at stake is the plausibility of alleged industrial, environmental, iatrogenic, or social harm.

- In occupational health, cases of work-related diseases and their consequences within the realm of assistance and compensation are discussed at various **worker compensation boards.**

- Various important health programs and policies are submitted for discussion, approval, legislation, and financing by various **governments at local, national, or international levels.**

- Discussions on health matters can occur in **interviews, statements, open-line radio and television programs, or other reports in electronic and print media.**

In all these environments, the topic most often discussed (and argued about) is some cause-effect relationship. Does passive smoking cause health problems in nonsmokers? Do outcomes of a complicated obstetric delivery represent malpractice? Does health evidence show strongly enough that increasing the speed limit on highways will not lead to an increase in fatal injuries? Are immunizing agents against an infectious disease effective enough, and the outcomes of this disease frequent and serious enough, to justify as cost-effective compulsory immunization paid from a governmental budget?

Sharing the same problem in an argumentative discussion occurs in different contexts with varying reasoning, knowledge, and experience of the parties involved, as shown in Table 7-1.

As this table illustrates, health professionals in the "outside world" must count on their interlocutors having somewhat similar reasoning, but different knowledge and different experience. They must adjust their argumentation accordingly.

In a patient-doctor relationship, reasoning, knowledge, and experience may all be different. In doctor-to-doctor communication, reasoning, knowledge, and experience are all more or less the same, or they should be.

In the world of medicine and law, a common understanding of reasoning and different experience must be amalgamated to solve health problems under scrutiny.

TABLE 7-1

Reasoning, knowledge, and experience in various settings of argumentation

Partners in dialogue	Reasoning	Knowledge	Experience
Physicians to patients	Different	Different	Different
Physicians to physicians (medical records, clinical rounds, research)	Similar	Similar	Similar enough
Physicians and "the outside world" (administrators, lawyers, politicians, media)	Similar (ideally)	Different	Different

Any expert advice, recount, or consult is a collection of arguments, not a simple demonstration of knowledge of the matter in question. In such arguments, the value or force of evidence is not the only thing that matters. How such evidence is used in an argumentative discourse also matters. Legal reasoning is an extension and application of the general rules of reasoning, as outlined in Chapter 2 and elsewhere.[1] Consequently, aren't logicians as important in litigations as biostatisticians or epidemiologists already are?[2]

7.2 Physicians in Courts of Law: Their Contributions to Decision-making in Tort Litigation

Individual patients and whole communities sometimes complain and sue when they doubt medical decisions, effects of industrial and other environmental factors, or their possible role in perceived poor health. Did a physician's care and decisions during a difficult labor lead to a newborn's brain damage? Did exposure of a population to air pollutants in an urban area lead to a high occurrence of respiratory problems? Does toxic waste disposal lead to leukemia outbreaks and clusters? Is cancer in military veterans due to exposure to chemical warfare agents?

The notion of "evidence" is important not only to physicians in times of evidence-based medicine (EBM), but equally, if not more broadly, in the field of law. A common language is currently being constructed.[3,4] Common understanding is vital wherever and whenever medical findings are used outside, "in the real world," such as in tort litigation in courts of law. Physicians and other providers of health information who may be potential expert witnesses must all know the fundamentals of doctor-lawyer interplay.

Historically, the world of law followed closely developments in medicine[5]: from its intuitive times to the times of epidemiology, clinimetrics, or EBM. It makes a wise distinction between the "evidence for groups" and the evidence for each particular patient, representing a "statistic of one." As clinimetrics develops in medicine, lawyers develop their own kind of "*iurimetrics*," such as the scoring systems for competency to stand trial.[6] We are living now in an era of increasing commonality of thinking and mutual understanding between the world of medicine and the world of law. Both these worlds, however, have their own specifics with which both parties must be familiar.

A health professional offers his or her testimony for or against a given proposition, but the court decides. The present **role of an expert witness** is defined among others by the following[7 (abridged)]:

- The court controls expert evidence.

- The expert's duty is to the court, not the solicitor.

- Instructions must be clear.

- Evidence must be in writing.

- Experts may request directions.

- Judges, barristers, solicitors, and experts are increasingly trained in report writing and witness skills.

Medicolegal expertise is becoming, for some, a prevalent and highly specialized activity.[8]

7.2.1 What to Expect When Dealing with Decision-Making Legal Bodies

Courts often deal with **tort litigation**. In the field of health, the typical case is one of a person (the **plaintiff**) reporting a health problem (silicosis, lead poisoning, etc) and its presumed cause (unhealthy working conditions). The **defendant** is the employer of the plaintiff. Malpractice suits in medicine are also tort litigations.

Medically and legally speaking, a **tort** is "*a wrongful act, other than a breach of contract, that results in injury to another person, property, reputation, or some other legally protected right or interest, and for which the injured party is entitled to a remedy of law, usually in the form of damages.*[9] A tort may be **intentional** or **nonintentional**.

Health professionals are now increasingly called as experts to help, through their testimonies, decision makers (judges, lawyers, politicians, or administrators) reach appropriate conclusions in dealing with health problems. We must be aware, among others, of analytic pathways necessary for testimonies.

For lawyers, an **expert** is "*a person who, through education or experience, has developed skills or knowledge in a particular subject, so that he or she may form an opinion that will assist the fact-finder.*"[10]

Black's Law Dictionary defines an **expert witness** as "*a witness qualified by knowledge, skill, experience, training, or education to provide a scientific, technical, or other specialized opinion about the evidence or a fact issue*"[10] or "*one who by reason of education or specialized experience . . . possesses a superior knowledge respecting subjects about which persons having no particular training are incapable of forming an accurate opinion or deducing correct conclusions.*"[11] In Clapp's[9] words, an expert is "*a person possessing the qualifications of education and experience to render service to an attorney or party in a specialized field or to testify as **expert witness**.*" Invited experts may expect that their training and experience will be scrutinized and must be considered acceptable for all parties involved. Rules of eligibility may be found in the overview of this topic by Norton.[7]

Two kinds of information are used. The simplest one is a **statement:** "*an oral or written assertion, or sometimes a nonverbal conduct intended as an assertion, such as nodding one's head or pointing.*"[9] For example, one may report that "*after the patient suffered a cardiac arrest at a shopping center, an emergency ambulance crew was called and a defibrillator was used in an attempt to reestablish the patient's heart function.*" It is a report of a fact; there is nothing to discuss. A special kind of statement is an **excited utterance,** "*a statement about a startling event* [eg, about a traffic accident and ensuing injuries] *or condition made in the excitement caused by the situation. Such utterances are usually admitted into evidence as an exception against hearsay.... Their perceptions may be distorted. . . ."*[9] Other information is obtained through **arguments,** as we already know them from logic. For example, *"Cardiac arrests require defibrillation as an emergency street procedure. This shopper has had a cardiac arrest. Therefore, he had to be defibrillated."* **Any expert witness's contribution relies both on the quality of evidence (statements) and the way in which it is handled through dialogue with other parties (argumentation).** In many cases, we are more prepared to deliver evidence than to handle it through arguments.

Lawyers and judges usually want to know about:

- The testability of a theory or technique (and if it was tested)

- Peer reviews and publication of facts

- Potential and real errors in analysis

- Acceptance of findings and knowledge by the professional and scientific community

- Overall quality of evidence (if any)

Two problems emerge now as challenges for argumentation:

1. The cause-effect relationship

2. Clinical guidelines

7.2.2 Cause-Effect Challenges: General and Specific

Most often, the statements and arguments of a medical expert witness focus on cause-effect relationships. Was the unsuccessful hip replacement using a new technique the cause of a patient's handicap? Were antipollution measures in a metallurgy plant effective enough to prevent respiratory problems in the employees?

Physicians and epidemiologists are called with greater frequency as expert witnesses to express their opinions about such kinds of cause-effect relationships by using criteria for good evidence, as partly outlined in Chapter 5 and in more detail elsewhere.[12] They are requested to answer two kinds of questions:

1. Is there a **general cause-effect relationship** between a presumed medical or nonmedical factor (treatment, pollution, etc) and a particular disease (eg, cancer)?

2. Did this particular factor cause a health problem **in this particular individual**?

General cause-effect considerations for a health problem under scrutiny

Any health professional called to testify in a court of law will encounter an even more expanded array of views of causation for the purposes of law and will then be expected to link it with considerations of causation as we know them from philosophy, epidemiology, or biostatistics. This health professional will enter a new world of many refined meanings that is unusual in a health setting. Nevertheless, he or she will be required to assist judges, lawyers, and juries in the world of meanings as follows:

CAUSES AND CONSEQUENCES

In law, **causation** is " *the fact that a certain action or event produced a certain result. This is an essential element to be proved in many kinds of cases; for example . . . to recover* [health] *damages in a tort or contract action, the plaintiff must prove that the claimed loss* [disease, handicap, incapacity] *was actually caused by a defendant's wrongful conduct* [eg, lack of work security measures].[9]

Dukelow and Nuse[13] see causation as "*an expression of the relationship that must be found to exist between the tortious act of the wrongdoer and the injury to the victim in order to justify compensation of the latter out of the pocket of the former.*"

It is up to the plaintiff to prove causation.[10]

The legal definition of a **cause** is more general than in medicine or philosophy: "*something that produces an effect or result (eg, the cause of an accident).*"[10]

Levin[14] defined a general approach to the legal proof of causation as follows: "*The standard of proof in the courtroom is similar to that in clinical medicine. To be indicted as a causative factor in an illness, an agent must be shown to a reasonable degree of medical certainty to cause or substantially contribute to that illness. This standard of proof is true for infectious and toxin-associated diseases in clinical medicine.*"

Norton[7] reviews in more detail possible court questions about causation. Chapter 5 of this book and other readings[12] already summarize these considerations. Legal professionals now know quite well how epidemiologists and physicians handle the cause-effect problem, and the bridging of legal and medical considerations is easy to establish. As a matter of fact, John Stuart Mill's general criteria for causation are already imbedded in epidemiologic thinking, as outlined in Chapter 5.

Lawyers and judges have a broader and often slightly different view of causation than do their medical counterparts.[15] In general, epidemiologic criteria of causation fit with those in the world of law. Some basic definitions from the world of law are worth quoting because it is expected that a health professional will contribute to the clarification of a cause-effect relationship in a way that is acceptable for both courts and epidemiology.[12 (Chap 5)] A health professional as a court witness should be familiar with the court's terminology, so as to contribute efficiently by cogent arguments to the solution of the problem under consideration. This terminology may, however, differ from one time or legal system to another, and the reader is encouraged to be familiar with both general and local meanings. A health professional as expert witness should agree with the court about the mutually acceptable meaning of wordings used in tort litigation. The domains of causation and evidence are worthy of attention, given their meanings in medicine and law. For lawyers:

A **cause** is "[e]*ach separate antecedent of an event. Something that precedes and brings about an effect or a result. A reason for an action or condition. A ground for legal action. An agent that brings something about. That which in some manner is accountable for a condition that brings about an effect or that produces a cause for the* *resultant action or state."*[11] In Clapp's[9] words, a cause is *"an action or event that brings about or contributes to a particular outcome."*

A **necessary cause** *(causa sine qua non)* is *"the cause without which the thing cannot be or the event could not have occurred."*[10]

A **direct cause** is *"the active, efficient cause that sets in motion a train of events which brings about a result without the intervention of any force* [that] *started* [from] *and* [is] *working actively from a new and independent source."*[11]

An **immediate cause** is *"the nearest cause in a point of time and space."*[16]

A **proximate cause** is *"that which in natural and continuous sequence unbroken by any new independent cause produces an event, and without which the injury would not have occurred."* [16] *". . . In tort cases, it is a wrongful conduct by a defendant leading to an injury complained of in a sufficiently direct way to justify holding the defendant liable for the plaintiff's damages. Also called **efficient cause** or **legal cause**."* [9] Also, *"a cause that directly produces an event and without which the event would not have occurred."*[10] Clapp[9] notes that *"to recover for a tort, it is not enough to show that the defendant did something wrong and that the plaintiff suffered from injury; it must be also shown that the wrong was a proximate cause of an injury."*

For Yogis,[17] it does not necessarily suffice for legal liability to establish the defendant's or defendants' negligence as a causal factor in the injury.

An **intervening cause** is *"an action or event that alters the course of a chain of events leading to the injury or loss that is the subject of a tort case. If the intervening event was foreseeable it would not relieve a person who set the chain of events in motion from liability."*[9] It is a later event after the negligence.[17] The intervening or supervening cause may or may not exonerate the defendant.[17] In occupational health and law, an **intervening efficient cause** is *"a new and independent force which breaks* [positively or negatively] *the causal connection between the original wrong and injury and itself becomes the direct and immediate cause of injury."*[11] It is *"one which comes into active operation in producing the result after the negligence of the defendant."*[16] In criminal law, an intervening efficient cause is *"a cause which comes between an antecedent and a consequence; it may be either independent or dependent, but in either case it is sufficient to negate criminal responsibility."*[11]

A **superseding** or **supervening cause** in tort law is *"an action or event that intervenes so dramatically and unexpectedly in a chain of causation, and changes its course so significantly, that the law regards it as a proximate cause of the injury or damage complained of."*[9] A superseding cause is one that is *"so substantially responsible for the ultimate injury that it acts to cut the liability of preceding actors regardless of whether their prior negligence was or was not a substantial factor in bringing about the injury complained of."*[17] A breakdown of a nuclear reactor is a superseding cause of a sudden high incidence of cancers in the surrounding community if some of the affected people would later have developed cancer anyway from other causes, such as air pollution from other industries. A traffic accident that kills a pedestrian recently released from the hospital is a superseding cause of the person's death, even if the patient would have died eventually from a piece of surgical equipment that the surgeon negligently left in the patient's abdomen. The surgeon cannot be blamed for this patient's death.

A **producing cause** (of an employee's death for which compensation is sought) is "*that cause, which, in a natural and continuous sequence, produces the death, and without which death would not have occurred.*"[11] Its meaning is close to the notion of necessary cause in epidemiology.[18]

A **remote cause** in tort law is "*an action or event that plays a role in bringing about an injury or loss, but is not a sufficiently direct cause to give rise to liability.*"[9]

A **probable consequence** is "*one that is more likely to follow its supposed cause than it is not to follow it.*"[11]

A **proximate consequence** is "*a result following unbroken sequence from some (especially negligent) event.*"[10]

The above definitions apply to the sense of "cause" as that which produces an effect. In law, however, the word cause has a second meaning. It also means "*a reason for taking certain action, especially a good or legally sufficient reason*" and "*a cause of action or civil case*"[9] as well as a reason for recovery. In this sense of cause, a **sufficient cause** is "*a cause that will hold a defendant to answer charges.*" It may be seen also as a "*reasonable and probable cause or the state of facts that would lead a man of ordinary caution to continuously entertain a strong suspicion of defendant's guilt.*" A **probable cause** means a "*reasonable cause; having more evidence for than against. . . . A set of probabilities grounded in the factual and practical considerations which govern the decisions of reasonable and prudent persons and is more than mere suspicion, but less than the quantum of evidence required for conviction.*"[11]

EVIDENCE

Evidence in law has a much broader sense than in EBM. It may be "*any species of proof or probative matter legally presented . . . for the purpose of inducing belief in the minds of the court or jury as to their* [the parties'] *contention.*"[17]

Evidence in law comes from a considerable array of sources.[19] Its purpose is to facilitate the introduction of all *logically relevant* facts (admissible evidence) without sacrificing any fundamental policy of the law, which may be of more importance than the ascertainment of truth.[17] Hearsay is generally not admissible as evidence.

Dukelow and Nuse[13] stress that evidence does not necessarily mean a proof of something. In law, **evidence** is "*an assertion of fact, opinion, belief or knowledge, whether material or not and whether admissible or not. . . . It . . . includes judgments, decisions, opinions, speeches, reports **and all other matters done or said before the court, including matters relating to the procedure**"* [including those of the judge]. This is quite different from evidence as defined in EBM or in philosophy. In other words, it means not only **what** is presented but also **how** it is presented. A proof of some cause-effect relationship may be an example of the former. A written report, recorded tape, or expert testimony falls into the latter category of evidence in the world of law. Hence, an exhibit itself also becomes evidence.[9]

Presumptive evidence is "*prima facie evidence, or evidence which is not conclusive and admits explanation or contradiction; evidence which must be received and treated as true and sufficient until and unless rebutted by other evidence.*"[11] It is "*[e]vidence deemed true and sufficient unless discredited by other evidence.*"[10] Sometimes such evidence is also called **probable evidence** from its foundation in probability.[11]

Sufficient evidence is *"that which is satisfactory for the purpose; that amount of proof which ordinarily satisfies an unprejudiced mind beyond a reasonable doubt. The term is synonymous with "**conclusive**" but it may be used interchangeably with the term 'weight of evidence'."* [11]

For courts, the **best evidence** is *"the evidence of the highest quality available, as measured by the nature of the case, rather than the thing being offered as evidence."* [10]

Expert evidence is evidence about a scientific, technical, or professional issue given by a person familiar with the subject or specially trained in the field. [10]

Scientific evidence is based on specialized knowledge that relies on scientific method for its evidentiary value. [10]

LEGAL DECISIONS ABOUT CAUSATION

The evidence that determines the judgment of the court is a **proof**. [10]

For courts, a cause means either the event as a **necessary condition** *(sine qua non)* or a condition that, along with others, is **sufficient** for the outcome. [20] For Mill, as put into the context of law by Greenberg, [21] the concept of cause should involve the *totality* of conditions (possible etiological factors, epidemiologically speaking) in which the event occurs.

In decisions about causation, two levels of decision must be distinguished. In **civil law**, it must be demonstrated that a particular agent or act is a **more probable than improbable cause** of a given health problem (in other words, "this one rather than any other one"). In **criminal law**, a balance of probabilities is not enough; proof beyond a reasonable doubt is required, and it must be demonstrated that a health problem in litigation (eg, paralysis, coma, death) is **unquestionably due to and only to** a given factor (cause). In other words, "it cannot (reasonably) be the other one".

Hoffman [22] summarizes this point as follows: *"Whereas scientific proof and statistical significance rest by convention on the demonstration of a 95 per cent or greater probability that the results of an experiment or investigation were not due to chance, in civil tort cases the most widely used standards of proof require a 'preponderance of evidence', 'more likely than not', a '50.1 per cent or more probability', 'but for', or 'reasonable medical certainty'. Probable is defined as 'having more evidence for than against'. 'Preponderance of evidence' is defined as 'evidence of greater weight or more convincing than the evidence which is offered in opposition to it. . . . [P]reponderance' denotes 'a superiority of weight'. In criminal cases, the usual standard of proof is 'beyond a reasonable doubt'. Therefore, quantitative epidemiologic data must be expressed more qualitatively in the courtroom."*

In general, proof must be drawn from up-to-date knowledge of specific evidence and research. The question of whether the criteria of causation (as reviewed in this chapter) were met [23,24] is also important. (Criteria of causation are not fixed, but they evolve with technology. [24])

First and foremost, were all variables (cause, effect, etc) well defined qualitatively and quantitatively? Was exposure well defined and quantified? Are health problems defined satisfactorily from the point of view of clinimetrics? What is fatigue? What is malaise? What is a lack of concentration? Frequently, very soft and nonspecific clinical data are presented as evidence, and only physicians can help the court make a "right" decision.

In the legal world, an **operational definition of both causes and consequences (outcomes)** remains an ongoing challenge. On the "cause" side, how can one define more precisely a "stressful factor"? On the "consequence" (outcome) side, how can one better define a "multiple chemical sensitivity"[21]? A syndrome that has multiple causes[12] poses an additional legal challenge[25] if it is presented as a cause for legal action.

Did the alleged cause really precede the effect? Did the plaintiff begin to lose weight before or after using a suspect household cleanser? Many cases are motivated by greed and come from poorly defined areas; others are much more substantial.

IS THE CAUSAL LINK UNDER REVIEW STRONG AND SPECIFIC ENOUGH?

In civil law, if one cause is known, its etiological fraction should be superior to 50%; if more etiological factors are known, the etiological fraction of the factor under scrutiny should be superior to any other known cause.

In criminal law, an absolutely specific relationship is sought in terms of an attributable fraction approaching 100%. For example, based on the review by Cole and Goldman,[26] while studying occupational exposure to vinyl chloride monomers as a cause of liver cancer, a 200.0 odds ratio (giving an approximate attributable fraction of 99.5%) was found. An odds ratio of 2 relating benzene occupational exposure to bone marrow neoplasia[27] giving a 50% attributable risk percent is less convincing than the former. Similar attention must be paid to **all other criteria of causation** as reviewed elsewhere,[12] not only to strength and specificity of a given cause-effect link.

The **temporal sequence** should be well understood. For example from the field of psychiatry,[25] a mental disease might be considered a cause of crime or a different outcome of sorts. In other cases, it might be viewed as a consequence (outcome) of some imputable factor or factors such as interpersonal relationships or drugs.

GENERAL AND INDIVIDUAL-FITTED CAUSE-EFFECT RELATIONSHIPS

Rose[27,28] rightly distinguishes causes of disease incidence, that is, causes of disease as a mass phenomenon in the community, and causes of a particular case. High national salt intake may be responsible for a high incidence of hypertension in the whole country, but what is the reason for the development of hypertension in a particular patient? This demonstration is more difficult. Causes of individual cases are less well known than causes of incidence. At present, conclusions must be based on rigorous judgment and inference from knowledge of causation at the community level.

It is essential to remember that **the burden of proof rests with the plaintiff**.[10,29] If this were generally known, there would be fewer court cases concerning health problems of individuals or communities.

CAUSATION IN HEALTH AND LAW

Both lawyers and health professionals are increasingly trying to reach a better mutual understanding of cause-effect relationships.[15] Judges and lawyers are now aware of epidemiology, and the issue of causal proof in health and disease is the

TABLE 7-2

Criminality and causality: parallels between reasoning in criminal law and reasoning in medical research*

Mayhem or murder and criminal law	Morbidity, mortality, and causality
1. Criminal present at the scene of the crime	Agent present in lesion of the disease
2. Premeditation	Causal events precede onset of disease
3. Accessories involved in the crime	Cofactors and/or multiple causality involved
4. Severity or death related to state of victim	Susceptibility and host response determine severity
5. Motivation: the crime must make sense in terms of gain to the criminal	The role of the agent in the disease must make biologic and common sense.
6. No other suspect could have committed the crime in the circumstances given	No other agent could have caused the disease under the circumstances given
7. The proof of guilt must be established beyond a reasonable doubt	The proof of causation must be established beyond reasonable doubt or role of chance

*Compiled with permission from Oxford University Press. (Evans AS. Causation and disease: a chronological journey. *Am J Epidemiol.* 1978;108:249–258.)

subject of attention in law and medicine[29-36] as well as in a growing body of literature. Surprisingly for many, the reasoning processes of people of law and medicine are very similar.

Table 7-2 represents Evans' postulated logical similarities between reasoning processes in the areas of health and law.[37]

Several basic questions emerge from this interface between epidemiologic considerations of cause-effect relationships and those in the realm of law[38]:

- Did the preponderance of evidence indicate that a presumed exposure led to more than 50% of the cases of the disease? (Look at the etiological fraction.)

- To what extent did that exposure (as opposed to other exposures) cause the disease? (Look at the attributable risk.)

- Was that particular exposure more likely than not the cause of that particular disease in that particular person? (**Consider a "phronetic" approach**, as outlined in more detail in Section 6.2.5.)

- Who was responsible for the exposure, and was the risk of disease foreseen?

- If the risk was foreseen, should the responsible person or institution be held accountable for *all* diseases following the exposure?

- The questions of costs go well beyond epidemiologic considerations. (The attributable risk concept may help.)

- Beyond epidemiologic considerations, courts will try to establish legal and administrative costs proportional to the cause-effect proof.

All health professionals, not just epidemiologists, must be cognizant of the rigor of causal proof in the face of the law. Considerable amounts of money and the health and well-being of subjects are at stake. Conclusions are made based on solid evidence and not on hearsay or demagogic statements from positions of authority, function, or qualification. Meta-analysis[39,40] will play an increasingly important role in such endeavors. Causal demonstrations in courts are challenging and difficult. The credibility, competence, and experience of all experts involved must be rebuilt from scratch before the judge. Everything is recorded, and the records become part of the public domain.

Inevitably, expert witnesses are brought to the court both by the plaintiff and by the defendant. They are recruited to one side or another, no matter their objectivity. Ethics must be scrupulously respected, as in all fields of epidemiology, and its rules are now available in the literature.[41]

The health professional can help the court reach the right decision but will never be in a position to decide. The decision is up to the jury (or judge).[25]

Causal considerations of a health problem in specific cases and individuals

Ultimately, physicians giving their expert opinions in court must realize that, although courts are certainly interested in general truths, for example, that a particular chemical causes cancer, **decisions are made for the specific and precise case of the plaintiff.** For example, was the lung cancer in this waitress who worked in these precise smoke-filled restaurants and bars caused by her working environment? So the issue goes from a general to a specific one. Do studies giving a general proof apply to a specific individual? This is similar to the question, "Does this research result apply to my patient?" General rules of admissibility have partly been listed in Chapter 6 and elsewhere,[12] mainly with respect to the theoretical eligibility of a particular individual for analytical studies brought to the attention of the courts as evidence.

The general legal thinking may be understood as follows: Yes, it is nice to know that this substance causes harm to people. But how did all this work in the case of this particular individual in this particular setting? The answer is not simple. An important consideration is whether the particular individual fits into the evidentiary proof brought to the court. Suppose, for example, that testimony is based on a well-designed clinical trial showing the effectiveness of the drug with which the patient in court was treated, with apparent success or failure. **Did this drug have an effect in this specific individual?** There are five points to ponder.

1. Is the patient under scrutiny **eligible to participate in a clinical trial showing the effectiveness of the drug under scrutiny** (demographic characteristics, stage, spectrum and gradient of disease, comorbidity, treatments for comorbidity, etc)?

2. Would the patient be **eligible for a phase III** (classic randomized, double-blind, controlled), **phase IV** (a postmarketing study of "clean" cases), or **phase V** (a postmarketing study of "dirty" patients, ie, as they come with comorbidities and cotreatments) **clinical trial?**

3. Eventually, do **the patient's characteristics correspond to those of the responders to treatment?** Unfortunately, this information is most often not available in space-limited research articles on clinical trials. Treatment responders may differ in their characteristics from the whole experimental group or from all patients enrolled in the trial.

4. What are the **characteristics of patients responding to a placebo or any other control treatment?**

5. Ultimately, are the **characteristics of responders and nonresponders within and between experimental and control groups comparable?**

In the search for causes of litigation-prone and other adverse drug reactions, similar cause-effect considerations apply, except that for ethical reasons evidence comes from observational analytical studies (based on surveillance) and not necessarily as some fringe information from clinical trials.

All five of these considerations are important, not only in court but also in the clinical practice of EBM, because they help answer the question, *"Does this apply to my patient?"*

In this way, clinical epidemiology makes more tangible and concrete the phronetic approach outlined in Section 6.2.5.

The problem of transferability of general knowledge to a particular patient or other individual was treated in greater detail by others, Rose[27,28] in particular.

Epidemiologic experience from the investigation of causes can be applied to such unusual "outbreaks" as a series of clinical complications or patient deaths in hospitals, which might be related to a cause, such as a mentally disturbed or criminal employee, or any other responsible "cause" of such a situation. Multiple cause-effect hypotheses (which employee might be related to the occurrence of cases) must be and have been successfully analyzed in courts as contributing evidence to strengthen final conclusions about the guilt of suspected individuals.[42-45]

7.2.3 Emergence of Clinical Guidelines and Their Role in Courts of Law

Besides the cause-effect relationship and its logical uses as a topic of litigation, a new element appears in courts of law: the **validity and uses of guidelines in cases under litigation and their consequences.**

Did the physician follow guidelines in caring for the patient? Was the doctor aware of existing guidelines? What is the validity of these guidelines? Did their use lead to benefits for the patient or to harm of some sort? Clinical guidelines themselves or their uses may become a subject of litigation. Do they function in given cases as a statutory standard of care?

Guidelines are defined in general as formal statements about a defined state or function.[46] More precisely, guidelines are considered "*a standardized set of information describing the best practices for addressing health problems commonly encountered either in clinical or public health practice.*"[47] In other words, from the American

Institute of Medicine, clinical guidelines are *"systematically developed statements to assist practitioner and patient decisions about appropriate health care for specific clinical circumstances."*[48,49] Information is based either on the best available research evidence or on the consensus opinion of medical and other health experts.

The reader may be aware of three types of guidelines:

1. **Practice guidelines based on evidence.** These most desirable guidelines are the fruit of an eight-step process,[50] in which the first is added by us:

    a. The values relevant to the health problem and other components of the guidelines under consideration are stated.

    b. The topic and the process for developing the guidelines are defined.

    c. A systematic review of evidence supporting guidelines is performed.

    d. Expert opinions are evaluated and integrated if necessary.

    e. Public policy is identified and taken into account.

    f. Recommendations are developed.

    g. A draft version of a report that includes guidelines in situations of varying complexity is written down.

    h. A final version is worked up in accordance with the results of an external review.

2. **Structured consensus-based guidelines** are the product of a methodologically well-defined step-by-step process.[51]

3. **Unstructured guidelines** are conclusions from an informal get-together of experts. The recipient of the guidelines does not know how the experts arrived at their proposal.

Different types of guidelines may have different inferential force in cases in which it must be decided if the use of guidelines (or not using them) has had some impact on patients' or community health. Evidence-based guidelines are more clearly founded on logical uses of evidence than are guidelines of obscure origin.

In any case, guidelines are meant as **advice**, and they do not have the power of law needed for them to be followed blindly.[52] Their users must argue properly for, and justify, their use *or* their nonuse.

For practical purposes, clinical guidelines may be developed as uses of the best evidence in a logical way, either as a **benefit to the patient** or as a **cost-cutting measure**.

Gevers[49] points out that *"guidelines do not replace medical responsibility and cannot completely reduce medical discretion. Therefore, compliance with a guideline never protects a practitioner from liability, particularly if he could and should have realized that acting in accordance with the guideline would not have the desired effect in the particular case."* Cogent arguments must justify their use.

7.2.4 Reflective Thinking in Courts of Law

For Aldisert,[53] logical thinking in court is a kind of reflective thinking, solving a problem in law by pondering a given set of facts in order to perceive their connection. The phrase *reflective thinking* here is practically synonymous with *critical thinking*. Hence, legal argumentation may focus on the variety of evidence brought to the attention of the court as well as on **how it is presented.** Apparently truthful premises based on good evidence are not enough. Were they well chosen? Are they related to the problem of interest? Are the inferences to the conclusions warranted? Are there exceptional circumstances in the particular case that override a usually applicable warrant? Poor logic in argumentation may harm the case as much as poor primary evidence itself. Conclusions stemming from arguments are taken as new evidence in the legal process and in further legal argumentation.

The knowledge and practice of basic rules of informal logic, as outlined in Chapter 3, must be coupled with attention to, avoidance of, and countering of numerous fallacies, which may occur throughout legal argumentation. More about this can be found later in this chapter, in Section 7.5.

7.3 ARGUMENTATION ABOUT CASES BEFORE WORKER COMPENSATION BOARDS AND OTHER CIVIC BODIES

In relation to logic, argumentation about occupational health before various civic bodies is not in its substance different from argumentation in courts of law. As a matter of fact, Worker Compensation Boards in many countries[54-56] were created to avoid costly litigation for plaintiffs (injured or sick workers) and defendants (companies). Industry receives protection from expensive litigation, and workers receive an agreed-on compensation faster by sacrificing their right to sue.[54]

Behind a legally and administratively streamlined procedure lies a similar basic logical argumentation. As in courts of law, decisions must often be made under a variable degree of uncertainty.

Again, the key problem is a demonstration of a cause (work)-effect (injury, disease) relationship in individuals and groups of individuals. Criteria for such relationships were already mentioned briefly in Chapter 5 and more extensively elsewhere[12,57] and were applied to work and environment issues.[57-59] All concerned parties must be aware of the philosophical, logical, and scientific reasoning underlying practical decisions.[56,60]

Epidemiologic considerations, however challenging and sometimes limited they might be, are crucial to establish work-related health effects.[60] Most decision makers are now aware of cohort, case-control, or experimental studies (trials); individual, relative, and attributable risks; etiological fractions (attributable risk percents); validity of diagnostic methods; and other probabilities.[12] Some specific adaptations may apply.

As in court cases, scientific evidence must be presented to help the tribunal or the compensation board decide about the guilt (causing the disease) or innocence (not causing it) of the suspect (working environment, company).[61] For example, the principle of likelihood ratios, well known to epidemiologists, may be linked with similar reasoning in the field of law, as outlined by Curran et al.[62] Two hypotheses are considered:

H_p: The suspect is the source (cause) of the health problem. Hypothesis is in favor of the plaintiff (worker), p.

H_d: Someone unrelated to the suspect (working environment, company) is the source (cause) of the health problem. Hypothesis is in favor of the defendant (company), d.

E: Evidence. The test result or diagnosis of disease relevant to the decision between H_p and H_d.

Pr: Probabilty.

The likelihood ratio, LR, is then:[62]

$$LR = \frac{Pr\ (E \mid H_p)}{Pr\ (E \mid H_d)}$$

This kind of likelihood ratio is used for genetic matches in paternity cases or in other forensic cases[62] in which the answer to the following question is sought: "How much does the evidence increase the probability that a given health problem was produced by a suspected cause?" We are close here to the notion of relative risks as we use and understand them in epidemiology.

The failure to produce evidence may itself be evidence, that is, evidence in favor of something else causing the problem. The absence of positive evidence, however, does not mean a negative conclusion. In practice, denial of a claim should not be based on this.

In causal proof, clinical and laboratory logic is strongly influenced now by Popperian refutation.[63]

In the case of a divergence of opinion, lack of evidence, and a high degree of uncertainty, consensus methods[51] may be considered.

Decision makers may sometimes be more aware of evidence itself than of the nature and quality of argumentation and the absence of major fallacies in it.

7.4 DEALING WITH HEALTH PROBLEMS IN THE MEDIA AND ON THE POLITICAL OR ENTERTAINMENT STAGE

Dealing with health problems in the media can be challenging because the considerable heterogeneity of triggers and motives for the topic and the ensuing information means that the customary rules of argumentation do not necessarily apply. Topics may be raised for four basic reasons:

1. Facts and evidence relevant to the question

2. Vested interests of some party (government, industry, academe)

3. Beliefs instead of facts and evidence

4. Simple attention grabbers without any other specific consideration

Any health professional in any of these four circumstances is brought into the discussion with one of two expectations. He or she will bring expertise (evidence and its logical uses) either to complete the discussion or to defend the position of some stakeholder. In either circumstance, the maxim "noblesse oblige" applies. Because "anything goes," the testimony of a health professional will not be accepted automatically. Sometimes, seemingly innocuous unsubstantiated remarks may be taken out of context and used elsewhere where more than the reader's or viewer's information is at stake.

In any of the four just-mentioned situations, the arguments of health professionals must proceed from **justified premises** (evidence-based), which include **all practically obtainable relevant information** to **relevant conclusions** in accordance with **justified warrants,** which have **no known overriding exceptions** in the particular case. Such virtues may sometimes be difficult to achieve, if the discussion is dealing with **beliefs instead of facts**.

As already discussed in previous chapters, a belief is not a fact. Belief means holding a proposition for a fact or truth. A belief may be substantiated to some degree by rational or irrational factors. It is defined in more than one way.

Belief has variously been defined as:

- *A dispositional psychological state in virtue of which a person will assent to a proposition under certain conditions*[64]

- *The acknowledgment that a proposition is true in the absence of demonstrable proof as required by scientific method*[65]

- *The power behind ideas* (Spanish philosopher José Ortega y Gasset, 1883 to 1955)[66]

- *A rather primary cognitive state as a precursor of reasoning towards evidence.*

In some cultures, beliefs may constitute an organized system and consequently a coherent organizing force.[65]

Health professionals are often disarmed if they try to handle beliefs through arguments containing justified (evidence-based) premises. Their greatest contribution in these kinds of discussion may be to give a sober account of both available and missing desirable evidence and their uses in justifying conclusions.

Beliefs in the media are often presented as statements on an equal footing with evidence-based information. Expert viewer and reader beware!

Fallacies and Rhetorical Ploys to Recognize, Avoid, or Correct

In the outside world, almost anything goes. In court, lawyers are there to win a case for their clients, not necessarily to unravel an absolute truth. Before occupational medicine boards, compensation is the main stake. In politics, winning the next election, being elected or reelected counts. In many media, attracting readership or viewership is the main goal. In advertising, selling products and services beats the most impeccable logical argument. Argumentation, if any, is subjected to these objectives.

Flows of thought may be fallacious, unintentionally or elsewhere intentionally, in order to reach these objectives. To reach such objectives, two kinds of persuasive devices may be used: rhetorical ploys and fallacies.[67] These must be identified and countered. **Fallacies**, as defined in Chapter 3, are faults in reasoning, argument, or argumentation. **Rhetorical ploys** are nonargumentative deficiencies in reasoning. For Bowell and Kemp,[67] rhetorical ploys are **nonargumentative sham reasonings** (whereas fallacies are of the argumentative type). For these authors, **rhetoric** is *"any verbal or written attempt to persuade someone to believe, desire or do something that does not attempt to give good reasons for the belief, desire or action, but attempts to motivate that belief, desire or action solely through the power of the words used."* A rhetorical ploy may be hard to crack by a logician who is relegated to the reading of the word. The logician may ignore the reasoning that may be dissociated intentionally from the verbal message.

Rhetorical ploys are *"commonly encountered instances of the rhetorical use of language."*[67] They may involve appeals to anything: novelty, sexiness, dignity, rights, logic, political correctness, morality, monetary matters, or even fear of harm, disease, or death.

A rhetorical ploy may look like a faulty argument, but correct reasoning may lie behind it. The opposite may also be true. The "ploy-master" may even be aware of this dissociation between mind and the spoken word. In this kind of rhetoric, the messenger wants his or her message to be accepted by readers, viewers, or listeners. The messenger does not necessarily and intentionally present the truth. Rhetorical ploys play most often on a recipient's feelings.

APPEAL TO NOVELTY

Appeal to novelty is used very often in drug marketing. A pharmaceutical company may develop the nth subtle chemical variant of an already existing minor tranquilizer or anxiolytic benzodiazepine or an over-the-counter nonprescription analgesic or antipyretic. "*Because it's new, it must be better!*" Compared with a placebo, the drug is effective. If a similarly impeccable clinical trial would use as a control treatment the most effective one currently available, the *relative* effectiveness of the new drug might prove less convincing.

APPEAL TO POPULARITY

In an **appeal to popularity**, a reference is made to some event, product, or person and linked to celebrities. Here is a caricatured example: "Get the best face-lift! Dr Cheeksmoother is the preferred plastic surgeon of stars. (Not to be confused with his competitor, Dr Cheeksmotherer!) Have you had your face-lift yet? If not, be a patient of Dr Cheeksmoother, and be a star! Roll your wrinkles back 20 years by calling the following phone number. . . ."

Rhetorical ploys play on our feelings, emotions, and perceived values.

Contrary to rhetorical ploys, **fallacies** may be somehow related to the content of premises and conclusions (**evidence or content-related**) or to the architecture and inference of the argument itself (**formal fallacies**).

The following serve as examples of fallacies. A quarter century ago, in occupational health, Ison[60] made a correct evidence-related point: "*On any question of employment causation, there appears to be a widespread feeling in the medical profession that the absence of positive data requires a negative assumption. Uncertainty about the cause of a disease can, therefore, lead automatically to the denial of a claim without any intermediate reference to the evidentiary criteria prescribed by law.*" His thought draws our attention to the fallacy *ad ignorantiam.*

FALLACY "AD IGNORANTIAM"

This fallacy occurs if the argument contends that some statement must be true (or false) because there is no evidence to disprove (or prove) it. It is used to convince the masses about the effectiveness of some alternative medicines. Nobody has proved that they do not work, so they must! In reverse, nobody has proved that they work, so they don't!

FALLACY OF AMBIGUITY AND AMPHIBOLY

A **fallacy of ambiguity** occurs if more than one meaning is given to a single word or sentence, the latter case being given the name **fallacy of amphiboly**. "*Our evaluation leads us to the conclusion that sudden acute respiratory syndrome (SARS) and the ongoing surveillance/prevention/cure program shall be subdued*" is a statement straight from a Delphic oracle. It may mean either the uncontrolled spread of SARS or the success of the control measures implemented by the health service.

FALLACY OF "ARGUMENTUM AD VERECUNDIAM"

The **fallacy of *argumentum ad verecundiam*** is very common in daily clinical life, as in the ecclesiastic doctrine of the infallibility of the pope. For example: "*Put Mrs Putrill in Room 218 on a course of corticosteroids. Why? The attending endocrinologist, Dr Smart, said so. He is quite knowledgeable in these things! Dr Clever thinks otherwise, but that's how it works in this place.*" Such appeals to authority are illegitimate when authorities disagree (as in this example), when the conclusion is not within the expertise of the supposed authority, when it is possible and desirable to work out the conclusion for oneself on the basis of evidence, or when the supposed authority has not applied her or his expertise carefully. On the other hand, appeals to authority may be unavoidable and necessary in other situations, such as those when some public health measure is prescribed by law: quarantine for some diseases, preventive leave of a pregnant worker, or exclusion by authority of a pedophiliac from contact with children. In other situations, *in extremis*, authorities in the matter are selected for interviews in the media because they hold a particular office, such as the coroner or public health officer. In such situations, there is a defeasible presumption that qualified experts speak the truth when they make statements in their field of expertise after having carefully considered the relevant evidence. With no opportunity to examine the evidence ourselves, we take their word for it, recognizing that they might turn out to be mistaken.

STATISTICAL OR CLINICOEPIDEMIOLOGICAL FALLACY (DANGLING RELATIVE)

Let us say that a television advertisement claims that *"Lipidator is 10 times better at lowering blood cholesterol! Ask your doctor about Lipidator!"* This ad commits a **statistical** or **clinicoepidemiologic fallacy** (**dangling relative**[68]), because a reference treatment in this comparison is not specified.

Things are even more complicated if the premises are correct and if equally correct conclusions do not emanate from them. Let us take a caricatured situation: *"Vitamin C is good for your health. . . . Preventing cancer requires proper nutrition. . . . Therefore, improve your lifestyle!"* In this situation, the premises may be good (truthful, evidence-based), but they may be totally unrelated to a poorly defined lifestyle.

7.5 CONCLUSIONS

For a health professional, communicating with the outside world does not mean having to lower or otherwise modify standards of evidence and its proper uses in cogent argumentation. Rather, communication should be directed according to the legal and political context, which is given by the commissioner of discussion (courts, stakeholders, media), the participants (professional and lay public), and the target population (beneficiaries of the endeavor).

Health professionals will use not only skills acquired in epidemiology, EBM, or basic and clinical sciences. They also will apply these skills in the framework of logic and critical thinking, as outlined in the previous chapters and adapted to the realm of law[1] and other domains of public life.

References

1. Toulmin S, Rieke R, Janik A. *An Introduction to Reasoning.* 2nd ed. New York, NY: Macmillan Publishing Co; 1984:281–311.

2. Kamm FM. The philosopher as insider and outsider. *J Med Phil.* 1986;11:347–374.

3. Havighurst CC, Hutt PB, McNeil BJ, Miller M. Evidence: its meanings in health care and in law. *J Health Politics Policy Law.* 2001;26.

4. Waller BN. *Critical Thinking: Consider the Verdict.* Englewood Cliffs, NJ: Prentice Hall; 1988.

5. Alpers A. Justice Blackmun and the good physician: patients, populations and the paradox of medicine. *Hastings Constitutional Law Q.* 1998;26:41–58.

6. Cruise KR, Rogers R. An analysis of competency to stand trial: an integration of case law and clinical knowledge. *Behav Sci Law.* 1998;16:35–50.

7. Norton ML. The physician expert witness and the U.S. Supreme Court—an epidemiologic approach. *Med Law.* 2002;21:435–449.

8. Stevenson JR. An expert experiment—medico-legal expert testimony. *Med Law.* 1999;18:47–53.

9. Clapp JE. *Random House Webster's Dictionary of the Law.* New York, NY: Random House; 2000.

10. Garner BA, ed. *Black's Law Dictionary.* 7th ed. St. Paul, Minn: West Group; 1999.

11. Black HC. *Black's Law Dictionary.* 6th ed. St. Paul, Minn: West Group; 1990.

12. Jenicek M. *Foundations of Evidence-Based Medicine.* New York, NY: The Parthenon Publishing Group; 2003.

13. Dukelow DA, Nuse B. *The Dictionary of Canadian Law.* 2nd ed. Toronto, Ontario: Thomson Professional Publishing; 1995.

14. Levin AS. Science in court. *Lancet.* 1987;2:1526.

15. Freckleton I, Mendelson D, eds. *Causation in Law and Medicine.* Burlington, Vt: Ashgate Publishing Co; 2002.

16. Gifis SH. *Law Dictionary.* Woodbury, NY: Barron's Educational Series Inc; 1975.

17. Yogis JA. *Canadian Law Dictionary.* 4th ed. Hauppauge, NY: Barron's Educational Series Inc; 1998.

18. Rothman KJ. Causes. *Am J Epidemiol.* 1976;104:587–592.

19. Burton WC. *Burton's Legal Thesaurus.* 3rd ed. New York, NY: McGraw-Hill; 1998.

20. Honoré A. Principles and values underlying the concept of causation in law. In: Clapp JE, ed. *Random House Webster's Dictionary of the Law.* New York, NY: Random House; 2000:3–13.

21. Greenberg P. The cause of disease and illness: medical views and uncertainties. In: Clapp JE, ed. *Random House Webster's Dictionary of the Law.* New York, NY: Random House; 2000:38–57.

22. Hoffman RE. The use of epidemiologic data in the courts. *Am J Epidemiol.* 1984;120:190–202.

23. Norman GR, Newhouse MT. Health effects of urea formaldehyde foam insulation: evidence of causation. *Can Med Ass J.* 1986;134:733–738.

24. Evans EA. Causation and disease: effect of technology on postulates of causation. *Yale J Biol Med.* 1991;64:513–528.

25. Slovenko R. Causation in law and psychiatry. In: Clapp JE, ed. *Random House Webster's Dictionary of the Law.* New York, NY: Random House; 2000:357–378.

26. Cole P, Goldman MB. Occupation. In: Fraumeni JF Jr, ed. *Persons at High Risk of Cancer.* New York, NY: Academic Press; 1975:167–184.

27. Rose G. Sick individuals and sick populations. *Int J Epidemiol.* 1985;14:32–38.

28. Rose G. *The Strategy of Preventive Medicine.* Oxford, England: Oxford University Press; 1992.

29. Brennan TA, Carter RF. Legal and scientific probability of causation of cancer and other environmental disease in individuals. *J Health Politics Law.* 1985;10:33–80.

30. Black B, Lilienfeld DE. Epidemiologic proof in toxic tort litigation. *Fordham Law Review.* 1984; 52:732–785.

31. Lilienfeld DE, Black B. The epidemiologist in court: some comments. *Am J Epidemiol.* 1986;123:961–964.

32. Teret SP. Litigating for the public's health. *Am J Public Health.* 1986;76:1027–1029.

33. Norman GR. Science, public policy, and media disease. *CMAJ.* 1986;134:719–720.

34. Cole P. Epidemiologist as an expert witness. *J Clin Epidemiol.* 1991;44:35S–39S.

35. Greater use of expert panels proposed as additional means of presenting epidemiologic evidence to the courts [editorial]. *Epidemiol Monitor.* 1989;10:1–3.

36. Holden C. Science in court. *Science.* 1989;243:1658–1659.

37. Evans AS. Causation and disease: a chronological journey. *Am J Epidemiol.* 1978;108:249–258.

38. Evans AS. *Causation and Disease: A Chronological Journey.* New York, NY: Plenum Medical Book Co; 1993.

39. Jenicek M. Meta-analysis in medicine: where are we and where we want to go. *J Clin Epidemiol.* 1989;42:35–44.

40. Jenicek M. *Méta-analyse en médecine: evaluation et synthèse de l'information clinique et épidémiologique. [Meta-analysis in Medicine. Evaluation and Synthesis of Clinical and Epidemiological Information].* Paris, France: EDISEM et Maloine; 1987.

41. Fayerweather WE, Higginson J, Beauchamp TL, eds. Industrial epidemiology forum's conference on ethics in epidemiology. *J Clin Epidemiol.* 1991;44.

42. Rothman KJ. Sleuthing in hospitals. *N Engl J Med.* 1985;313:258–259.

43. Istre GR, Gustafson TL, Baron RC, Martin DL, Orlowski JP. A mysterious cluster of deaths and cardiopulmonary arrests in a pediatric intensive care unit. *N Engl J Med.* 1985;133:205–211.

44. Buehler JW, Smith LF, Wallace EM, Heath CW Jr, Kusiak R, Herndon JL. Unexplained deaths in a children hospital: an epidemiologic assessment. *N Engl J Med.* 1985;313:211–216.

45. Sacks JJ, Stroup DF, Will ML, Harris EL, Israel E. A nurse-associated epidemic of cardiac arrests in an intensive care unit. *JAMA.* 1988;259:689–695.

46. Last JM, ed. *A Dictionary of Epidemiology.* 4th ed. Oxford, England: Oxford University Press; 2001.

47. Brownson RC, Baker EA, Leet TL, Gillespie KN. *Evidence-Based Public Health.* Oxford, England: Oxford University Press; 2003.

48. King JY. Practice guidelines and medical malpractice litigation. *Med Law.* 1997;16:29–39.

49. Gevers S. Clinical practice guidelines; legal aspects. *Med Law.* 1996;15: 671–675.

50. Woolf SH, George JN. Evidence-based medicine: interpreting studies and set-ting policy. *Hematol Oncol Clin North Am.* 2000;14:761–784.

51. Murphy MK, Black NA, Lamping DL, et al. Consensus development methods, and their use in clinical guideline development. *Health Technol Assess.* 1998;2:i–iv,1–88.

52. Hulst E. Clinical guidelines and their civil law effects. *Med Law.* 2002;21:651–660.

53. Aldisert RJ. *Logic for Lawyers: A Guide to Clear Legal Thinking.* 3rd ed. Notre Dame, Ind: National Institute for Trial Advocacy; 1997.

54. Plumb JM, Cowell JWF. An overview of workers' compensation. *Occup Med.* 1998;13:241–272.

55. Harte D, Smith DA. Workers' compensation appeals systems in Canada and the United States. *Occup Med.* 1998;13:423–428.

56. Richman SI. Why change? A look at the current system of disability determina-tion and workers' compensation for occupational lung disease. *Ann Intern Med.* 1982;97:908–914.

57. Weed DL. Epidemiologic evidence and causal inference. *Hematol Oncol Clin North Am.* 2000;4:797–807.

58. Kaufman JS, Poole C. Looking back on causal thinking in the health sciences. *Annu Rev Public Health.* 2000;21:101–119.

59. Ricci PF, Rice D, Ziangos J, Cox JA Jr. Precaution, uncertainty and causation in environmental decisions. *Environ Internat.* 2003;29:1–19.

60. Ison TG. The dimensions of industrial disease. Part II. The compensation boards. *Can Med Assoc J.* 1978;118:317–322.

61. Guidotti TL. Applying epidemiology to adjudication. In: Guidotti TL, Cowell JWF, eds. *Occupational Medicine: State of the Art Reviews.* April-June 1998;13, No 2.

62. Curran JM, Robertson B, Vignaux GA. Genetic matches and the logic of the law. *Genetica.* 1999;105:211–213.

63. Federspil G, Vettor R. Clinical and laboratory logic. *Clin Chim Acta.* 1999;280:25–34.

64. Blackburn S. *Oxford Dictionary of Philosophy.* Oxford, England: Oxford University Press; 1996.

65. Trombley S. Belief. In: Bullock A, Trombley S, eds. *The New Fontana Dictionary of Modern Thought.* 3rd ed. London, England: HarperCollins Publishers; 1999:70.

66. Reese WL. *Dictionary of Philosophy and Religion: Eastern and WesternThought.* Expanded Ed. Amherst, NY: Humanity Books; 1999.

67. Bowell T, Kemp G. *Critical Thinking: A Concise Guide.* London, England: Routledge; 2002.

68. Hitchcock D. *Critical Thinking: A Guide to Evaluating Information.* Toronto, Ontario: Methuen Publishing; 1983.

Concluding Remarks

*Deficiency in judgment is just what
is ordinarily called stupidity, and for
such a failing, there is no remedy.*

IMMANUEL KANT, 1781

NOT QUITE, PROFESSOR KANT!

THERE IS, IN FACT, ONE REMEDY: LOGIC AND CRITICAL THINKING.

*Evidence-based Medicine is still considered by many
as the most discomforting paradigm of medicine
devised by the wit of man, except for all the others.*

PARAPHRASING WINSTON SPENCER CHURCHILL,

1947, ON DEMOCRACY

*It is easy to be certain.
One has only to be sufficiently vague.*

CHARLES SANDERS PEIRCE, 1902

*If clinical common sense
is not pragmatically evaluated
to the same extent as trial evidence,
then no possible advance or sharpening
of clinical reasoning is possible.*

ROSS UPSHUR, 1997

For decades, clinical and community medicine
have greatly benefited from epidemiology, biostatistics,
sociology, anthropology, and management-related disciplines
such as health administration or health economics.
Given this, shouldn't logic and critical thinking
be additional ingredients to master and practice,
and guide the inquisitive mind of the health professional
in his or her reasoning and decision-making?

Here ends our exploration of logic and critical thinking in medicine and other health sciences. The reflections and proposals in this writing are part of a trend in medicine and other health sciences to bridge philosophy, scientific method, and human experience in an effort to improve medical reasoning and decisions. Such an ongoing modern stream of thought may be seen across the medical literature during the last 30 years.[1-8] The initiatives are different, but they reflect a common line of thought that has only just begun.

This is an exciting time for health sciences. On the one hand, evidence-based medicine (EBM) strikes a better balance between evidence and experience in medical decision making. On the other, a new challenge emerges: how can we put into practice the best evidence and experience available?

Evidence-based medicine and critical thinking are an interwoven complex. Critics complain that the EBM movement makes of research evidence a golden calf to venerate.[9] Much criticism also stems from a reductionist view of EBM by those who regard it as limited solely to cause-effect evaluations instead of viewing its principles, techniques, and methods as relevant to solving all problems in clinical and community medicine. Most often, those who restrict EBM in this way are its recipients rather than its authors.

From a logical standpoint, there are two opposing perspectives on EBM. The first is based on Kurt Gödel's view that, in the simplest of terms, there is always a part (data, theories, hypotheses, and so on) that cannot be proved, such as the effectiveness or ineffectiveness of some treatment. For Sleigh,[10] this means that one must solve the problem by "jumping outside" the system (research studies) and applying "common sense." From this perspective, EBM is unworkable. The second perspective relies on Charles Sanders Peirce's concept of abduction, which for Upshur[11] makes EBM workable.

The production and evaluation of evidence are methodologically much more advanced than "using evidence in medical practice" as the ultimate and final step of EBM. Uses of evidence require as much understanding, methodological development, and testing in practice as producing evidence. Such uses are erratic and their results are uncertain if they are applied uncritically and with poor logic.

Critical thinking is a much more elusive domain than biostatistics, clinical epidemiology, or laboratory measurement. The reader should notice, however, that behind it lie, as anywhere else, many complex and well-structured methods and techniques. The mastery of this domain requires formal training comparable to that required in basic or clinical research, or in clinical skills. Present challenges to the clinical research enterprise[12] should benefit from it.

The logic behind critical thinking is focused either on its symbolic and mathematical structure (formal logic)[13] or on its practical uses in everyday life. This text was about the latter, which enriches daily reflection and work and rewards for good results. The former is reserved only for a select few.

Behind the ubiquitous reflection on the "art and science of medicine" stand the essential knowledge (*episteme*), know-how (*techne*, or practical skills and experience in those skills), and long-forgotten *phronesis* of the ancient Greek philosophers, clinical judgment, and decision making in the ever-changing practical and concrete situations of our times. Like the basic sciences (*episteme*) learned theoretically and the medical art (*techne*) acquired by clinical training, *phronesis* is learned through both theory and practice, and this book aspires to contribute to it.

Challenges to clinical judgment are increasing, with competing paradigms of the more traditional Aristotelian logic of excluded middle on the one hand and fuzzy theory and its product, fuzzy logic,[14] on the other.

Are critical thinking and logic different in public health and community medicine than in clinical medicine? They are not.

Instead of a bedridden patient, we deal in public health and community medicine with "community-ridden" groups of individuals sharing similar characteristics, ways of life, and purposes. Critical thinking and logic as they relate to community health problems are the same as in clinical medicine; only the premises and ensuing conclusions are different. They go beyond a single individual, beyond a disease case to the disease itself, and they try to provide the best answer to different problems and questions about them. The *phronesis* of public health or community medicine judgment just drags the same logic and critical thinking from the bedside to the street.

For Pellegrino,[15] "*evidence-based medicine is the newest name for a very old idea. The best physicians have always sought the best empirical evidence available on which to base diagnoses and therapeutic decisions. What is new today is the availability of a much broader array of empirical data and far more sophisticated methods for validating and interpreting them. . . . [R]ational medicine is impossible without a sense of the moral obligations required to make evidence based medicine possible.*" These virtues are not emotions or knowledge, but states. A virtue in Aristotle's *Nicomachean Ethics* is a "*state concerned with choice, lying in a mean relative to us, this being determined by reason and in the way in which the man of practical wisdom would determine it.*" The present textbook should contribute to making these 2000-year-old virtues flourish in our present millennium.

Zarkovich and Upshur[16] conclude for us: "*Evidence represents a way to justify or validate propositions. We use evidence as a means of supporting conclusions we have drawn. Medically speaking, physicians use evidence to justify their beliefs about illness and disease. In this sense, EBM provides a vast quantity (and quality) of related evidence both in a personal and [in] a scientific context. . . . While it is true that evidence is conceived in a scientific context, it is also conceived through a human context, therefore possessing a social and human dimension.*" In a two-step and two-component path, general evidence joins a physician's past experience, views, and values within the concrete context of a specific case: "our stuporous patient lying in the third bed of Room 12 on the third floor of this hospital" or "This index case of sudden acute respiratory syndrome at the Happy Traveler Hotel is a potential trigger of a community outbreak of this new entity in this city."

Can we practice good medicine without evidence, logic, and critical thinking? We can't! Not only logic but also several other domains of philosophy are increasingly present in all medical domains of evidence as shown in Table 1.

TABLE 1

Domains of evidence and related aspects of philosophy

Domain of evidence	Related aspects of philosophy
Gathering clinical material as grounds for evidence	Techne/episteme/phronesis, inductive, deductive logic
Producing evidence	Logic, epistemology, logical positivism
Evaluating evidence	Logic, hermeneutics, epistemology, pragmatism
Using evidence	Logic, phronesis, pragmatism, instrumentalism, ethics
Evaluating practice based on evidence	Logic, pragmatism

Logical positivism was perhaps one of the first important bridges between analytical and experimental aspects of science and philosophy as well as other philosophical movements.

Pragmatism (as espoused by William James and Charles Sanders Peirce) as a method of solving and evaluating intellectual problems and a theory about the kinds of logic we are capable of acquiring[17] offers a necessary look at values of propositions and statements if they are true ("cash value"). It is an apprehension of an independent universe through purposive interaction such as clinical encounters or experiments.[11]

With application to medicine, John Dewey's **instrumentalism** sees knowledge in terms of the biological and psychological role that the knowing process plays in human affairs (patient-physician interaction in our case) and in the ways of employment of this conception as a guide of application to and direction of health professionals' activities to solve health problems.

The streams of thought—logical positivism, pragmatism, and instrumentalism—illustrate how much we depend in medicine on the increasing interface between science and philosophy. It is only logical that philosophical foundations of medicine are becoming an important element in integrative medical education and a comprehensive curriculum.[18] Logic and critical thinking deserve to be part of the medical curriculum.

This book is not intended to bring definitive answers to every question about logic and critical thinking in the health sciences. It emphasizes various ways of thinking: presumptive warrants with the need to be aware of exception-making circumstances; induction and deduction as an iterative process; linear thinking in the Western tradition (logical reasoning, categorization, cause-effect link); fuzzy logic and chaos theory as an alternative to either-or concepts and probability theory; and Eastern associative thinking, which makes connections rather than choices and has a greater tolerance for ambiguity and contradiction.[19]

Now, let us put logic and critical thinking in practice. Let us apply them in a learned, organized, and focused manner. We are not alone anymore.[20] The evaluation of such an initiative should reveal stimulating results for us as health professionals and, last but not least, major benefits for the well-being of our patients and communities.

We are now just at the starting point of many exciting developments.

References

1. Murphy EA. *The Logic of Medicine.* Baltimore, Md: The Johns Hopkins University Press; 1976.

2. Elstein AS, Shulman LS, Sprafka SA. *Medical Problem Solving: An Analysis of Clinical Reasoning.* Cambridge, Mass: Harvard University Press; 1978.

3. Wulff HR, Pedersen SA, Rosenberg R. *Philosophy of Medicine: An Introduction.* Oxford, England: Blackwell Scientific Publications; 1986.

4. Albert DA, Munson R, Resnik MD. *Reasoning in Medicine: An Introduction to Clinical Inference.* Baltimore, Md: The Johns Hopkins University Press; 1988.

5. Bradley GW. *Disease, Diagnosis and Decisions.* New York, NY: John Wiley & Sons; 1993.

6. Phillips CI, ed. *Logic in Medicine.* London, England: BMJ Publishing Group; 1995.

7. Higgs J, Jones M, eds. *Clinical Reasoning in the Health Professions.* Oxford, England: Butterworth Heinemann; 1995.

8. Jenicek M. *Foundations of Evidence-Based Medicine.* New York, NY: The Parthenon Publishing Group; 2003.

9. Shahar E. A Popperian perspective of the term 'evidence-based medicine'. *J Eval Clin Pract.* 1997;3:109–116.

10. Sleigh JW. Logical limits of randomized controlled trials. *J Eval Clin Pract.* 1997;3:145–148.

11. Upshur R. Certainty, probability and abduction: why we should look to C.S. Peirce rather than Gödel for a theory of clinical reasoning. *J Eval Clin Pract.* 1997;3:201–206.

12. Sung NS, Crowley WF Jr, Genel M, et al. Central challenges facing the national clinical research enterprise. *JAMA.* 2003;289:1278–1287.

13. Vickers JM. Logic, probability and coherence. *Phil Sci.* 2001;68:95–110.

14. Kosko B. *Fuzzy Thinking: The New Science of Fuzzy Logic.* New York, NY: Hyperion; 1992.

15. Pellegrino ED. Medical evidence and virtue ethics: a commentary on Zarkovitch and Upshur. *Theor Med Bioeth.* 2002;23:397–402.

16. Zarkovich E, Upshur RE. The virtues of evidence. *Theor Med Bioeth.* 2002;23:403–412.

17. Popkin RH, Stroll A. *Philosophy Made Simple.* 2nd ed, rev. New York, NY: Broadway Books; 1993.

18. Maizes V, Schneider C, Bell I, Weil A. Integrative medical education: development and implementation of a comprehensive curriculum at the University of Arizona. *Acad Med.* 2002;77:851–860.

19. Mole J. The geography of thinking. *Clin Med.* 2002;2:343–345.

20. Gibbs L, Gambrill E. Measuring skills and reasoning scientifically and critically about practice. In: *Evidence-Based Practice Manual: Research and Outcome Measures in Health and Human Services.* Roberts AR, Yeager KR, eds. Oxford, England: Oxford University Press; 2004:219–226.

Glossary

Definitions of terms in this glossary reflect primarily the meaning given to them in this reading. A delicate balance between meanings in philosophy, medicine, and law was attempted. Besides logic, the following definitions also follow closely the meanings given to them in current major general, medical, epidemiologic, and legal dictionaries as well as in textbooks of epidemiology, clinical epidemiology, and evidence-based medicine. Some additional terms from philosophy, which the reader might find elsewhere in the health-related literature, complete this glossary. The glossary does not replace the above-mentioned sources, but rather complements them, faithful to the message of this book.

Abduction: A form of reasoning in which one reasons from observed phenomena to a hypothesis that would explain them. Usually, abductive reasoning shows only that the hypothesis is a possible explanation, and further observation or experiment and reasoning are required to determine whether the hypothesis is justified.

Algorithm (clinical): A step-by-step written protocol or flowchart drawn for management of a health problem. Each step (consideration, decision) depends unequivocally on the preceding one. Often confused with a decision tree. See *decision tree.*

Alternative medicine: A label for a heterogeneous collection of clinical maneuvers, whose efficacy and safety are generally not scientifically tested, which are not used in mainstream medicine and which are intended to replace conventional medical treatments. See also *complementary medicine*, a label for maneuvers intended to supplement conventional medical treatments.

Argument: A set of statements, some of which, the premises, are offered as reasons for another statement, the conclusion. *Example*: You have a streptococcal infection, so you must start taking antibiotics. *Premise*: You have a streptococcal infection. *Conclusion*: You must start taking antibiotics.

Argumentation: Discussion between two or more people in which at least one of them advances arguments. *Example*: *Patient*: "I prefer natural remedies like herbs to chemicals manufactured by pharmaceutical companies. Chemicals have side effects." *Physician*: "So do herbal remedies." (Here the patient advances an argument supporting her preference for natural remedies. The physician replies by questioning the strength of support given by the patient's stated reason.)

Art: The application, or the principles of application, of skill, knowledge, and so on, in a creative effort to produce something. The art of medicine, for example, contributes to producing (or preserving) health. Fine art, in particular, produces works that have a form of beauty, aesthetic expression of feeling, and so forth, as in music, painting, sculpture, literature, architecture, and the dance. Beyond its scientific basis, a good part of plastic and reconstructive surgery is fine art.

Art of medicine: Systematic application of sensory skills, creative imagination, faithful imitation, innovation, intuition, knowledge in speech, reasoning, or motion in the care of the health of patients and communities.

Association: A tendency of two variables to be systematically related in a group of individuals. As thus defined, association is not the same as causation. *Association* is one of the most nebulous terms in medicine and epidemiology. Across the literature and in medical talk, it may mean a statistical (probabilistic) association (as defined here), a causal association, or any other parallel observation of two or more phenomena. Reader beware!

Atomization of a problem: Bringing a problem to its manageable parts.

Attributable fraction: Same as *attributable risk percent*.

Attributable risk: In cohort studies, the difference between the risk of an outcome of interest in subjects exposed to a suspected causal factor and the risk in unexposed subjects. Both groups compared share presumably the same web of causes except the factor under study. Also called *risk difference*.

Attributable risk percent: In etiological studies, it is the proportion of all observations (morbid events) which may be explained by the causal factor under study (from the whole web of causes). Synonyms: *etiological fraction, attributable fraction*.

Backing: One of the six elements in the contemporary layout of arguments due to Toulmin. Backing is the body of experience and evidence that supports the warrant. See *warrant*.

Belief: A dispositional psychological state in virtue of which a person will assent to a proposition under certain conditions. More narrowly, the acknowledgment that a proposition is true in the absence of demonstrable proof as required by scientific method. As such, it is a rather primary cognitive state as a precursor for reasoning toward evidence

Best research evidence: The most valid clinically relevant research from the available options.

CAM: Abbreviation for *complementary and alternative medicine*. See separate entries for *complementary medicine* and *alternative medicine*.

Categorical statement: A statement that affirms or denies that some predicate belongs to all or some members of some subject class. Simple affirmative or negative statements about an individual ("Mrs. Fitzpatrick is critically ill") can also be regarded as categorical statements by treating them as statements about all members of the class consisting just of that individual. *Examples*: "All patients in our intensive care unit require continuous monitoring of their vital signs." "Mrs Fitzpatrick requires continuous monitoring of her vital signs." (universal affirmative or A statement—*affirmo*) "None of the patients in our intensive care unit should be transferred to another ward without a thorough assessment of their needs, risks, and prognosis." "Mrs Jones does not require continuous monitoring of her vital signs." (universal negative or E statement—*nego*). "Some patients in the coronary care unit can be transferred to other wards without a thorough assessment of their prognosis and needs." (particular affirmative or I statement—*affirmo*) "Some patients with a respiratory distress syndrome should not be transferred to other wards without a thorough assessment of their care needs and prognosis." (particular negative or O statement—*nego*).

Categorical syllogism: Reasoning or argument consisting of two premises and a conclusion, all of which are *categorical statements* (see the preceding entry). The predicate of the conclusion occurs in one premise, the subject of the conclusion in the other, and a common middle term occurs in both premises. *Example*: All patients in the intensive care unit are critically ill; all critically ill patients require continuous monitoring of their vital signs; therefore, all patients in the intensive care unit require continuous monitoring of their vital signs. (In this example, which is deductively **valid**, the subject of the conclusion, "patients in the intensive care unit," occurs in the first premise; the predicate of the conclusion, "require continuous monitoring of their vital signs," occurs in the second premise; and the middle term, "critically ill patients," occurs in both premises.) *Second example*: Not all patients in ward 17 require continuous monitoring of their vital signs; Mrs Fitzpatrick is a patient in ward 17; therefore, Mrs Fitzpatrick does not require monitoring of her vital signs. (In this example, which is deductively **invalid**, the subject of the conclusion, "Mrs Fitzpatrick," occurs in the second premise; the predicate of the conclusion, "require continuous monitoring of vital signs," occurs in the first premise; and the middle term, "patients in Ward 17," occurs in both premises.)

Causality: Relationship between a presumed cause and its effect. Path from a cause to an effect. *Causation* is a preferred term to causality in this book (see below).

Causation: A relation between two events that holds when, given that one occurs, it produces or brings forth, or determines, or necessitates a second. See *causality.*

Causation in civil law: Demonstration that a particular agent or act is a more probable than improbable cause of a given state of affairs (eg, a health problem).

Causation in criminal law: Proof beyond a reasonable doubt that a given state of affairs (eg, a health problem) is due to and only to a given factor.

Cause (in general): An event without which some subsequent event would not have occurred or because of which it occurred. An agent or act that produces some phenomenon (the effect). Example: *Clostridium tetani* as cause of tetanus. See also *necessary cause* and *sufficient cause.*

Cause (at courts of law): Each separate antecedent of an event. That which in some manner is accountable for a condition that brings about an effect or that produces a cause for the resultant action or state.

Chance: An uncalculated, and possible incalculable, element of existence: the contingent as opposed to the necessary aspects of existence. Also, a probability of an event.

Chaos (chaos theory, chaotic behavior in biological systems): An aperiodic, seemingly random, and unpredictable behavior in systems governed by deterministic laws that exhibits a sensitive dependence on initial conditions.

Circle diagram: See *diagram (circle diagram)*.

Claim: One of the six elements in the contemporary layout of arguments due to Toulmin. The claim or conclusion is the proposition at which we arrive as a result of our reasoning, or which we defend in argument by citing our supporting grounds.

Clinical: Pertaining to the care of the individual patient both in the hospital and in outside-hospital settings (eg, medical practice office). See *paraclinical*.

Clinical expertise: The ability to use clinical skills and experience at any stage of clinical work with the patient.

Clinical guidelines: A standardized set of information describing the best practices for addressing health problems commonly encountered either in clinical or public health practice.

Clinical judgment: Capacity to make and choose data and information and to use them to produce useful (true or false) claims in clinical practice and research. It means also critical thinking in the practice of medicine based on the "patient/evidence/setting" fit.

Clinical sign: See *sign (clinical)*.

Clinical symptom: See *symptom (of disease)*.

Clinimetrics: A domain of observation, measurement, classification, and categorization of clinical phenomena. A medical equivalent to biometrics, econometrics, and other metrics in their respective domains.

Cogent argument: A compelling argument. One that justifies its conclusion to its addressee or addressees. It must meet four conditions, which are jointly sufficient. First, both the argument's author and the addressee must be justified in accepting the premises. Second, the premises must include all good relevant information obtainable by either. Third, the conclusion must follow in virtue of a general warrant, which both author and addressee are justified in using. Fourth, if the warrant is not universal, both author and addressee must be justified in assuming that in the particular case there are no exceptional circumstances (rebuttals) that rule out application of the warrant. *Example*: "This patient has group A streptococcal pharyngitis, so she should take penicillin for 10 days. She informed me that she is not allergic to penicillin." (The premise that the patient has group A streptococcal pharyngitis is assumed to be justified by laboratory test of a throat culture. Given what is already stated in the premises, no further practically obtainable information is relevant to the conclusion. The warrant is that penicillin is the drug of choice for the treatment of group A streptococcal pharyngitis, except in individuals with a history of penicillin allergy; this warrant is justified by the best available evidence as of June 2003. The statement of the patient is taken to justify the belief that there is no contraindication in this case to treatment by penicillin.)

Common knowledge: A shared knowledge between individuals.

Common sense: Both sensation and certain intuitively known general truths or principles that together yield knowledge of external objects. In the layperson's mind, common sense means logic. It does not! It is a mental faculty that all people are supposed to possess "in common" for knowledge of basic everyday truths.

Competent layperson: A non-expert who has generic intellectual abilities to delve into areas of specialization. In medicine, a patient who is able, because of his or her intellectual abilities, experience, and judgment broader than the medical field, to assist the physician by proper questions and other information to direct even better clinical decisions in his or her case.

Complementary medicine: A heterogeneous ensemble of often poorly defined traditional, popular, or new health trends parallel to mainstream medicine. It includes proven and mostly unproven clinical maneuvers to add to accepted mainstream medical practices.

Complete information (condition of): The premises include all practically obtainable good information relevant to the question.

Conclusion: The ending point of reasoning or argument, that which is drawn from the premise or premises. *Examples*: See entries for *argument* and *reasoning*.

Conclusion indicator: A word or phrase that indicates that an immediately following phrase, clause, or sentence is the conclusion of an argument or piece of reasoning. *Examples*: therefore, thus, so, hence, shows that, accordingly, it can be concluded that. *Warning*: Most of these words and phrases can also be used to indicate other roles of the immediately following phrase, clause, or sentence, especially the role of being an effect. Attention to context is needed to determine whether a word or phrase is actually functioning to indicate a conclusion.

Connectives (connectors): Expressions (words) connecting various parts of statements. *Examples*: if, or, and, only if.

Connotation: One of two dimensions of meaning. A single set of characteristics that a person grasps who understands what a term means. Synonyms: intension, comprehension, sense. See *denotation*.

Consult: Conferring with another physician about a case.

Copula: A connector between subject and predicate terms. It binds together subject (S) and predicate (P) terms, most often by some form of the verb "be" (with "not" in negative propositions). *Example*: This psychiatric patient (S) is suicidal (P).

Correct reasoning: See *good reasoning.*

Critical thinking: Reasonable reflective thinking that is focused on deciding what to do or believe. *Contrast concept*: dogmatic, unreflective thinking. Critical thinking has several components, whose sequencing varies with the situation. (1) **Identify** and if necessary **analyze** the problem. (2) **Clarify** meaning. (3) **Gather** evidence.

(4) **Assess** evidence. (5) **Infer** conclusions. (6) **Consider** other relevant information. (7) **Judge** how to solve the problem. Critical thinking requires both abilities and dispositions, the latter combining attitudes and inclinations.

Data: Facts or figures from which conclusions may be drawn. Rough quantitative (measured and quantified) and qualitative first-line observations, which enter the reasoning process. *Example:* Blood pressure of 120/80 mm Hg, blood glucose value, or any cell count. (See *information*.)

Decision analysis (in medicine): A method to find the best solution among available multiple options (choices, actions, outcomes, and their values) derived from operations research and game theory. Risks, diagnoses, treatments, disease outcomes, burdens, and costs may represent components of decision analysis.

Decision tree (in medicine): A graphical representation of various options in health and disease evolution and management. Their analysis leads to the best option (most beneficial, most effective, etc) between multiple choices. Hence, a decision tree is not direction-giving; *algorithms* are (see earlier definition). It is a direction-seeking device.

Deduction: A form of reasoning in which one reaches a conclusion by a deductively valid inference. It often proceeds from the general to the particular.

Deduction (in epidemiology): Intellectual process from an a priori formulated hypothesis to data collection, analysis, and hypothesis confirmation or rebuttal leading to and depending on the result of the study. Hypothesis precedes its ground. Generalization accepted or refuted by observation (data).

Deductively valid inference: An inference in which it is impossible for the premises to be true and the conclusion false, because of their meaning. Typically, one premise will be an unqualified warrant. *Example*: "My patient has a streptococcal infection. Patients with streptococcal infections must be treated with antibiotics. Therefore, my patient must be treated with antibiotics."

Defeasible warrant: A warrant with a modal qualifier other than "necessarily," which can be defeated by a rebuttal, an exceptional circumstance in which the conclusion is false. *Example*: In general, an antibiotic may be prescribed for treatment of a bacterial infection—but not if the patient is allergic to it.

Delusion: A false belief that cannot be corrected by reason. It is logically unfounded and cannot be corrected by argument or persuasion or even by the evidence of the patient's own senses.

Denotation: One of two dimensions of meaning. The denotation of a term means the individual objects to which the term applies. Synonyms: extension or reference. See *connotation*.

Diagram (circle diagram): An outline figure using circles intended to represent sets. The relative arrangement or marking of the circles indicates relationships (overlap, proper inclusion, nonoverlap) between the sets. See *Venn diagram* and *Euler diagram*.

Differential diagnosis: Making choices between various diagnostic options that might apply to the same patient or clinical situation.

Discourse: A continuous stretch of language containing more than one sentence: conversations, narratives, arguments, speeches.

Discussion (section in medical articles): A section of a medical research article in which the author or authors explain the nature, meaning, strengths, weaknesses, possible remedies for errors, and directions for the future pertaining to the raw findings as reported in the Results section preceding it.

Dispositional reasoning (in fuzzy logic): Reasoning based on propositions that are fuzzy, hence not always true. *Example*: *Heavy* alcohol drinking is a *leading cause* of liver cirrhosis.

Enthymeme: Reasoning or argument that is not deductively valid but which can be made deductively valid by adding one or more premises. Typically, the added premise will be a warrant that licenses the original inference. *Example*: The sphygmomanometer shows a reading of 200/120 mm Hg, so the patient has high blood pressure. (This piece of reasoning would become deductively valid if one added as a premise the warrant: Anyone with a sphygmomanometer reading of 200/120 mm Hg has high blood pressure.)

Epistemology: The theory of knowledge.

Etiological fraction: See *attributable risk percent*.

Euler diagram: A diagram that represents the relation between sets by the spatial relationship of circles representing the sets. Two partially intersecting circles represent partial overlap between the sets; for example, a partial intersection of circles for melancholia and delusional depression indicates that some people have both conditions, that some have melancholia but not delusional depression, and that some have delusional depression but not melancholia. One circle completely inside another indicates that the set represented by the first circle is a proper subset of the set represented by the second one; for example, a circle for persons with acquired immunodeficiency syndrome (AIDS) inside a circle for persons infected by the human immunodeficiency virus (HIV) indicates that all persons with AIDS have been infected by HIV, but not all persons infected by HIV have AIDS at a given moment. Sometimes the extent of overlap or inclusion indicates proportional relationships; for example, a diagram with 60% of the delusional depression circle inside the melancholia circle indicates that 60% of people with delusional depression have melancholia. Euler diagrams (often falsely called Venn diagrams) can be used to test a categorical syllogism for deductive validity, by trying to diagram the premises in a single diagram so as to depict the conclusion as false. If this **cannot** be done, the syllogism is valid: the information in the premises forces one to represent the conclusion as true. If this **can** be done, the syllogism is invalid: it is possible for the premises to be true and the conclusion false.

Evidence in law: (1) Any species of proof or probative matter legally presented for the purpose of inducing belief in the minds of court or jury as to the contention of a party to a case. (2) An assertion of fact, opinion, belief, or knowledge, whether material or not and whether admissible or not. It includes judgments, decisions, opinion, speeches, and all other matters done and said before the court, including matters relating to the procedure. (The second definition is much broader than the definition of evidence in medicine and philosophy by including as "evidence" procedural matters at courts.)

Evidence in medicine: Any data or information, whether solid or weak, obtained through experience, observational research, or experimental work (trials), relevant either to the understanding of a health problem or to decision making about it. *Examples*: Clinical case observations as proof of effectiveness of treatment (weak evidence) or randomized double-blind controlled clinical trials (strong evidence that the treatment works, ie, that there is a cause-effect relationship between treatment and cure). Other types of evidence may concern disease history and course, disease occurrence, its causes, prognosis, and other topics of interest in health sciences.

Evidence-based medicine (EBM): *Original definition:* The process of systematically finding, appraising, and using contemporaneous research findings as the basis of clinical decisions. *Current definition:* The integration of best research evidence with clinical expertise and patient values. *Comment:* It is an application of critical thinking in medical practice. Its components are as follows: (1) formulation of the question concerning the patient which has to be answered (*identifying need for evidence*), (2) search for the evidence (*producing the evidence*), (3) appraisal of evidence (*evaluating the evidence*), (4) selection of the best evidence available for clinical decision making (*using the evidence*), (5) linking evidence with clinical knowledge, experience, and practice and with the patient's values and preferences (*integrated uses of evidence*), (6) using evidence in clinical care to solve the patient's problem (*uses of evidence in specific settings*), (7) evaluation of the effectiveness of the uses of evidence in this case (*weighing the impact*), (8) teaching and expanding EBM practice and research (*going beyond what was already achieved*).

Evidence-based public health (community medicine): Three definitions currently prevail: (1) The process of systematically finding, appraising, and using contemporaneous clinical and community research findings as the basis for decisions in public health. (2) The conscientious, explicit, and judicious use of current best evidence in making decisions about the care of communities and populations in the areas of health protection, disease prevention, and health maintenance and improvement (health promotion). (3) The integration of best research evidence with public health (community medicine) expertise and community (population) values.

Fallacy: A type of mistake in reasoning, argument, or argumentation. *Medical example*: In diagnostic reasoning, ignoring possible diagnoses consistent with the patient's observed signs and/or symptoms, such as failing to consider the possible appendicitis, peritonitis, or internal bleeding in a patient complaining of abdominal pain.

Falsity: The opposite of truth. The property of a statement (belief, proposition) of asserting what is not really the case.

Formal logic: A branch of logic that builds a formalized system of reasoning, using abstract symbols for the various aspects of natural language.

Fuzzy (fuzziness): An adjective identifying any phenomenon without clear and well-specified borders and distinctions between its presence and absence.

Fuzzy decision making: Decision making based on fuzzy premises.

Fuzzy logic: A kind of formal logic based on *fuzzy set theory.*

Fuzzy predicates, probabilities, or **quantifiers:** Semiquantitative identifiers of a degree in fuzzy set theory. *Example:* "Moderately" elevated blood pressure, "advanced" atherosclerosis.

Fuzzy set theory: A kind of set theory that replaces the two-valued set-membership function with a real-valued function; that is, membership is treated as a probability, or as a degree of truthfulness. Likewise, one assigns a real value to assertions as an indication of their degree of truthfulness; 0 is definitely false, 1 is definitely true, 0.6666 repeating is two thirds true. The theory reflects the view that phenomena around us are not necessarily dichotomous and that many things are a matter of degree. *Example:* Blood pressure is a matter of degree rather than being either normotensive or hypertensive.

Fuzzy syllogism: A syllogism based on one or more fuzzy premises. Its conclusion will necessarily be fuzzy.

Gestalt: A German term meaning pattern or configuration. See *pattern recognition of a health problem*.

Good argument: An argument that serves its function well. If the function of the argument is to justify the conclusion to one or more addressees, then it must meet four conditions, which are jointly sufficient. First, both the argument's author and the addressee or addressees must be justified in accepting the premises. Second, the premises must include all good relevant information obtainable by either. Third, the conclusion must follow in virtue of a general warrant which both author and addressee (addressees) are justified in using. Fourth, if the warrant is not universal, both author and addressee (addressees) must be justified in assuming that in the particular case there are no exceptional circumstances (rebuttals) that rule out application of the warrant. If an expert in some field addresses an argument to a nonexpert (eg, physician to patient, automobile mechanic to customer), then the nonexpert's justification may be acceptance of the authority of the expert. See *cogent argument*.

Good argumentation: Argumentation that serves its function well. If the function is to rationally resolve a conflict of opinion, then argumentation must be addressed to the issue in dispute and any argument advanced must justify its conclusion to all parties in the discussion.

Good reasoning: Reasoning that justifies the conclusion to the reasoner. The reasoner must be justified in accepting the premises; that is, they must be evidence-based. The premises must include all good practically obtainable relevant information. The conclusion must follow in virtue of a justified general warrant. If the warrant is not universal, the reasoner must be justified in assuming that in the particular case there are no exceptional circumstances (rebuttals) that rule out application of the warrant. *Example*: This patient has a pulsating abdominal mass, so she may have an aneurysm of her abdominal aorta. It is assumed that the reasoner has felt the pulsating abdominal mass, thus justifying the premise by direct observation, and that no other practically obtainable information is relevant to the conclusion that the patient *may* have an aneurysm of her abdominal aorta. The warrant is that a pulsating abdominal mass may indicate an aneurysm of the abdominal aorta. Since the warrant is qualified by the word *may,* the conclusion is quite weak and there are no rebuttals. Further investigation is needed to arrive at a definite diagnosis.

Grounds: One of the six elements in the contemporary layout of arguments due to Toulmin: the basis from which we reason and argue. They are the specific facts relied on to support a given claim or conclusion.

Guidelines: See *clinical guidelines.*

Hard data: Any data that can be well defined in operational terms and/or measured. *Example:* Body weight, blood glucose level, electrocardiogram reading. See also *soft data*.

Hardening of soft data (in clinical epidemiology): Defining in operational terms and giving dimension to clinical and paraclinical observations.

Hazard (in medicine and epidemiology): Probabilities studied in the domain of prognosis (once the patient gets the disease). A similar concept to *risk* of getting the disease (see *risk*). Elsewhere, a factor or exposure that may adversely affect health or disease.

Hermeneutics: The practice or theory of interpretation. Once closely associated with the interpretation of the Bible, it is now used more generally as a method, art, or technique of understanding and interpretation. In medicine, taking a patient history may be seen as falling into the domain of hermeneutics.

Heuristics: Quick and dirty mental shortcuts to discovery, which sometimes err. A heuristic approach uses heuristics to simplify our thinking in arriving at the solution of a problem. It can also be used in artificial intelligence to reduce the complexity of computational tasks. Such an approach is expected to save time, memory, attention, and other requirements for a given mental or computational process. Making a diagnosis at the bedside or in a medical office is often a heuristic process (eg, reducing the number of diagnostic options in differential diagnosis). So is computer-assisted diagnosis.

Hypothesis: A proposition to be confirmed or rejected by scientific inquiry.

Induction (in epidemiology): Any method of logical analysis that proceeds from the particular to the general. Intellectual process in which hypotheses are generated, confirmed, or refuted on the basis of previously gathered data. Hypothesis follows its ground. Generalization from observations.

Inductive generalization: A form of reasoning in which one concludes that all cases of a specified kind have a specified property on the basis of observation that all examined cases of that kind have the property. The strength of support for the conclusion, assuming that the examined cases have been correctly observed to have the property, depends on the qualification of the justified warrant that applies. *Example*: The sphygmomanometer shows a reading of 130/90 mm Hg. So the patient's blood pressure is approximately 130/90 mm Hg. Here the generalization is from one instance to all instances over an unspecified time interval. The word *approximately* is an appropriate qualification, since blood pressure fluctuates according to time of day, stress, exercise, and other factors. A series of readings under different conditions gives a better estimate of blood pressure than does a single reading.

Inductive strength: The probability that the conclusion of an inference is true given that the premises are true. Often qualitative or comparative rather than quantitative. The probability is relative to the information in the premises; it can change with additional relevant information. *Example*: A patient in the emergency department reports that he fell recently, landing on his right hand, and that his wrist has been feeling sore. This provides somewhat strong support for the conclusion that there is a broken bone in the wrist. Examination of the wrist showing swelling, and painfulness to the touch gives stronger support for this conclusion. Radiographs for a definitive diagnosis are indicated. See *inductively strong inference.*

Inductively strong inference: An inference whose conclusion is probable (in the absence of further information) given that the premises are true. Typically, one premise will be a warrant with a modal qualifier like "probably" or "generally." *Example*: This patient's nodular melanoma is 5 mm thick (in depth). Patients with melanoma tumors more than 4 mm in depth have a high risk of melanoma developing elsewhere in the body. So probably, this patient will develop melanoma elsewhere in the body. Here the second premise is the warrant, which could also have been expressed as the statement, "Most patients with melanoma tumors more than 4 mm in depth develop melanoma elsewhere in the body."

Inference: The drawing of a conclusion from one or more premises. In reasoning, inference is a mental activity, which may or may not be verbalized, either to oneself or to others. In argument, inference is a linguistic activity expressed in speaking or writing.

Inference indicators: Words identifying premises and conclusions in reasoning and arguments expressed in natural language. See *premise indicator* and *conclusion indicator*.

Informal logic: A branch of logic that uses methods and techniques to identify, analyze, interpret, and evaluate reasoning and argument as it happens in the context of natural language used in everyday life. Contrary to formal, symbolic, or mathematical logic, informal logic deals directly with reasoning and argument in natural (everyday) language.

Information: Knowledge acquired or derived. Some conclusion drawn from raw data as a second-line subject to reason about. *Examples:* Hypertension, diabetes (as conclusions drawn from blood pressure or blood glucose observations for the purposes of treatment and prognostic considerations).

Integrative medicine: An attempt to make a coherent ensemble from various trends in traditional, complementary, and alternative medicine.

Intervening cause (in law): An action or event that alters the course of a chain of events, leading to the injury or loss that is the subject of a tort case. If the intervening event was foreseeable, it does not relieve a person who set the chain of events in motion from liability.

Intervening efficient cause (in occupational health and law): A new and independent force that breaks (positively or negatively) the causal connection between the original wrong and the injury, and itself becomes the direct and immediate cause of injury.

Judgment: The act or faculty of affirming or denying a proposition, whether based on a direct comparison of objects or ideas or derived by a process of reasoning. The evaluation of the nature and soundness of some information, giving it a value for subsequent decision making.

Knowledge: Justified true belief. Alternatively, true belief that has been acquired by a generally reliable process.

Layout of arguments: Graphical representation of components of arguments and their interrelationships.

Logic: The normative science that investigates the principles of valid reasoning and correct inference.

Logic in medicine: A system of thought and reasoning that governs understanding and decisions in clinical and community care, research, and communication. It defines valid reasoning, which helps us to understand the meaning of medical phenomena and leads us to the justification of the choice of clinical and paraclinical decisions on how to act on such phenomena.

Logical operators: Words or phrases that indicate logical properties or relations. They include quantifiers ("some," "all," "no," "at least two"), sentence connectives ("and", "or," "if"), indicators of identity or negation ("equals," "not"), and modal qualifiers ("necessarily," "possibly").

Logical positivism: A position in philosophy, advocated by the Vienna Circle in the 1920s and 1930s. Its central doctrine was the verification principle, that a sentence is meaningful if and only if it is either "analytic" or empirically verifiable. The verification principle is self-refuting and has been discredited as anything more than a prejudice.

Major term (in categorical syllogisms): The predicate of the conclusion.

Medical ethics: Study of values of health, disease, and care and the morality of physicians' actions, behavior, and conduct.

Medicine: The art and science of diagnosis, treatment, and prevention of disease and the maintenance of good health. Applies both to the care of individual patients and to that of communities.

Meta-analysis in medicine: Statistical integration of original research studies focusing on a similar problem and question, leading to a quantitative summary of the pooled results. It is a quantitative component of research synthesis; systematic review is its qualitative one. See *systematic review of evidence.*

Meta-cognition: Thinking about our own thinking.

Meta-language: A language used to talk about another language, which is known correlatively as the "object language." *Example*: If you explain in English the meaning of a French word, English is your meta-language and French your object language. Discourse in English about the meaning of English words (*hypertensive, schizophrenia, diabetic*) takes place in a meta-language with respect to the statements that use those words to describe reality.

Metaphysics: Any inquiry that raises questions about reality that lie beyond or behind those capable of being tackled by the methods of science.

Middle term (in categorical syllogisms): The term that appears in each premise but not in the conclusion.

Minor term (in categorical syllogisms): The subject of the conclusion.

Modal logic: A branch of logic that focuses on logical operators that are modal qualifiers, principally "necessarily" and "possibly."

Modal qualifier: An adverb indicating the scope of a warrant, and thus the degree to which the conclusion of some reasoning or argument is supported by the premises, if they are true. *Examples*: probably, presumably, necessarily, possibly.

Necessary cause: Within a web of causes, a causal factor whose presence is required for the occurrence of some effect. See also *necessary condition* and *sufficient cause.*

Necessary condition: A condition that is required for something else to occur. If the necessary condition is not present, then the other thing does not occur. *Contrast concept*: sufficient condition. *Example*: Infection by the tuberculosis bacillus (*Mycobacterium tuberculosis*) is a necessary condition for getting tuberculosis. A necessary condition need not be a sufficient condition. *Example*: The tuberculosis bacillus is not a sufficient condition for getting tuberculosis; many people infected by this bacterium do not get clinically manifest tuberculosis. On the other hand, it is a necessary condition: a person who has not been infected by the bacterium will not have tuberculosis. Many necessary conditions are necessary causes, but not all are. *Example*: Pain in the chest is a necessary condition for a diagnosis of angina pectoris, but this is a necessity of definition; the pain does not cause the angina pectoris but is part of the condition. See also *necessary cause* and *sufficient condition.*

Nocebo effect: Any negative effect such as causation of sickness or death by a pill, potion, or procedure, but not due to its pharmacodynamic or specific properties. Harm due to the power of suggestion. *Example:* Voodoo in Caribbean health culture.

Object language: A language used to talk directly about (nonlinguistic) reality, as contrasted with the meta-language used to talk about an object language. See *meta-language.*

Ockham's razor: See *parsimony* (the *principle of parsimony*).

Odds ratio: In case-control studies, the ratio of the odds in favor of exposure to a supposed causal factor among cases of a disease to the odds in favor of exposure among noncases. Like relative risk from cohort studies, the odds ratio is a useful estimation of the strength of cause-effect relationships.

Paraclinical: Activities and services beyond bedside care but related to it and most often vital for it. Examples: Clinical laboratory, diagnostic imaging sites, and diagnostic technology. See *clinical.*

Paradigm: A theoretical framework for scientific or philosophical endeavors and investigations of problems. A way in which we look at things. *Example:* Medicine is probabilistic. The universe is infinite.

Parsimony (principle of parsimony, Ockham's razor): Keeping things (hypotheses, studies, data, analyses, or interpretations) as simple as possible. Not complicating things beyond a strict necessity. Parsimony, or Ockham's razor, is a useful rule of thumb in formulating hypotheses for investigation, whether in general causal research or in diagnosis of individual patients. However, it is not an infallible guide; sometimes the truth is complicated.

Patient values: Each individual's unique preferences, concerns, and expectations related to clinical decisions.

Pattern recognition of a health problem: A mental process of finding characteristics of a health problem corresponding or identical to a previously lived and/or learned experience. Diagnosis relies often (sometimes too often) on pattern recognition.

Philosophy: Systematic analysis and critical examination of fundamental problems and nature of being, reality, thinking, perception, values, causes, and choices underlying principles of physical and ethical phenomena. Traditionally, its fundamental branches are metaphysics, epistemology and logic, and ethics.

Philosophy in medicine: Use and application of philosophy to health, disease, and medical care. Its aim is to study and understand general principles and ideas that lie behind views, understanding, and decisions about health, disease, and care. Use of the formal tools of philosophical inquiry to examine medicine itself as a subject of study, the place of patients and health professionals within it, and establishment of the rule of their conduct in the domain of health, disease, and care.

Philosophy of medicine: Formal inquiry into the structure of medical thought. Philosophical inquiry on the nature of medicine as medicine and subsequent development of some general theory of medicine and its activities. It pays a lot of attention to medicine's own contributions to philosophy, such as clinical trials or the methodology of observational analytical studies in the domain of cause-effect proof.

Philosophy of science: Systematic philosophical study of the workings and functioning of science, of the extent of its ability to gain access to the truth about the material world, and of concepts used in scientific inquiry, such as laws of nature, causality, probability, and explanation.

Phronesis in medicine: A label given by some authors to the process of knowing and doing, experiencing and acting, undertaken by a physician on behalf of a particular patient in a specific clinical situation and setting. Practical wisdom in dealing with particular individuals, specific problems, and the details of particular cases or actual situations.

Placebo effect: Any healing, suffering-alleviating, or comforting effect attributable to a pill, potion, or procedure but not to its pharmacodynamic or specific properties. Effect due to the power of suggestion.

Post hoc ergo propter hoc: A Latin term for "After this, therefore because of this." The fallacy of inferring a causal relationship from mere temporal sequence of a presumed cause and its expected effect instead of from its plausible causal proof. *Example*: After more storks arrived, more babies were born; therefore, storks bring babies.

Postulate: In philosophy and mathematics, a proposition that forms a starting point of inquiry but which is neither definition, nor provisional assumption, nor so certain that it can be taken as axiomatic. Such postulates are laid down as true and used without demonstration. Postulates **in medicine** bear often many of these above-mentioned properties. *Examples:* A working diagnosis of a new phenomenon such as sudden acute respiratory syndrome (SARS). "Gastric ulcer is a stress-produced disease" before the demonstration of its infectious etiology. An absolutely necessary assumption in contrast to the conjectural nature of hypothesis. Often, an equivalent of **posit**, as something put forward as a useful assumption or starting point, but not necessarily regarded as known to be true.

Premise: A starting point of reasoning or argument, that from which the conclusion is drawn, possibly in combination with other premises. *Examples*: See entries for *argument* and *reasoning*.

Premise indicator: A word or phrase indicating that an immediately following phrase, clause, or sentence is the premise of an argument or piece of reasoning. *Examples*: since, as, because, given that, given. *Warning*: Most of these words and phrases can also be used to indicate other roles of the immediately following phrase, clause, or sentence, especially the role of being a cause. Attention to context is needed to determine whether a word or phrase is actually functioning to indicate a premise.

Presumptive evidence (in law): *Prima facie* evidence or evidence that is not conclusive and admits of explanation or contradiction; evidence that must be received and treated as true and sufficient until and unless rebutted by other evidence. Evidence deemed true and sufficient unless discredited by other evidence.

Probable cause (in law): A "reasonable cause," having more evidence for than against. A set of probabilities grounded in the factual and practical considerations that govern the decisions of reasonable and prudent persons and is more than mere suspicion but less than the quantum of evidence required for conviction in a criminal case.

Producing cause (in law and occupational health): That cause which, in a natural and continuous sequence, produces an effect (eg, a death), and without which the effect (eg, death) would not have occurred. See *necessary cause.*

Prognosis: The art of foretelling the course of disease, or the application of this art to a particular case, or the result of such an application. The prospect of survival and recovery from a disease as anticipated from the usual course of that disease and indicated by special features of the case in question.

Proximate cause (in law): That which in natural and continuous sequence, unbroken by any new independent cause, produces an event, and without which the injury would not have occurred. In tort cases, it is a wrongful conduct by a defendant leading to an injury complained of in a sufficiently direct way to justify holding the defendant liable for the plaintiff's damages.

Qualifier: One of the six components in the modern layout of arguments due to Toulmin. A word or phrase that indicates the strength conferred by the warrant on the inference from grounds to claim, and thus the strength of support given to our conclusion by the grounds we offer (assuming those grounds are true). See *warrant, grounds,* and *claim.*

Qualitative reasoning (in fuzzy logic): Reasoning based on fuzzy "if-then" rules in which premises and conclusions involve linguistic variables, which may themselves be fuzzy.

Quantifiers: Words that indicate the quantity of some phenomenon: *how often, how much, how many,* and so on. They give dimension to our observations and statements, even when given in fuzzy terms. See *fuzzy logic* and *fuzzy set theory*. *Example:* An "occasional" dyspnea; "profuse" bleeding; "frequent" hemoptysis; "all" patients with streptococcal pharyngitis; "some" pulsating abdominal masses.

Rational thought: According to Henrik Wulff, an analysis of reasons given for different statements and a determination how these reasons are related in justifying and/or understanding other statements.

Rational: Conformable to reason; judicious; sensible. *Example*: This patient is rational, and that one is irrational.

Reasoning: Thinking leading to a conclusion. Ideally, thinking enlightened by logic. *Example*: (Said to oneself) This patient of mine has a streptococcal infection, so he must be treated with antibiotics immediately. *Premise*: This patient of mine has a streptococcal infection. *Conclusion*: He must start taking antibiotics. See *good reasoning*.

Reconstruction of an argument: A process giving a structured, analyzable, interpretable, and evaluable argument on the basis of its conversion from natural language into a standard form with a clearly identified premise or premises and conclusion.

Rebuttals: One of the six elements in the contemporary layout of arguments due to Toulmin. Exceptional circumstances which show that a warrant does not apply in the particular case. *Example*: A patient's allergy to penicillin, which rebuts the conclusion that the patient, who has a bacterial infection, may be treated with penicillin. Rebuttals may or may not be specified in the warrant. *Examples*: Patients with a bacterial infection may be treated with penicillin, unless they are allergic to penicillin or there is reason to believe that the bacterium is resistant to penicillin. Patients with a bacterial infection may generally be treated with penicillin or some other antibiotic.

Reflective thinking (in law): Solving a problem in the law by pondering a given set of facts in order to perceive their connection.

Relative risk: In cohort studies, the ratio of risk of an outcome in exposed subjects to its risk in unexposed subjects. It is a measure of the strength of a cause-effect relationship.

Rhetorical ploys (in law): Nonargumentative deficiencies in reasoning. *Example:* Appeals to novelty or to fear.

Risk (in medicine and epidemiology): Absolute or relative probability of the occurrence of an event (eg, disease occurrence or its cure) over a specified time period in relation to its determining factors.

Risk difference: Same as *attributable risk*.

Rounds, clinical rounds, floor rounds: Reviewing cases with other physicians and health professionals focusing on laying out elements of arguments and defending them. Analysis and consensus for plans for care.

Science: The study of the material universe of physical reality in order to understand it.

Science of medicine: Discovery, implementation, and evaluation of evidence in understanding human health, disease, and care.

Scientific method: Method of study of nature involving problem definition, hypothesis formulation, observation, measurement, analysis and interpretation of findings, and subsequent generation of new hypotheses. This "hypothetico-deductive" method is one of many methods used in science.

Semiotic or semeiotic (in medicine): Pertaining to the signs or symptoms of disease. Pathognomonic.

Semiotics: The general study of symbolic systems, including signs and language. Study of the interpretation of signs, as a part of hermeneutics. General science of signs and languages. The subject is divided into three areas: *syntax*, or the abstract study of the signs and their interrelationships; *semantics,* the study of the relation between the signs and those objects to which they apply; and *pragmatics* as the relationship between users and the system.

Set: A collection of defined, distinct, or somehow related items. *Examples:* Human races, ethnic groups, types of blood cells, series of measurements in an experiment.

Sign (clinical): Objective manifestations of disease. Those disease manifestations that are perceived by a third person. *Examples:* Exanthem, external bleeding, diarrhea.

Soft data: Any observation that cannot be adequately defined in precise operational terms and/or measured. *Example:* Sorrow, anger, nausea. See also *hard data.*

Specificity of an association: Magnitude of how a particular suspected causal factor of interest prevails among other possible causes. See *attributable risk* and *attributable risk percent.*

Strength of association: The distance between two or more series of observations. This is appropriately expressed by *relative risk* in cohort studies and by the *odds ratio* in case-control studies.

Stochastic process: A process that incorporates some degree of randomness.

Sufficient cause: In a web of causes, a set of conditions, factors, or events that will produce a given outcome, regardless of what other conditions are present or absent. A complete causal mechanism that does not require the presence of any other determinant in order for the outcome, such as disease, to occur. See also *sufficient condition* and *necessary cause.*

Sufficient condition: A condition that is enough by itself for something else to occur. If the sufficient condition is present, then the other thing occurs. *Contrast concept:* necessary condition. *Example:* Irreversible cessation of heartbeat and respiration is a sufficient condition for death. A sufficient condition need not be a necessary condition. *Example:* Irreversible cessation of heartbeat and respiration is not a necessary condition for death in many legal jurisdictions. In New York State, for example, a person may be declared dead if his or her heartbeat and respiration are being maintained by "extraordinary mechanical means" provided that there is "an irreversible cessation of all functions of the entire brain, including the brain stem." (*People v Eulo*, 63 N.Y. 2d 341 at 357–358 [1984]). Many sufficient conditions are sufficient causes, but not all are. *Example:* Angina pectoris is a sufficient condition for pain in the chest, but this is a matter of definition; angina pectoris *is* a certain sort of pain in the chest. See also *sufficient cause* and *necessary condition.*

Sufficient evidence (in law): That which is satisfactory for the purpose.

Superseding or supervening cause (in tort law): An action or event that intervenes so dramatically and unexpectedly in a chain of causation, and changes its course so significantly, that the law regards it as a proximate cause of the injury or damage complained of. See *proximate cause.*

Syllogism: Defined by Aristotle as a discourse or argument in which certain things have been laid down (eg, A and B) and something other than what has been laid down (C) follows by necessity from their being so. See *categorical syllogism.*

Symbolic logic: See *formal logic.*

Symptom (of disease): Manifestation of disease as perceived subjectively by the patient. Often hidden to other people. *Examples:* Hot flashes, itching (unless the patient scratches himself), pain, feeling of persecution.

Systematic review of evidence (in evidence-based medicine): The application of strategies that limit bias in the assembly, critical appraisal, and synthesis of all relevant studies on a specific topic. Meta-analysis may be, but is not necessarily, used as a part of this process. Also, overview of qualitative characteristics of original studies of a given problem, "epidemiology of results."

Theory: A set of ideas, concepts, principles, or methods used to explain a wide set of observed facts. A theory may or may not have been confirmed by scientific inquiry, explanation, and proof. *Examples:* The theory of evolution (of biological species), the germ theory of disease, the theory of special relativity, Newtonian mechanics, plate tectonics, thermodynamics.

Thinking: Mental action, which, if verbalized, is a matter of combining words in propositions. Not all thinking is able to be verbalized. Visual imaginings in daydreaming, for example, cannot be completely verbalized.

Tort (in law): A wrongful act, other than a breach of contract, that results in injury to another person and for which the injured party is entitled to a remedy of law, usually in the form of damages. Tort may be intentional or nonintentional.

Tort litigation: Evaluation by courts of law of harm, its causes, responsibility, and compensation.

Tree diagram (in logic): The graphical representation of the structure of reasoning or argument from premises to conclusions in a spoken or written text.

Truth: The property of a statement (belief, proposition) of asserting what is really the case.

Uncertainty: Any situation in which probabilities of different possible phenomena or outcomes are not known. Due mostly to chance and our poor knowledge and understanding of the phenomenon under consideration.

Validity (of an inference): See *deductively valid inference.*

Venn diagram: A diagram that represents the relations between sets by shading out subsets that are empty (ie, with no members) and putting an *x* in subsets that are not empty (ie, with at least one member). Venn diagrams can be used to test whether a categorical syllogism is deductively valid. *Example:* Diagram the information that all patients in the intensive care unit are critically ill and that all critically ill patients need continuous monitoring of their vital signs. Three sets are mentioned: patients in the intensive care unit (ICU), critically ill patients (CIP), patients who need continuous monitoring of their vital signs (CMVS). Draw three circles, one for each set, with the circles overlapping so that all possible combinations are represented by a segment. Shade out the part of the ICU circle that is *outside* the CIP circle, to represent the information that all patients in the intensive care unit are critically ill. Shade out the part of the CIP circle that is *outside* the CMVS circle, to represent the information that all critically ill patients need continuous monitoring of their vital signs. Notice that all parts of the ICU circle that are outside the CMVS circle are now shaded out, thus showing that this subset is empty; that is, all ICU patients need continuous monitoring of their vital signs. The diagram thus shows that the inference from the given information to the latter proposition is deductively valid: if the information is correct, the conclusion *must* be correct. *Note*: In the medical literature, the phrase *Venn diagram* is often used for what is in fact a Euler diagram. See *Euler diagram*.

Warrant: One of the six elements of the contemporary layout of arguments due to Toulmin. A general rule that permits us to infer a claim of the given type from grounds of the type we have adduced. See *grounds. Example*: Given that a patient has a streptococcal infection, you may conclude that the patient must be treated with antibiotics. Warrants may be expressed as general statements. *Example*: Patients with streptococcal infections must be treated with antibiotics. Warrants are usually implicit (ie, unstated) in reasoning and arguments; if the warrant is added as an explicit premise, the inference becomes deductively valid, provided that any modal qualifiers are removed. *Example*: My patient has a streptococcal infection. Patients with streptococcal infections must be treated with antibiotics. Therefore, my patient must be treated with antibiotics.

Warranted inference: An inference with a justified warrant.

Web of causes (in epidemiology): An ensemble (set) of causes of a health phenomenon (health, disease, cure, etc) with all their interaction and relationship in time and space.

Web of consequences (in epidemiology): An ensemble or set of outcomes (health problems) with all their interaction and relationship in time and space as produced by their cause or causes.

Workers' compensation board: An organization established by a government to provide compensation to workers who suffer a work-related injury or disease. Courts of law as sites for litigation are replaced for ease of settlement by various health and civic stakeholders whose mandate is to evaluate risk, harm, prognosis of occupation-related health problems, and for particular workers financial compensation and health and social needs. These settings may vary from one country to another.

About the Authors

Milos Jenicek, MD, PhD is Professor of Clinical Epidemiology and Evidence-Based Medicine and Public Health at McMaster University in Hamilton, Ontario, Canada. He is also Professor Emeritus at the Université de Montréal, Adjunct Professor at McGill University, and Fellow of the Royal College of Physicians and Surgeons of Canada.

David L. Hitchcock, PhD is Professor of Philosophy at McMaster University in Hamilton, Ontario, Canada and author of *Critical Thinking: A Guide to Evaluating Information,* published by Methuen Publishing in 1983. He is a member of the Canadian Philosophical Association, Association for Informal Logic and Critical Thinking, Society for Ancient Greek Philosophy, and International Society for the Study of Argumentation.

Index

A

A statement (universal affirmative), 69, 74, 75
Abdomen, tender, and appendicitis 74–75; [figure], 75
Abdominal mesothelioma, 200–201
Abduction, 66–68; [table], 67
    definitions of, 67
    glossary term, 259
    hypotheses and, 67–68
    uncertainty and, 68
Abstraction (hypostatization), 171
Accent, fallacy of, 211, 217
Accident, fallacy of, 169, 198
Acupressure, 122, 125
Acupuncture, 122, 125
Ad ignorantiam fallacies, 245
Ad populum, 171
Affective disorders, suicide attempts and suicide [figure], 72
Affirmative propositions, 214
    particular, description of, 69, 71–72
    universal, description of, 69, 71
Age, prognostic markers, 201
Aggregation bias, 169
Agreement, method of, 154
Air pollution, lung cancer mortality rate in developing country (fictitious example), 163–166
Al-Farab, 25
Alcohol, risk factors versus prognostic factors, 201
Algorithm
    clinical (glossary term), 259
    diagnostic, 191–193; [figure], 192
Alternative medicine, *see* Complementary and alternative medicine
Ambiguity, 245, 256
Amphiboly, 245
Analogies, false, 218
Analysis
    complementary and alternative medicine and critical thinking, 120–121

Analysis—*cont.*
    critical thinking skills, 108; [table], 107
    logical, and critical thinking, 108
    multivariate, 158
    problem identification and (critical thinking checklist), 109, 110–111, 136; [table], 110
Analytic statements, 27
Analytical studies, demonstrating, refuting cause-effect relationships, 157–158
Anecdotal evidence, 126
Antecedents, (if ... then reasoning), 55–56
Antibiotics, streptococcal infections (examples) 73; [figure], 74, 75–76, 90, 92
Antineoplastons, 122
Appendicitis, tender abdomen and, 74–75; [figure], 75
Application, Tarka methodological reasoning in Indian philosophy, 79
Arborization (diagnostic path), 191
Argumentation
    definition of, 28
    glossary term, 259
    good, 51
    good (glossary term), 267
    patient persuasion, 184
Arguments
    causal, fallacies in, 167–172
    circular, 55
    cogent (glossary term), 262–263
    complementary and alternative medicine and critical thinking, 125–128
    components and architecture of, 29–41
    components identified, in rounds as dialogue [table], 213
    convincing, 49, 50
    criteria in communications, 219
    deficiencies in medical articles, 173
    definition of, 28
    differing, in outside world [table], 228
    evaluation of, 41–52
    evidence and inference in [figure], 113
    glossary term, 259